Baillière's
CLINICAL
OBSTETRICS
AND
GYNAECOLOGY
INTERNATIONAL PRACTICE AND RESEARCH

Baillière's

CLINICAL OBSTETRICS AND GYNAECOLOGY

INTERNATIONAL PRACTICE AND RESEARCH

Volume 3/Number 4
December 1989

Psychological Aspects of Obstetrics and Gynaecology

M. R. OATES MB, ChB, DPM, MRCPsych
Guest Editor

Baillière Tindall
London Philadelphia Sydney Tokyo Toronto

This book is printed on acid-free paper. ∞

Baillière Tindall   24–28 Oval Road,
W.B. Saunders   London NW1 7DX

The Curtis Center, Independence Square West,
Philadelphia, PA 19106–3399, USA

55 Horner Avenue
Toronto, Ontario M8Z 4X6, Canada

Harcourt Brace Jovanovich Group (Australia) Pty Ltd,
30–52 Smidmore Street, Marrickville, NSW 2204, Australia

Harcourt Brace Jovanovich Japan, Inc,
Ichibancho Central Building,
22-1 Ichibancho, Chiyoda-ku, Tokyo 102, Japan

ISSN 0950–3552

ISBN 0–7020–1387–0 (single copy)

Baillière's Clinical Obstetrics and Gynaecology is published four times each year by Baillière Tindall. Annual subscription prices are:

TERRITORY	ANNUAL SUBSCRIPTION	SINGLE ISSUE
1. UK	£40.00 post free	£18.50 post free
2. Europe	£50.00 post free	£18.50 post free
3. All other countries	Consult your local Harcourt Brace Jovanovich office for dollar price	

The editor of this publication is Margaret Macdonald, Baillière Tindall, 24–28 Oval Road, London NW1 7DX.

Baillière's Clinical Obstetrics and Gynaecology was published from 1983 to 1986 as *Clinics in Obstetrics and Gynaecology*.

Typeset by Phoenix Photosetting, Chatham.
Printed and bound in Great Britain by Mackays of Chatham PLC, Chatham, Kent.

Contributors to this issue

ELIZABETH M. ALDER BSc, PhD, Lecturer in Psychology, Department of Management and Social Science, Queen Margaret College, Clerwood Terrace, Edinburgh EH12 8TS, UK.

STANFORD BOURNE MB, MRCP, FRCPsych, Consultant Psychotherapist, Perinatal Bereavement Unit, Tavistock Clinic, 120 Belsize Lane, London NW3 5BA, UK.

JOHN L. COX DM, FRCPE, FRCPsych, Department of Postgraduate Medicine and Biological Sciences, University of Keele, Thornburrow Drive, Hartshill, Stoke on Trent ST4 7QB, UK.

SANDRA A. ELLIOTT BSc, MPhil, PhD, Postnatal Project Director, National Unit of Psychiatric Research and Development, Lewisham Hospital, London SE13 6LH, UK.

TREVOR FRIEDMAN BSc, MB BS, MRCPsych, Lecturer and Honorary Senior Registrar, University Department of Psychiatry, Floor A, South Block University Hospital, Clifton Boulevard, Nottingham NG7 2UH, UK.

DENNIS GATH DM, FRCP, FRCPsych, Clinical Reader in Psychiatry, University of Oxford, University Department of Psychiatry, Warneford Hospital, Oxford OX3 7JX, UK.

N. L. HOLDEN MA, MB, BS, MRCP, MRCPsych, Senior Lecturer, Nottingham University Medical School, Professorial Unit, Department of Psychiatry, Mapperley Hospital, Porchester Road, Nottingham NG3 6AA, UK.

SUSAN ILES DPhil, MRCPsych, Wellcome Research Fellow in Mental Health, University Department of Psychiatry, Warneford Hospital, Oxford OX3 7JX, UK.

R. KUMAR MD, PhD, MPhil, FRCPsych, Reader, Institute of Psychiatry, De Crespigny Park, London SE5 8AF; Honorary Consultant Psychiatrist, Bethlem Royal and Maudsley Hospitals, London SE5, UK.

EMANUEL LEWIS MB, MRCP, FRCPsych, Consultant Psychotherapist, Perinatal Bereavement Unit, Tavistock Clinic, 120 Belsize Lane, London NW3 5BA, UK.

LYNNE MURRAY MA, PhD, Winnicott Research Fellow/Senior Research Associate, University of Cambridge, Child Care and Development Group, Free School Lane, Cambridge CB2 3RF, UK.

MARGARET OATES MB, ChB, DPM, MRCPsych, Senior Lecturer and Consultant in Psychiatry, Department of Psychiatry, 'A' Floor, South Block, University Hospital, Clifton Boulevard, Nottingham NG7 2UH, UK.

GWYNETH A. SAMPSON MB, ChB, DPM, MRCPsych, Consultant Psychiatrist, Honorary Clinical Lecturer, University of Sheffield, Whiteley Wood Clinic, Woofindon Road, Sheffield S10 3TL, UK.

ALAN STEIN MB, BCh, MRCPsych, Wellcome Trust Lecturer and Honorary Senior Registrar in Child Psychiatry, Department of Psychiatry, University of Oxford; The Park Hospital for Children, Old Road, Heddington, Oxford OX3, UK.

ANGELIKA WIECK MRCPsych, Senior Research Registrar Institute of Psychiatry, De Crespigny Park, Denmark Hill, London SE5 8AF; Honorary Senior Registrar, Bethlem and Maudsley Hospitals, London SE5, UK.

Table of contents

Foreword

This volume of *Baillière's Clinical Obstetrics and Gynaecology* covers those syndromes and procedures where psychological issues are of particular importance in aetiology, management and outcome. There is one topic included, 'Eating Disorders', which is not conventionally covered in books on gynaecology. This has been done because of the increased awareness of these problems and the frequency with which they present to the gynaecologist, either as menstrual problems or as a significant finding in infertility clinics. Not included is a specific chapter on sexual dysfunction, although the issue of sexual problems arising in context of other procedures and situations is frequently addressed throughout the volume. The issue of sexual functioning after childbirth is given particular attention as there is a great deal of misunderstanding, not only in women and their partners but also in health care professionals, about what is normal. It is hoped that this chapter will help those giving advice to women and their partners and bring about realistic expectations. The second part of the volume is particularly related to obstetric practice, to the emotional changes and psychiatric disorders associated with childbirth, the loss of a baby and the impact of emotional disorders on the children.

Throughout the book the chapters have been written by researchers, who in the main are deeply clinically involved in their area of interest. The emphasis is not only on recognising the vulnerable few who have adverse reactions to the gynaecological or obstetric events, but also on recognising the valid psychological needs and normal emotional reactions to these events. This volume aims to help the clinician reduce the psychological hazards of obstetrics and gynaecology and to increase the satisfaction of the women in their care.

Childbirth and the puerperium represents a major psychological hazard for women in terms of a high incidence of all forms of mental illness and a particularly high risk of serious mental illness. In addition to this, a substantial proportion of women suffer emotional discomfort and problems. The devotion of half of this volume to the puerperium reflects the concerns of the editor and her contributors (most of whom are members of the Marce Society, an International Scientific Society, founded in 1980 to study the prevention and detection of postnatal mental illness) that psychiatric disorder following childbirth is a major health hazard, largely undetected, causing needless morbidity and suffering not only for the woman but for her family. It is hoped that this volume will help obstetricians detect postnatal mental illness more easily, and include the possibility of psychiatric disorder in their management of the puerperium.

Special thanks are due to my secretary, Mrs Elizabeth Jeffrey, without whose patience and forebearance this work would never have been completed, and to those colleagues, obstetricians, midwives and psychiatric nurses, whose views and advice have influenced this volume but who do not appear in print.

MARGARET OATES

1

Premenstrual syndrome

GWYNETH A. SAMPSON

Premenstrual syndrome, formerly called premenstrual tension, is a comparatively modern phenomenon in terms of medical and scientific literature. There was a paucity of literature until the 1980s but in the last decade the relationship between symptoms, behaviour and menstruation has been assessed by clinicians, endocrinologists, psychologists, sociologists and physiologists.

One major problem which has bedevilled all this research is that of analysing whether symptoms are related to premenstruation, postmenstruation or menstruation itself. At a simplistic level if one assesses the premenstrual phase as one week and menstruation as one week then 50% of a menstruating woman's life is paramenstrual and half of all random symptoms would occur paramenstrually. This encourages sceptics to doubt the existence of a group of women who have symptoms which are episodic and which have a consistent time relationship to the onset of menstruation. However, even sceptical research workers consistently find a group of women who do have premenstrual syndrome (Steiner et al, 1980; Rubinow et al, 1984; Metcalf and Hudson, 1985). These and other workers demonstrate that women complaining of premenstrual syndrome are not a homogeneous group and that premenstrual syndrome needs to be clearly defined.

DEFINITION OF PREMENSTRUAL SYNDROME

Dalton (1984) states that 'the symptoms that can occur in the syndrome are of extraordinary diversity and include many of the commonest symptoms in each medical speciality'. Symptoms are often simplistically grouped into psychological (e.g. irritability, depression, tension, problems of concentration) and physical (e.g. bloatedness, breast tenderness), although many symptoms (e.g. headache, loss of energy) could be perceived as both psychological and physical. There are semantic difficulties as one woman's 'irritability' may be another's 'frustration' or 'anger'. Different subgroups or types of premenstrual symptoms have been postulated by various workers (Moos, 1985). Unfortunately the majority of the symptoms of premenstrual syndrome are also symptoms of other disorders and can also be experienced by men and postmenopausal women.

It is the timing not the type of symptoms which is important to the definition and diagnosis of premenstrual syndrome. By definition symptoms must occur premenstrually; the debate is then 'when is premenstrually' and whether symptoms occur *only* premenstrually or at other times in the cycle as well.

As well as the type of symptoms and their timing in relation to menstruation the severity of the symptoms and their effect upon the woman and those around her has to be considered.

The general population's definition

For women today the dilemma 'Do I have premenstrual syndrome?' is a real one. The media have given subjects such as premenstrual syndrome and the menopause wide publicity but have rarely clearly defined what they are. A message many women and their families receive is 'if you are irritable, tense and angry with your husband you may have premenstrual syndrome—so go and see your doctor'. This has at least three consequences: it may bring women to their doctors who believe they have and do have premenstrual syndrome, it may bring women to doctors who have another disorder but call their disorder premenstrual syndrome, and it may make husbands (whose wives are angry with them for good reason) attribute all anger and irritability to 'period trouble'.

Many women and men accept the physiological and psychological changes of the menstrual cycle as normal and expect women to be irritable before and have pain with menstruation; they would not consider such phenomena as illness nor use a medical model to alleviate them. Other people consider such changes pathological and seek 'treatment'.

The scientific research definition (pure premenstrual syndrome)

A consensus definition amongst research workers is now becoming clearer, and although there may be variations there is general agreement with most aspects of Dalton's definition (Dalton, 1984).

Premenstrual syndrome is 'the recurrence of symptoms in the premenstruum with absence of symptoms in the postmenstruum'. Many workers agree with the following criteria:

1. Symptoms are cyclical, occurring only during the second half of the menstrual cycle.
2. Symptoms increase in severity as the cycle progresses.
3. Symptoms must be relieved by the onset of the full menstrual flow, with complete absence of symptoms within two to three days after the onset.
4. There must be an absence of symptoms in the postmenstruum, with a symptom-free time lasting at least seven clear days and often nine to ten days.
5. Symptoms must have been present for at least three consecutive cycles; there may be variation between cycles in degree of severity of symptoms.
6. The symptoms interfere with work or with usual social activities or relationships with others.

In careful surveys of women who believe they have premenstrual syndrome, and who are then asked to keep prospective diaries of symptoms so the timing and intensity of these in relation to menstruation is recorded, only around one in four has premenstrual syndrome fulfilling the above criteria (Steiner et al, 1980; Sampson and Prescott, 1981; Rubinow et al, 1984; Metcalf and Hudson, 1985).

Although this definition is currently accepted, many research publications, especially in the past, did not adopt such strict criteria. This is demonstrated in Table 1 which lists figures for the incidence of premenstrual syndrome. The wide discrepancies are related to the different definitions of premenstrual syndrome used, although in many cases the definitions are not precisely stated and in few cases is there any diary-keeping of symptoms. It is therefore advisable when reading articles on premenstrual syndrome to ascertain what diagnostic criteria the authors are using.

Table 1. Reported incidence of premenstrual syndrome (PMS).

Authors	Year	Group	Number	% with PMS
Rees	1953	'Normal women' (UK)	61	21
Kessel and Coppen	1963	GP practices (UK)	500	25
Sutherland and Stewart	1965	Hospital personnel and students	150	33
Clare	1977	GP practices (UK)	521	75
Van Keep and Lehert	1981	Community survey (France)	2501	85
Hargrove and Abraham	1982	Gynaecology clinic	1395	50

The clinician's definition

Clinicians often feel that they are trapped between patients insisting they have premenstrual syndrome and an awareness of a more scientific definition of premenstrual syndrome. The majority of women most doctors see do not fulfil all the criteria described above. For example, in some women symptoms continue through menstruation, others are irritable at times throughout the cycle and many of them have low grade symptoms all the time with an exacerbation of these paramenstrually.

To many researchers a further definition is needed to describe women who have a premenstrual component to their symptoms but who have symptoms at other times in the menstrual cycle. Dalton (Dalton, 1984) coined the term 'menstrual distress' to describe the presence of intermittent or continuous symptoms throughout the cycle which increase in severity during the premenstruum or menstruation. Dennerstein et al (1984) define 'menstrual distress' as the presence of symptoms of a diagnosable psychiatric disorder which are of at least moderate intensity throughout the cycle with exacerbation in the premenstrum. Harrison (1985) uses the term 'premenstrual magnification' to describe a similar condition to Dalton (Dalton, 1984). Bäckström (1988) uses the term 'premenstrual aggravation' and Sampson 'perimenstrual distress'.

Figure 1 highlights the differences between pure premenstrual syndrome

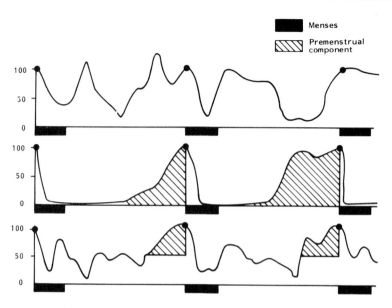

Figure 1. A graphical representation of a generalized anxiety state with mood fluctuations unrelated to menstruation (top), classical premenstrual syndrome (middle) and perimenstrual distress (bottom). All cycles score 100 on day 1 of menstruation. The premenstrual component of symptoms is highlighted.

and perimenstrual distress; the premenstrual component of complaining is highlighted.

It is likely that in a clinical setting the majority of patients experience perimenstrual distress. Watts et al (1980) reassessed women selected by gynaecologists as having premenstrual syndrome and excluded 17 out of 42 when using a pure definition.

It is important in a clinical setting to distinguish between pure premenstrual syndrome and perimenstrual distress, as their management will differ. Clinicians will also see women complaining of premenstrual syndrome who have symptoms with no time relationship to the menstrual cycle. Conversely they may identify women as having premenstrual syndrome who do not complain of it.

A clinician's premenstrual definition could include both pure premenstrual syndrome and perimenstrual distress.

AETIOLOGICAL HYPOTHESES

Premenstrual syndrome, including perimenstrual distress, encompasses a broad aetiological spectrum; it is now clear that it is not a simple biological phenomenon. It is helpful to view it as a psychosomatic disorder with biological, psychological, social and cultural components.

A major dilemma which affects not only aetiological hypotheses but diagnosis and management is 'Is premenstrual syndrome a spectrum disorder, or is it an ill/well phenomenon?'

As with incidence studies, papers on aetiology are often unclear about definitions; many are describing emotional distress related to the menstrual cycle rather than clinical premenstrual syndrome.

Biological hypotheses

The menstrual cycle is a highly complicated, finely balanced series of events taking place in a context of many other biological functions. Asso (1988) in a review of the physiology of the normal menstrual cycle points out that, although the rhythmic fluctuation in oestrogen, progesterone, follicle-stimulating hormone and luteinizing hormone are well documented, it is increasingly clear that they are part of a larger pattern of cyclical changes which have far-reaching effects. More details are emerging of a number of neurophysiological variables which change systematically through the cycle; it is likely that many of the effects of cyclical hormone change are mediated through the nervous system.

During the last decade there have been many studies assessing endocrine profiles (oestrogen, progesterone, follicle-stimulating hormone, luteinizing hormone, aldosterone, testosterone, sex hormone binding globulin, prolactin) throughout the cycle in women complaining of premenstrual syndrome compared with controls (although in some cases controls also showed cyclical mood changes) (Andersch et al, 1978; O'Brien et al, 1980; Dalton, 1981; Munday et al, 1981; Bäckström et al, 1983). No consistently abnormal pattern of hormones has been found, a fact which becomes more understandable as the complexities of the menstrual cycle unfold. There is still debate as to whether premenstrual syndrome can occur in an anovulatory cycle.

There is a wide range of evidence that oestrogen increases and progesterone decreases central nervous system activity. There are probably individual differences in the reactivity of the nervous system to hormone levels. During the menstrual cycle central arousal rises probably during the follicular phase to a peak around ovulation and thereafter falls and remains low to the end of the cycle (Asso, 1983). This pattern corresponds temporally with the increasingly positive buoyant mood of the first half of the cycle through the quieter more contented luteal phase to the reported negative mood at the end. Prostaglandins and endorphin are likely to be relevant (Reid and Yen, 1981), as well as neurotransmitters involved in the control of hypothalamic hormone-releasing mechanisms and mood and behaviour. Asso (1988) reports that it appears that certain aspects (not all) of autonomic reactivity (as opposed to levels) and certain other indices of autonomic functioning are high premenstrually and low at mid cycle. She hypothesizes that these changes and probably individual perception often play an important part in other manifestations of the cycle.

Psychological hypotheses

Several studies of normal women show a cyclical variation in mood throughout the menstrual cycle, which is hypothesized as being related to the primarily reproductive role of the cycle. Little and Zahn (1974) conclude that normal women suffer premenstrually and at the beginning of menstruation, not so much from pronounced shifts in negative feeling as from a lack of positive energy and 'warmth'. Asso (1988) hypothesizes that this is a biological by-product of the events in the second half of a non-fertilized reproductive cycle. However, other workers (Slade, 1984) found that although cyclical physical symptoms were reported there were no significant mood changes. Others (Halbreich and Endicott, 1987) describe a group of women who have increased feelings of well-being and more energy premenstrually. Negative feelings during the menstrual phase have been considered a response to the pain and discomfort experienced (Golub and Harrington, 1981).

If there is a normal cyclical mood variation through the cycle this supports the concept of a spectrum disorder with premenstrual syndrome at one end of the spectrum.

When studies are made of women complaining of premenstrual syndrome it is found that these women are more likely to complain of intrapersonal conflicts and marital disharmony (Clare, 1983), and are more likely to have high trait anxiety scores indicating a predisposition to suffer from anxiety (Watts et al, 1980). They also score a higher level on tests of neuroticism (Slade and Jenner, 1980; Sampson, 1983). This group of women is likely to consist of both women with pure premenstrual syndrome and those with perimenstrual distress. It is therefore possible that the findings are related to 'complaining' rather than the presence of premenstrual syndrome in a broader population. Laws (1985) claims that many women focus on premenstrual syndrome instead of facing and dealing with other problems such as stressful relationships or adverse circumstances. Consequently she feels they find it more difficult to cope with otherwise unobtrusive premenstrual alterations in mood.

Psychoanalytically there are studies voicing often disparate views that premenstrual syndrome is the manifestation of one or more unresolved psychological conflicts. However, there are many methodological problems in assessing these studies (Parlee, 1982), and these hypotheses have not been supported by recent studies.

In assessing psychological hypotheses we need to distinguish between premenstrual syndrome and 'complaining'. The aetiology of 'complaining' is complex.

The environment

Diet, either in terms of its nutritional value, possible toxicity or sensitivity to additives, has been postulated as an aetiological factor, especially in the lay press (Rea, 1988). Many articles have a broad-based concept of premenstrual syndrome and may relate more to general well-being than premenstrual syndrome specifically. Rea (1988) also cites air pollution as an aetiological factor.

Many allergic conditions are aggravated premenstrually so factors which diminish the allergic component will help diminish the perimenstrual exacerbation. This is not classical premenstrual syndrome.

Culture and society

A WHO examination of the worldwide patterns of beliefs, practices and symptoms associated with menstruation (Snowden and Christian, 1984) found that in the UK 75% of women reported experiencing mood changes premenstrually, 50% menstrually and 33% intermenstrually. In the USA one-half to one-third reported mood swings in the premenstrual and menstrual phases with only 20% intermenstrually. However, in other nations the biggest shift in moods corresponds to the onset of menstrual bleeding and not the premenstruum. In Egypt and the Philippines there was no menstrual shift in moods, although between one-half and one-third of women reported high levels of mood changes throughout the cycle. In virtually all nations women with heavier and/or longer menstrual bleeds are significantly more likely to report mood shifts with menstruation; heavier bleeding is not significantly related to premenstrual moods.

This global study suggests that premenstrual syndrome is a Western 'civilized' phenomenon, unlike dysmenorrhoea and menstrual mood changes which appear to be universal. The aetiological hypothesis as to why the West has premenstrual syndrome are many and often highly conjectural.

CLINICAL PRESENTATION AND ASSESSMENT

Only a small percentage of women with premenstrual syndrome seek medical help. Hallman (1986) estimates only 7.5% of women with pre-menstrual syndrome feel they need to see a physician. There is a consider-able market in over-the-counter preparations of dietary supplements, there are agencies which offer advice about diet and general life-style manage-ment, and self-help books. As with many reproductive disorders, 'word of mouth' advice from other women is most important, as is media coverage of the symptoms and their management. Many women seeking medical help have already tried other remedies, although they may not have persisted with them over several cycles.

We do not know if the women seeking medical help are typical of the majority of premenstrual syndrome sufferers. Hallman (1986) describes the group requesting help as being older (30–40 years), they evaluate their own symptoms as being more serious and different, they are more likely to have children, more likely to have seen a physician or taken anxiolytics, and are more likely to have symptoms which affected family life and relationships. Anxiety and depression were more pronounced and they showed variations in spring and autumn. Other authors find them more likely to score higher on tests of neuroticism and tests indicating a predisposition to anxiety. Although they may present with similar case histories, when they are investigated with daily prospective diaries they become a very hetero-geneous group (Hammarbäck and Bäckström, 1985).

History taking

A full menstrual, pregnancy, postpartum, contraceptive and gynaecological history should be recorded in chronological order, noting the presence of any groups of symptoms in relation to these.

The present symptoms, their duration, intensity and timing in relation to the onset and cessation of bleeding should be identified. The commonest symptoms are irritability, anergia, poor concentration, emotional lability, a loss of or fear of losing control, breast tenderness and abdominal bloating. All other disorders, e.g. headache, which can be exacerbated premenstrually should be noted. As well as noting negative symptoms it is important to record positive symptoms, e.g. feeling good, affectionate, energetic.

Having obtained a list of the type of symptoms it is their timing in relation to bleeding which is important. The times of onset, peak intensity and loss of each symptom should be noted.

In order to clarify the differential diagnosis it is important to take a personal history, including a previous psychiatric history. The latter is not likely to involve psychiatric admission but should include all previous episodes of emotional distress and depression lasting more than a month (including postpartum episodes), and should identify whether help was sought for these episodes from a GP or other agency and if medication was prescribed. A family history including information on the patient's mother's menstrual history and an appraisal of the patient's current life situation (relationships, stresses) is helpful.

Prospective diary keeping

It is now well accepted that it is impossible to formulate an accurate diagnosis of premenstrual syndrome without information from prospective diary keeping. This is required to note the nature but especially the timing and intensity of symptoms; it is therefore important to have a diary for a minimum of two cycles and ideally for three. As premenstrual syndrome is a chronic condition, although the patient may demand that something be done 'urgently' it is especially important to have a correct diagnosis so correct management may be discussed with the patient.

There are many ways of asking the patient to keep a diary. The diary produced by the Drug and Therapeutic Bulletin for the Consumers' Association and advocated by Dalton (1984) with a space for every day allows timing and type of symptoms but not their intensity to be recorded for a year. Several pharmaceutical companies provide similar diaries, although they do not allow a long-term appraisal of symptoms. Several research diaries are available (Moos, 1977; Halbreich and Endicott, 1987). It is often feasible to ask the patient to produce her own diary in which she lists her commonest symptoms, their intensity and duration on a 0 to 3 scale as well as medication and life stresses. An example is shown in Figure 2.

Differential diagnosis

It is impossible to have a differential diagnosis without a full history and

SYMPTOMS **DATES**

		1	2	3	4	5	6	7	8	9	10	11	May 1980
1	Irritability	1	0	1	2	3	3	3	2	2	1	1	
2	Loss of control	0	0	0	0	1	2	1	1	0	0	0	
3	Depression	0	0	0	1	2	1	1	1	1	1	1	
4	Bust tenderness	3	3	3	3	3	3	2	1	0	0	0	
5	Bloating	2	3	2	2	3	2	1	0	0	0	0	
6	Overeating	0	3	0	2	0	3	0	0	0	0	3	
7	Headache	0	1	2	0	0	3	2	0	0	0	0	
8	Spots	0	1	0	0	0	0	0	2	2	0	0	
MENSTRUAL BLEED		0	0	0	0	S	M	M	M	M	M	S	
MEDICATION							A	A					
PROBLEMS				√	√								

Symptoms are to be rated as: 0 = absent
1 = mild
2 = moderate
3 = severe, disabling

Menstrual bleed is to be rated as: 0 = none
S = spotting
M = menstrual bleed

Medication is to be rated as: A = analgesics (pain killers)
V = vitamins
T = tranquillisers

Problems to be marked √ if symptoms are of an intensity to cause disruption to daily living

Figure 2. An example of a menstrual cycle diary allowing space for patient to list eight major symptoms and then record their intensity and duration.

prospective diaries—this will therefore entail two clinic visits, or the facility to send out diaries two months before the first visit. The differential diagnosis includes:

1. *Premenstrual syndrome*—patient only has symptoms premenstrually and is symptom-free for the remainder of the cycle.
2. *Perimenstrual distress*—patient has an increase in symptoms peri-menstrually but they are present at other times in the cycle.
3. *General anxiety state or depression*—if psychological symptoms persist or are intermittent throughout the cycle with no significant perimenstrual exacerbation.
4. *Fluid retention syndrome*—if bloating and swelling persists or is inter-mittent throughout the cycle (Dunnigan, 1983).
5. *Dysmenorrhoea.*
6. *Cyclical benign breast disease*—cyclical breast pain, usually in the luteal phase of the cycle (Mansel, 1988).

Natural history of premenstrual syndrome

There are few epidemiological studies using the general population and most information is from specialized subgroups of women.

The age of onset of the disorder is unclear, but many do not 'complain' until in their 30's. Sampson (unpublished observation) found only 20% of a sample reported symptoms before 19 years of age, whilst 64% had symptoms by 30 years. Most reports indicate that symptoms increase in duration and intensity with time, lasting until the menopause.

Several authors comment on the relationship between various pregnancy and puerperal factors and premenstrual syndrome. Dalton (1984) found that two out of five premenstrual sufferers attribute the onset of symptoms to a pregnancy; Sampson (unpublished observation) found one in five. Depression occurring postpartum (not puerperal psychosis) is related to later premenstrual symptoms but this is a complex indirect relationship more likely to be related to sociological rather than endocrine factors.

Prognosis

There are no long-term studies assessing prognosis either with or without therapy. Classical premenstrual syndrome will cease at the menopause; those women with perimenstrual distress will lose their premenstrual component but continue to experience distress.

MANAGEMENT

As premenstrual syndrome is a complex psychosomatic problem it is important:

1. To have an accurate diagnostic formulation both of the premenstrual symptoms and intercurrent gynaecological, contraceptive, social, psychological or emotional problems.
2. As management is of a chronic disorder to consider long- as well as short-term goals, i.e. a management strategy with a low incidence of side-effects that is capable of continuation until the menopause.
3. To identify the patient's expectations of both medical consultation and therapy.

Whatever management strategies are tried it is important to be aware of the high placebo response rate in premenstrual syndrome. Placebo response is itself a complex phenomenon and is usually predicted in disorders with psychological symptoms, although physical symptoms may respond as well to placebo as psychological symptoms. Placebo rates are often around 50% (Sampson, 1988).

Reassurance

Many women may only require that the diagnosis of premenstrual syndrome be confirmed and that other pathology is excluded. 'Talking to a doctor who understands' is often perceived as helpful.

Techniques to improve the ability to manage symptoms

Stress and premenstrual syndrome are closely related (Sampson, 1983). For some women stress is a precipitating or maintaining aetiological factor; for the majority of women stress is a consequence of premenstrual syndrome, especially when they have symptoms for over a week every month (this is over 84 days per annum and could continue for ten or more consecutive years). Techniques for diminishing stress and improving symptom coping are effective in premenstrual syndrome. Such techniques could include:

1. Reducing or avoiding stressful situations premenstrually, e.g. avoid driving tests, arrange child care to provide the woman with a 'break'.
2. Improving ability to cope with stressful situations, e.g. help from a health visitor with child management skills, attending an Anxiety Management Group.
3. Helping the woman alter her perception of herself and events so she becomes more confident at coping, e.g. cognitive therapy (Morse and Dennerstein, 1988).
4. Methods of altering the physiological response to stress and symptoms e.g. yoga, relaxation therapy.

Techniques to improve general well-being

It is appropriate to give dietary advice as to weight control, an adequate regular diet (avoiding hypoglycaemia) and, for headache patients, eliminating caffeine, chocolate, etc. to see if it diminishes symptoms.

Exercise has long been advocated and a prospective controlled six-month trial of exercise training demonstrated decreased premenstrual symptoms in two groups who trained, with no change in symptoms in a non-training group. The decrease in symptoms did not correlate with documented hormones, menstrual cycle or weight changes. Sedentary women increased the distance they ran from 0 to 76 km/menstrual cycle (Prior et al, 1987)—so patients should be advised to run ten miles per week!

If the patient has other life stresses or anxiety symptoms she could be referred for counselling; marital or sexual difficulties may be helped by couple counselling. 'Common sense' advise is often appropriately provided by health visitors, practice nurses or community psychiatric nurses.

Information and education

Many women, despite the inclusion of 'reproduction' in school curricula still have a poor and often incorrect understanding of the physiology and anatomy of menstruation. Improved knowledge reduces anxiety about symptoms.

This information can be provided by medical or nursing staff (as in antenatal clinics). There are self-help books available, although some are written by authors who firmly believe in one aetiological model and whose therapeutic strategies are based on this model. It is therefore important that doctors read the book before recommending it, as they may not be able to justify the concepts in it to their patients.

Symptomatic relief

Treatment may be aimed at the relief of symptoms once they are present.

Pain symptoms

Analgesics are appropriate for headache, abdominal pain and breast tenderness. Prostaglandin inhibitors may be tried after simple analgesics.

Breast tenderness and abdominal bloating

Although there is no clear evidence that women gain weight premenstrually, the majority of women experience breast tenderness and abdominal bloating. Initially dietary manipulation aimed at reducing the intake of refined carbohydrates and salt should be tried. There have been several uncontrolled studies of the benefits of diuretics. O'Brien et al (1979) found spironolactone better than placebo. The long term use of spironolactone in young patients requires careful consideration of the benefits and potential hazard involved.

Mood symptoms

Many women use alcohol or food for short-term relief of mood symptoms, but both lead to long-term problems. Minor tranquillizers have been used, but there have been no controlled studies of their use. Meprobamate, an anxiolytic, combined with the diuretic bendrofluazide (Tenavoid) has been advocated. One controlled study found 66% patients responded to Tenavoid and 48% to placebo. However, meprobamate usage may lead to dependence.

There is little evidence that antidepressant drugs are useful in true premenstrual syndrome. However, if there is persistent lowering of mood with associated biological symptoms and a premenstrual exacerbation their use may be indicated.

Correcting the hypothetical underlying aetiological causes

There are several differing aetiological models for premenstrual syndrome, most of which hypothesize a disorder or deficiency. The rationale for several therapies is that they correct or alter the hypothetical underlying disorder.

Vitamins, essential fatty acids and minerals

Pyridoxine (vitamin B_6) has been widely recommended for the treatment of premenstrual syndrome; its use is based on aetiological theories of its function as a cofactor in the metabolism of dopamine, noradrenaline (norepinephrine) and serotonin. Numerous uncontrolled studies suggest it is helpful. Controlled studies are less clear; Abraham and Hargrove (1980) found it better than placebo in a 500 mg daily dose. Recent work (Schuambergh et al, 1983) suggests that large doses (500 mg day or more) taken continuously produce a risk of neuropathy.

Many women buy evening primrose oil which is hypothesized as being effective because of its high content of linolenic acid which is a key intermediary in the n6 series of essential fatty acids and a precursor of prostaglandin E_1. Essential fatty acid deficiency states appear to correlate with some types of breast disease. Mansel (1988) reports a double blind study of evening primrose oil for treatment of cyclical mastalgia which found it better than placebo but less effective than danazol or bromocriptine. Open studies suggest it is helpful for mood symptoms, but controlled studies are lacking. It is available as an over-the-counter preparation which is expensive to buy.

There have been no controlled studies of magnesium or zinc in the treatment of premenstrual syndrome although they are sold over the counter for this condition.

Prostaglandin inhibitors

Prostaglandin levels fluctuate in response to changing levels of oestradiol and progesterone, and they exert sedative and other effects on the central nervous system. Uncontrolled studies suggested mefenamic acid (which blocks the production of the 2 series prostaglandins) was helpful and a double-blind randomized placebo-controlled cross-over study found it significantly better than placebo for physical and mood symptoms, especially fatigue, general aches and pains, and headache (Mira et al, 1986).

Endocrine therapies

It is now accepted that there is no simplistic endocrine cause of premenstrual syndrome, but the clear link between the luteal phase and premenstrual symptoms indicate that hormones are relevant. Endocrine therapies could theoretically alter premenstrual symptomatology by:

1. Hormonal replacement, although there is no consistent evidence of any deficiency.
2. Having a direct pharmacological effect.
3. Manipulating the endocrine profile of a cycle so the abnormal 'premenstrual cycle' is more like a normal 'non-premenstrual cycle'.
4. Ablating the menstrual cycle and its cyclical hormonal fluctuations.

Combined oral contraception. Several studies (Herzberg and Coppen, 1970; Royal College of General Practitioners, 1974) suggest oral contraceptives help premenstrual symptoms and it has been suggested that the more progestogenic formulations are more effective. Oral contraceptives 'manipulate' or can be used to ablate the cycle, although they also have a pharmacological effect.

Oestradiol implant. Magos et al (1986) hypothesize that suppression of ovulation should abolish premenstrual symptoms. In a parallel but not cross-over study comparing oestradiol implants with placebo implants, with a progestogen added for seven days to induce bleeding, they found a significant superiority of oestrogen over placebo. There appeared to be pharmacological effects due to the progestogen, and also an initial placebo response of 94%. Oestradiol implants should be given in a specialist clinic with close supervision and monitoring of symptoms by daily diaries to ascertain when a further implant is required.

Progesterone. The initial rationale for progesterone therapy appears to have been to provide hormonal replacement for the luteal phase. Dalton (1984) advocates progesterone based on clinical experience and open studies. Several double-blind cross-over studies of progesterone and placebo have been reported. Sampson (1979), Van der Meer et al (1983) and Maddocks et al (1986) report that, although progesterone was effective, it was no more so than placebo. Dennerstein et al (1985) using oral micronized progesterone found it more effective than placebo for some symptoms. Smith (1975) compared intramuscular progesterone with placebo and found no significant benefit. Progesterone is given as suppositories or pessaries which many women find unacceptable. Dalton (1984) reports use of high doses intramuscularly (up to 100 mg daily) and it is likely that this usage not only ablates the cycle but has a pharmacological effect on cerebral function.

Progestogens. Several progestogens have been used in the treatment of premenstrual syndrome; dydrogesterone has been the most widely evaluated. Its initial usage was as hormone replacement in the luteal phase and uncontrolled and single-blind studies reported great success (Taylor, 1977). Double-blind studies find placebo and dydrogesterone equally effective (Sampson et al, 1988). Williams et al (1983) found dydrogesterone and placebo equally effective for two months but in the third treatment month patient and physician indicated a significant preference for dydrogesterone over placebo. Lenton (1984) demonstrates that using the same dosage of dydrogesterone at different times in the cycle will produce differing endocrine profiles (and can act as a cycle 'manipulator' or ablator). Sampson (1988) describes cases where a different symptom profile is related to different dosage regimens. Keye (1985) used progestogens for cycle ablation.

Bromocriptine. The rationale for bromocriptine therapy is the aetiological hypothesis of high prolactin levels. There have been several double-blind studies using different dose levels; the majority report an improvement in breast but not mood symptoms (Anderson et al, 1977; Andersch et al, 1978; Mansel et al, 1978).

Danazol. The rationale for treatment with danazol (an androgen) is cycle ablation. Two preliminary reports of placebo-controlled double-blind studies show a higher percentage response to danazol than placebo (Gilmore et al, 1985; Watts et al, 1987). In both studies adverse side-effects caused those patients on active medication rather than placebo to withdraw. As premenstrual syndrome is a chronic condition and medication may be required for several years the longer term side-effects of danazol (which include hirsutism and acne) should be discussed with the patient before initiating therapy.

Gonadotrophin releasing hormone agonists. The rationale for gonadotrophin releasing hormone (GnRH) use is cycle manipulation/ablation. Muse et al (1984) reported that physical and behaviour symptoms were improved compared with placebo, and Bancroft et al (1985) found most convincing results in women who showed follicular suppression.

General comments. The endocrine therapy of premenstrual syndrome is a complex area. For each therapeutic agent the correct dosage, timing of dosage, the endocrine parameters it alters, the symptom factors it changes and its short- and long-term side-effects have to be appraised. The majority of endocrine therapies currently available are beneficial, although controlled studies suggest only as beneficial as placebo. The more effective therapies seem to manipulate or ablate the cycle, but also have the most side-effects. If it is considered appropriate to use an endocrine agent for treatment it is wise to commence with an oral contraceptive, progesterone or a progestogen (using the last two from early in the cycle e.g. day 5 to 26). Such treatment should be monitored by daily diaries for at least six consecutive cycles to assess its value. Other endocrine agents could then be reserved for more severe premenstrual syndrome when other therapies have not produced sufficient improvement.

SUMMARY

The term premenstrual syndrome is often used to describe several clinical conditions. Only a full history covering not only reproductive but also psychological and social factors, combined with daily diaries which are kept prospectively for at least two months, can help clarify the problems the patient experiences. As it is the timing rather than the type of symptoms which is essential to a diagnosis, diaries are used to assess symptoms, make a diagnosis and monitor the effectiveness of therapy. Patients with premenstrual syndrome should therefore always keep a diary and bring it to every consultation.

We do not know if patients complaining of premenstrual syndrome are at one extreme of a spectrum disorder or if they are a 'specific group'. Such patients may have classical premenstrual syndrome, perimenstrual distress, benign idiopathic oedema, dysmenorrhoea, cyclical benign breast disease or mood symptoms which are not significantly related to the menstrual cycle.

There are many aetiological theories—biological, psychological, environmental and social, the syndrome being a complex psychosomatic disorder.

For appropriate management an accurate diagnostic formation is required. Reassurance, stress management techniques, an improvement in general mental and physical well-being, information and education are the mainstays of therapy. Symptomatic relief of symptoms is often helpful. Many other managements have been tried with the aim of correcting the underlying aetiological case. These include vitamins, prostaglandin inhibitors and endocrine therapies. As the disorder is long-term, the safety of treatments should be carefully considered.

Acknowledgements

I wish to thank Jennifer M. Woodward for secretarial help and Gill Gill for library assistance.

REFERENCES

Abraham GE & Hargrove JT (1980) Effect of vitamin B6 on premenstrual symptomatology in women with premenstrual tension syndrome. *Infertility* **3**: 155–165.

Andersch B, Abrahamsson L, Wendestam C, Ohman R & Hann L (1978) Hormone profile in premenstrual tension. Effects of bromocriptine and diuretics. *Clinical Endocrinology* **11**: 657–664.

Anderson AN, Larsen JF, Steenstrup OR, Svendstrup B & Nielson J (1977) Effect of bromocriptine on the premenstrual syndrome: a double blind clinical trial. *British Journal of Obstetrics and Gynaecology* **84**: 370–374.

Anderson B, Hahn L, Wendestam C & Abrahamsson L (1978) Treatment of premenstrual syndrome with bromocriptine. *Acta Endocrinologica* **88 (supplement 216)**: 165–174.

Asso D (1983) *The Real Menstrual Cycle*. Chichester: John Wiley.

Asso D (1988) Physiology and psychology of the normal menstrual cycle. In Brush MG & Goudsmit EM (eds) *Functional Disorders of the Menstrual Cycle*, pp 15–36. Chichester: John Wiley.

Bäckström T (1988) Endocrine factors in the aetiology of premenstrual syndrome. In Brush MG & Goudsmit EM (eds) *Functional Disorders of the Menstrual Cycle*, pp 87–96. Chichester: John Wiley.

Bäckström T, Sanders D, Leask R et al (1983) Mood, sexuality, hormones and the menstrual cycle II. Hormone levels and their relationship to the premenstrual syndrome. *Psychosomatic Medicine* **45**: 503–507.

Bancroft J, Boyle H, Davidson DW, Gray J & Fraser HM (1985) The effects of an LH-RH agonist on the premenstrual syndrome: a preliminary report. In Schmidt-Gollwitzer M (ed.) *LH-RH and its Analogues. Fertility and Anti-fertility Aspects*, pp 307–319. Berlin: Walter de Gruyter.

Clare AW (1977) Psychological profiles of women complaining of premenstrual symptoms. *Current Medical Research and Opinion* **4 (supplement 4)**: 23–28.

Clare AW (1983) Psychiatric and social aspects of premenstrual complaint. *Psychological Medicine Monograph Supplement* **4**: 1–58.

Dalton K (1984) *The Premenstrual Syndrome and Progesterone Therapy* 2nd edn, pp 291. London: Heinemann.

Dalton ME (1981) Sex hormone binding globulin concentrations in women with severe premenstrual syndrome. *Postgraduate Medical Journal* **57**: 560–561.

Dennerstein L, Spencer-Gardner C, Brown JB, Smith MA & Burrows GD (1984) Premenstrual tension—hormonal profiles. *Journal of Psychosomatic Obstetrics and Gynaecology* **3**: 35–51.

Dennerstein L, Spencer-Gardner C, Gotts G et al (1985) Progesterone and the premenstrual syndrome: a double blind cross over trial. *British Medical Journal* **290**: 1617–1621.

Dunnigan MG (1983) The recognition and management of the fluid retention syndrome of women. In Taylor RW (ed.) *Premenstrual Syndrome*, pp 25–32. London: Medical News Tribune.

Gilmore DH, Hawthorn RJS & McKay-Hart J (1985) Danol for premenstrual syndrome: a preliminary report of a placebo controlled double blind study. *Journal of International Medical Research* **13**: 129–130.

Golub S & Harrington DM (1981) Premenstrual and menstrual mood changes in adolescent women. *Journal of Personality and Social Psychology* **41**: 961–965.

Halbreich MD & Endicott J (1987) Dysphoric premenstrual changes: are they related to affective disorders? In Ginsberg BE & Carter BF (eds) *Premenstrual Syndrome. Ethical and Legal Implications in a Biomedical Perspective*, pp 351–367. New York: Plenum Press.

Hallman J (1986) The premenstrual syndrome—an equivalent of depression? *Acta Psychiatrica Scandinavica* **73**: 403–411.

Hammarbäck S & Bäckström T (1985) Premenstrual tension—diagnostical aspects and classification of patients. *Archives of Gynaecology* **237 (supplement)**: 205.

Hargrove JT & Abraham GE (1982) The incidence of premenstrual tension in a gynecologic clinic. *Journal of Reproductive Medicine* **27**: 721–724.

Harrison M (1985) *Self Help with PMS*, p 210. London: Optima MacDonald.

Herzberg B & Coppen A (1970) Changes in psychological symptoms in women taking oral contraceptives. *British Journal of Psychiatry* **116**: 161–164.

Kessel N & Coppen A (1963) The problems of common menstrual symptoms. *Lancet* **ii**: 61–66.

Keye WR (1985) Medical management of premenstrual syndrome. *Canadian Journal of Psychiatry* **30**: 483–488.

Laws S (1985) Who needs PMT? A feminist approach to the politics of premenstrual tension. In Law S, Hey V & Eagan A (eds) *Seeing Red. The Politics of Premenstrual Tension*, pp 16–64. London: Hutchinson.

Lenton EA (1984) The effect of dydrogesterone on the mid cycle gonadotrophin surge in regularly cycling women. *Clinical Endocrinology* **20**: 129–135.

Little BC & Zahn TP (1974) Changes in mood and autonomic functioning during the menstrual cycle. *Psychophysiology* **11**: 579–590.

Maddocks S, Hahn P, Moller F & Reid R (1986) A double blind placebo controlled trial of progesterone vaginal suppositories in the treatment of premenstrual syndrome. *American Journal of Obstetrics and Gynecology* **154**: 573–581.

Magos AL, Brincat M & Studd JWW (1986) Treatment of the premenstrual syndrome by subcutaneous oestradiol implants and cyclical oral norethisterone: placebo controlled study. *British Medical Journal* **292**: 1629–1633.

Mansel RE (1988) Investigation and treatment of cyclical benign breast disease. In Brush MG & Goudsmit EM (Eds) *Functional Disorders of the Menstrual Cycle*, pp 191–198. Chichester: John Wiley.

Mansel RE, Preece PE & Hughes LE (1978) A double blind trial of the prolactin inhibitor bromocriptine in painful benign breast disease. *British Journal of Surgery* **65**: 724–727.

Metcalf MG & Hudson SM (1985) The premenstrual syndrome. Selection of women for treatment trials. *Journal of Psychosomatic Research* **29**: 631–638.

Mira M, McNeil D, Fraser IS, Vizzard J & Abraham S (1986) Mefenamic acid in the treatment of premenstrual syndrome. *Obstetrics and Gynecology* **68(3)**: 395–398.

Moos RH (1977) *Menstrual Distress Questionnaire Manual*. California: Social Ecology Laboratory, Stamford University.

Moos RH (1985) *Perimenstrual Syndromes: A Manual and Overview of research with the Menstrual Distress Questionnaire*. California: Social Ecology Laboratory, Stamford University.

Morse CA & Dennerstein L (1988) Cognitive therapy for premenstrual syndrome. In Brush MG & Goudsmit EM (eds) *Functional Disorders of the Menstrual Cycle*, pp 177–190. Chichester: John Wiley.

Munday M, Brush MG & Taylor RW (1981) Correlations between progesterone, oestradiol and aldosterone levels in the premenstrual syndrome. *Clinical Endocrinology* **14**: 1–19.

Muse KN, Catel NS, Futterman LA & Yen SSC (1984) The premenstrual syndrome. Effect of medical ovariectomy. *New England Journal of Medicine* **311**: 1345–1349.

O'Brien PMS, Craven D, Selby C & Symonds EM (1979) Treatment of premenstrual syndrome by Spironolactone. *British Journal of Obstetrics and Gynaecology* **86**: 142–147.

O'Brien PMS, Selby C & Symonds EM (1980) Progesterone, fluid and electrolytes in premenstrual syndrome. *British Medical Journal* **i**: 1161–1163.

Parlee MB (1982) The psychology of the menstrual cycle. Biological and psychological aspects. In Friedman RC (ed.) *Behaviour and the Menstrual Cycle*, pp 77–79. New York: Marcel Dekker.

Prior JC, Vigna Y, Sciarretta D, Alojado N & Schulzer M (1987) Conditioning exercise decreases premenstrual symptoms: a prospective controlled 6-month trial. *Fertility and Sterility* **47(3)**: 402–408.

Rea WJ (1988) Inter-relationships between the environment and premenstrual syndrome. In Brush MG & Goudsmit EM (eds) *Functional Disorders of the Menstrual Cycle*, pp 135–157. Chichester: John Wiley.

Rees L (1953) Psychosomatic aspects of the premenstrual tension syndrome. *Journal of Mental Science* **99**: 62–73.

Reid RL & Yen SSC (1981) Premenstrual syndrome. *American Journal of Obstetrics and Gynecology* **139**: 85–104.

Royal College of General Practitioners (1974) *Oral Contraceptives and Health*. London: Pitman Medical.

Rubinow DR, Roy-Byrne P, Hoban C, Gold PW & Post RM (1984) Prospective assessment of menstrually related mood disorders. *American Journal of Psychiatry* **141**: 684–686.

Sampson GA (1979) Premenstrual syndrome. A double blind controlled trial of progesterone and placebo. *British Journal of Psychiatry* **135**: 209–215.

Sampson GA (1983) Stress and premenstrual syndrome. In Taylor RW (ed.) *Premenstrual Syndrome*, pp 44–49. London: Medical News Tribune.

Sampson GA (1988) Endocrine treatment of premenstrual syndrome. In Brush MG & Goudsmit EM (eds) *Functional Disorders of the Menstrual Cycle*, pp 97–115. Chichester: John Wiley.

Sampson GA & Prescott P (1981) The assessment of the symptoms of premenstrual syndrome and their response to therapy. *British Journal of Psychiatry* **138**: 399–405.

Sampson GA, Heathcote PRM, Wordsworth J, Prescott P & Hodgson A (1988) Premenstrual syndrome. A double blind cross over study of treatment with dydrogesterone and placebo. *British Journal of Psychiatry* **153**: 232–235.

Schaumbergh H, Kaplan J, Windebank A et al (1983) Sensory neuropathy from pyridoxine abuse: a new mega vitamin syndrome. *New England Journal of Medicine* **309**: 445–448.

Slade P (1984) Premenstrual emotional changes in normal women: fact or fiction? *Journal of Psychosomatic Research* **28**: 1–7.

Slade P & Jenner FA (1980) Attitudes to female roles, aspects of menstruation and complaining of menstrual symptoms. *British Journal of Social and Clinical Psychology* **19**: 109–113.

Smith SL (1975) Mood and the menstrual cycle. In Basher EJ (ed.) *Topics in Psychoendocrinology*, pp 19–58. New York: Grune and Stratton.

Snowden R & Christian B (1984) *Patterns and Perceptions of Menstruation*. New York: St Martins Press.

Steiner M, Haskett RF & Carroll BJ (1980) Premenstrual tension syndrome—the development of research diagnostic criteria and new rating scales. *Acta Psychiatrica Scandinavica* **62**: 177–190.

Sutherland H & Stewart I (1965) A critical analysis of the premenstrual syndrome. *Lancet* **i**: 1180–1183.

Taylor RW (1977) The treatment of premenstrual syndrome with dydrogesterone (Duphaston). *Current Medical Research and Opinion* **4 (supplement 4)**: 35–40.

Van der Meer YG, Benedeck-Jaszmann LJ & Van Loenen AV (1983) Effect of high dose progesterone on the premenstrual syndrome: a double blind cross over study. *Journal of Psychosomatic Obstetrics and Gynaecology* **2**: 220–222.

Van Keep PA & Lehert P (1981) The premenstrual syndrome—an epidemiological and statistical exercise. In Van Keep PA & Utian WH (eds) *The Premenstrual Syndrome*, pp 31–42. Lancaster: MTP Press.

Watts JF, Butt WR & Edwards RL (1987) A clinical trial using danazol for the treatment of premenstrual tension. *British Journal of Obstetrics and Gynaecology* **94**: 30–34.

Watts S, Dennerstein L & Horne DJ de L (1980) The premenstrual syndrome. A psychological evaluation. *Journal of Affective Disorders* **2**: 257–266.

Williams JGC, Martin AJ & Hulkensberg-Tromp TEML (1983) PMS in four european countries. Part 2. A double blind placebo controlled study of dydrogesterone. *British Journal of Sexual Medicine* **10**: 8–18.

2

Eating disorders

NEIL L. HOLDEN

The eating disorders, anorexia nervosa and bulimia nervosa, though now accepted as psychological disorders, have a relevance to both medicine and gynaecology beyond that of many other aspects of mental health. This is reflected in the history of the conditions. Although first described by Richard Morton in 1689, anorexia nervosa was named by William Gull in 1874. At this time there seemed little controversy about the psychological nature of the condition, but when in 1914, Simmonds, the German pathologist, described pituitary lesions leading to cachexia, the scene was set for 40 years of confusion. Anorexia nervosa became regarded as pituitary cachexia, and psychological aspects were ignored. It was not until 1949, when Sheehan and Summers clarified that cachexia was not a feature of hypopituitarism, that attention returned to the psychological nature of the disorder, leading to the growth in understanding of anorexia nervosa as the product of an interaction between psychological stress and physiological mechanisms.

Bulimia nervosa has more recent origins. It was recognized by Russell (1979) as an 'ominous variant' of anorexia nervosa, and during the last decade cases have been recognized with increasing frequency. It can be regarded as either a separate, but related, entity to anorexia nervosa, or part of an eating disorder spectrum which can be widened still further to include obesity.

In spite of the above progress in the classification of the nature of the disorder, it remains a fact that many cases of eating disorders are referred to physicians or gynaecologists in the first instance because of the predominance of physical symptomatology and signs. Patients and relatives often reinforce this pathway of referral by ignoring the psychological aspects for reasons of denial and guilt. Since good prognosis is partially related to duration and early psychological treatment, it is extremely important that eating disorders are recognized and dealt with appropriately.

THE CLINICAL PICTURE OF ANOREXIA NERVOSA

Anorexia nervosa is at least ten times more common in women than men. Its peak age of onset is between 14 and 17 years of age, but it will occasionally affect prepubertal or mature adult females. It may be preceded by childhood emotional disturbances or food fads, but more often than not there is no previous history.

There is a core group of symptoms, essential to the diagnosis of anorexia nervosa. Amenorrhoea must be present in those who would normally have menstruation, with the exception of those receiving oral contraceptive medication. There must be severe self-induced weight loss or failure to gain weight during growth. In addition the patient must have the typical psychopathology of anorexia nervosa, consisting of a morbid fear of fatness together with a distortion of the body image in which they feel fat in spite of being emaciated.

Onset is variable, both in terms of the tempo and the order of occurrence of symptoms. It may be insidious or sudden in response to a precipitant (such as examinations, a sexual relationship or a severe infection). Amenorrhoea may be the first symptom, or may occur later following severe weight loss. Usually the patients will purposefully decrease calorie intake whilst at the same time increase activity, and from a premorbid weight often slightly above normal their weight is drastically reduced (by over 25% in many). Weight loss is accompanied by the associated psychological symptoms of restlessness, irritability and preoccupation with their studies. Libido and sexual activity is decreased and relationships with boyfriends may cease. Further progression leads to insomnia, depression, sensitivity to cold and decreased concentration.

Associated with anorexia nervosa are the classical physical symptoms of starvation. There is severe wasting and marked proximal weakness of limbs. Peripheries become cold and chilblains occur. The skin becomes dry and possibly purpuric. Lanugo, a fine downy hair, normal in childhood, returns, and is most prominent over the face, forearms, nape of the neck and down the spine. Secondary sexual characteristics, including hair, are preserved. The heart rate is decreased to around 50–60 beats/min and the blood pressure is low (systolic 90 mmHg, diastolic 60 mmHg). Ankle oedema may occur.

According to Crisp et al (1980), 45% of patients will have episodes of gross overeating when they experience craving for food and loss of control. Such episodes of bulimia may be followed by increased restriction of intake or by artificial methods of weight control. These methods include self-induced vomiting (43%), laxative abuse (58%), excessive exercise (36%), rumination and spitting, and appetite suppressants. Some patients will use these methods at other times when they cannot be considered to have been bulimic. Often patients with access to drugs will abuse diuretics and thyroxine, and diabetic patients have been known to develop a variant of anorexia when they independently decrease their insulin injections to lose weight. It is usual for most of these activities to be surrounded by secrecy and deception.

The mental state of those with anorexia nervosa is dominated by the fear of becoming fat. This fear has the nature of an overvalued idea, at times almost reaching delusional intensity. The patients will be particularly sensitive about the shape or size of parts of their body, especially hips, abdomen or thighs, which they irrationally regard as fat in spite of recognizing their low overall weight. Patients have a fear of losing control of their food intake and strive to achieve an increasingly strict ideal target weight. Paradoxically patients are usually hungry, though some claim that they have true anorexia.

In addition to the above issues, the patients may also be able to recognize their concern about other aspects of their life. They may be worried about the prospect of leaving home, sexual relationships, parental disharmony and the general responsibilities of adulthood. At times they may have obsessional thoughts relating both to food and to general aspects of life such as washing, dressing and tidiness. Some patients will indulge in associated maladaptive behaviour such as stealing, alcohol abuse and deliberate self-harm.

Nutritional state

Although dietary restrictions associated with food fads and vegetarianism can occasionally lead to nutritional deficiencies, this is not common. Anorectic patients differ from those with involuntary starvation who have protein malnutrition, which is often associated with deficiencies of essential nutrients and vitamins. Instead, those with anorexia nervosa have an adequate protein intake and good knowledge about nutrition and vitamin supplements. Only isolated cases of water-soluble vitamin deficiency (B complex, C, B_{12} and folic acid) have been reported. Low levels of fat-soluble vitamins (A, D and K) are more commonly found. Iron deficiency is rare. Copper and zinc levels tend to be low but rarely have clinical significance.

Neurophysiological changes

The electroencephalogram (EEG) in anorexia nervosa can be abnormal. There may be generalized slowing of the dominant frequency and unstable responses to hyperventilation. When fits have occurred the EEG is likely to show spike and wave complexes. The causal mechanism of these changes is unknown.

Neuroradiological changes in some of the brains of anorectic patients have been observed on computerized axial tomography (CAT). It seems likely that cortical atrophy occurs in 91% of patients, ventricular enlargement in 77% and cerebellar atrophy in 49%. It is uncertain as to whether weight gain reverses this change in all patients.

Laboratory findings in anorexia nervosa may reveal a hypokalaemic alkalosis (with latent tetany) in those who purge and vomit, and a cyclical neutropenia with a relative lymphocytosis. Hypercholesterolaemia is very common, as is hypercarotenaemia.

THE CLINICAL PICTURE OF BULIMIA NERVOSA

The nature of the relationship of bulimia nervosa to anorexia nervosa has been the subject of controversy since it was discussed by Russell (1979), who felt that a previous history of overt or cryptic anorexia nervosa was necessary for a diagnosis to be made. Other authors, conversely, will only consider a diagnosis of bulimia nervosa if a previous diagnosis of anorexia nervosa has been excluded. Additionally, alternative diagnostic terms have existed in different countries, the USA, until recently, using the diagnosis bulimia (DSM-III) with different diagnostic criteria. A revision of these criteria (DMS-III R) has now made the diagnosis of bulimia nervosa broadly acceptable internationally. These criteria are:

1. Recurrent episodes of binge eating (the rapid consumption of a large amount of food in a discreet period of time).
2. A feeling of lack of control over eating behaviour during the eating binges.
3. The person regularly engages in self-induced vomiting, use of laxatives or diuretics, strict dieting or vigorous exercise in order to prevent weight gain.
4. A minimum average of two binge eating episodes per week for at least three weeks.
5. Persistent overconcern with body shape and weight.

The usual age of onset for bulimia nervosa lies between 16 and 40 years, with a peak at 20 years. Patients complain of deceased control of their eating associated with a preoccupation with thoughts of food. Life is centred around attempts to mitigate against the fattening effects of their overeating. A study of the clinical features of patients with bulimia nervosa was reported by Fairburn and Cooper (1984a). A quarter of the patients had previously had anorexia nervosa and 60% had precipitated their problems by strict and rigid dieting. Average weight was only slightly below that of the mean population's matched weight (MPMW). Seventeen per cent of patients were binge eating twice per day, 74% were inducing vomiting at least daily and 40% were vomiting twice per day, 31% abused laxatives and 37% used rumination and spitting of food. Forty-six per cent of patients were taking oral contraceptive medication. Of the remainder, 21% had amenorrhoea, 37% had very irregular menstruation and only 5% had regular menses.

Bulimic behaviour usually occurs in response to some trigger feature such as stress, dysphoria or the availability of trigger foods. Often patients are unaware of these factors. Some patients describe perverse pleasure during the eating phase and regard it as 'comfort eating'. Binges can be variable in size, governed by availability of food (which may be purposefully bought or stolen), interruptions by others or abdominal distension. Cessation of eating is followed by dysphoria or panic at having departed from the strict dietary regimen, and then by vomiting, laxative abuse or other chosen mechanism to mitigate the fattening effects. Elation may follow vomiting or purgation, but this is usually short lived, giving way to further dysphoria.

The mental state examination of a patient with bulimia nervosa may reveal sadness and depression, irritability and decreased concentration. At times suicidal ideas can occur and be acted upon. There is a preoccupation with food (craving), with dietary restriction, and with the fear of being or becoming fat. Sometimes there is a distortion of body image similar to that of anorexia nervosa.

Physical state

Patients are frequently of normal weight, but can be over- or underweight by variable degrees. The weight of an individual can vary rapidly and widely. Other physical problems can be present and relate to the adopted bulimic mechanisms. Recurrent vomiting causes painless swelling of the parotid glands, hoarseness of the voice and dental caries (through perimolysis). Where fingers are used to stimulate the throat, ulcers or calluses may be present on the dorsum of the hand. Gastrointestinal reflux may be a problem, and occasionally acute dilation of the stomach may occur.

Metabolic state

Electrolyte disturbance with low serum potassium and elevated serum bicarbonate may be present, giving a hypokalaemic alkalosis. This may lead to tetany, muscle weakness, cardiac arrhythmia and ileus. Creatinine clearance may be reduced secondary to reversible renal impairment. The EEG may show small sharp waves or epileptiform discharges. Laxative abuse may also cause similar electrolyte disturbances, but in addition may cause steatorrhoea, finger clubbing and dehydration with rebound water retention. Colonic atony may occur after prolonged usage.

EPIDEMIOLOGY

Although anorexia nervosa and bulimia nervosa are easily recognized in terms of clinical symptoms or research criteria, there are difficulties for epidemiological studies because of the small proportion of the general population at risk (mainly young females) and the large number of sub-clinical cases which do not reach medical attention. Kendell et al (1973) reviewed three separate psychiatric case registers and found the rates of anorexia nervosa per 100 000 population to be 0.37 for Monroe County, New York, (1960–1969), 1.6 for north-east Scotland (1966–1969) and 0.66 for Camberwell (1965–1971). He found the rates to be increasing annually and that girls from higher socioeconomic class families were more at risk.

Looking at populations at risk for anorexia nervosa, much higher rates are seen. One in 250 state schoolgirls are affected, increasing to one in 100 schoolgirls from independent or boarding schools (Crisp et al, 1976); 3.5% of fashion students and 7.6% of professional ballet students were affected (Garner and Garfinkel, 1980).

Obtaining prevalence figures for bulimia is again difficult and dependent on the population studied. Halmi et al (1981) studied students in New York and found that 19% of female students fulfilled criteria for bulimia. Similarly Pyle et al (1983) obtained rates for male and female students of 0.5% and 4.5% respectively from a total number of 1300 given questionnaires. In a

British study, Cooper and Fairburn (1983) found a rate of 1.9% for bulimia nervosa amongst women attending a family planning clinic.

Subclinical disorders

Mild cases of anorexia nervosa are not easily recognized as such and therefore may not present to their general practitioner or be referred to a psychiatrist. Button and Whitehouse (1981) administered rating scales to 578 students (446 female) and compared them with 14 'control' students with anorexia nervosa. Of the students 6.3% had high scores and it was concluded, after interviewing this group, that 5% of the total had a subclinical form of anorexia nervosa.

Bulimia nervosa has the potential of being present subclinically in even larger numbers. In a study of bulimia nervosa giving questionnaires to those responding to an advert in *Cosmopolitan*, a women's magazine, Fairburn and Cooper (1982) identified 620 subjects with eating disorders. Of these, 3.1% had anorexia nervosa whilst 83% fulfilled criteria for bulimia nervosa. Of this bulimic group 56.1% had daily bulimic behaviour and most were of normal body weight, 68.1% had psychiatric morbidity and 89% had profoundly disturbed attitudes towards food and eating, and 56.4% felt they needed help but only 30.1% had discussed their problems with a doctor. A similar study by Fairburn and Cooper (1984b) used a television documentary to identify 579 women fulfilling a self-report diagnostic criteria for bulimia nervosa, and similar results were revealed.

The question of what is subculturally normal behaviour must be considered. It is clear that the spectrum of social dieting merges with that of anorexia nervosa and in some dieters menstruation will be disrupted. Similarly 'hedonistic binge-eating' followed by self-induced vomiting has been described in the normal population (Bearn and Robinson, 1985), differing from true bulimia nervosa by the absence of significant dysphoria. Bulimic behaviour is often reported by patients as having been learned from other 'bulimics' or from the media. Anorexia and bulimia nervosa also form a spectrum with each other.

Changing rates of the disorders

Given that it is difficult to estimate the incidence and prevalence rates of eating disorders, it does appear that the rates are increasing. Russell (1985a) outlined the changing nature of anorexia nervosa over time suggesting that in addition to an increased incidence there was also an alteration in the psychopathology, with increased body-image disturbance and morbid fear of fatness, and a change in the form, with more prominent vomiting and purging (and the emergence of bulimia nervosa as a distinct variant). Although eating disorders usually affect high social classes, there is some evidence that the incidence is increasing down the social scale. Similarly the previously low incidence in immigrant groups appears to be increasing (Holden and Robinson, 1988) with westernization.

MEASUREMENT OF WEIGHT

Although body weight and its loss are measured in metric or imperial absolute weights, comparisons with premorbid weights and the norms for the population are essential. Therefore weights are estimated as percentages of the mean population matched weight (MPMW) derived from actuarial tables of height and weight (see Table 1; Metropolitan Life Insurance

Table 1. 1983 Metropolitan height and weight tables for men and women on metric basis (according to frame, ages 25–59).

	Men Weight in kilograms (in indoor clothing)*				Women Weight in kilograms (in indoor clothing)*		
Height (cm) (in shoes)†	Small frame	Medium frame	Large frame	Height (cm) (in shoes)†	Small frame	Medium frame	Large frame
158	58.3–61.0	59.6–64.2	62.8–68.3	148	46.4–50.6	49.6–55.1	53.7–59.8
159	58.6–61.3	59.9–64.5	63.1–68.8	149	46.6–51.0	50.0–55.5	54.1–60.3
160	59.0–61.7	60.3–64.9	63.5–69.4	150	46.7–51.3	50.3–55.9	54.4–60.9
161	59.3–62.0	60.6–65.2	63.8–69.9	151	46.9–51.7	50.7–56.4	54.8–61.4
162	59.7–62.4	61.0–65.6	64.2–70.5	152	47.1–52.1	51.1–57.0	55.2–61.9
163	60.0–62.7	61.3–66.0	64.5–71.1	153	47.4–52.5	51.5–57.5	55.6–62.4
164	60.4–63.1	61.7–66.5	64.9–71.8	154	47.8–53.0	51.9–58.0	56.2–63.0
165	60.8–63.5	62.1–67.0	65.3–72.5	155	48.1–53.6	52.2–58.6	56.8–63.6
166	61.1–63.8	62.4–67.6	65.6–73.2	156	48.5–54.1	52.7–59.1	57.3–64.1
167	61.5–64.2	62.8–68.2	66.0–74.0	157	48.8–54.6	53.2–59.6	57.8–64.6
168	61.8–64.6	63.2–68.7	66.4–74.7	158	49.3–55.2	53.8–60.2	58.4–65.3
169	62.2–65.2	63.8–69.3	67.0–75.4	159	49.8–55.7	54.3–60.7	58.9–66.0
170	62.5–65.7	64.3–69.8	67.5–76.1	160	50.3–56.2	54.9–61.2	59.4–66.7
171	62.9–66.2	64.8–70.3	68.0–76.8	161	50.8–56.7	55.4–61.7	59.9–67.4
172	63.2–66.7	65.4–70.8	68.5–77.5	162	51.4–57.3	55.9–62.3	60.5–68.1
173	63.6–67.3	65.9–71.4	69.1–78.2	163	51.9–57.3	56.4–62.8	61.0–68.8
174	63.9–67.8	66.4–71.9	69.6–78.9	164	52.5–58.4	57.0–63.4	61.5–69.5
175	64.3–68.3	66.9–72.4	70.1–79.6	165	53.0–58.9	57.5–63.9	62.0–70.2
176	64.7–68.9	67.5–73.0	70.7–80.3	166	53.6–59.5	58.1–64.5	62.6–70.9
177	65.0–69.5	68.1–73.5	71.3–81.0	167	54.1–60.0	58.4–65.0	63.2–71.7
178	65.4–70.0	68.6–74.0	71.8–81.8	168	54.6–60.5	59.0–65.5	63.7–72.4
179	65.7–70.5	69.2–74.6	72.3–82.5	169	55.2–61.1	59.7–66.1	64.3–73.1
180	66.1–71.0	69.7–75.1	72.8–83.3	170	55.7–61.6	60.2–66.6	64.8–73.8
181	66.6–71.6	70.2–75.8	73.4–84.0	171	56.2–62.1	60.7–67.1	65.3–74.5
182	67.1–72.1	70.7–76.5	73.9–84.7	172	56.8–62.6	61.3–67.6	65.8–75.2
183	67.7–72.7	71.3–77.2	74.5–85.4	173	57.3–63.2	61.8–68.2	66.4–75.9
184	68.2–73.4	71.8–77.9	75.2–86.1	174	57.8–63.7	62.3–68.7	66.9–76.4
185	68.7–74.1	72.4–78.6	75.9–86.8	175	58.3–64.2	62.8–69.2	67.4–76.9
186	69.2–74.8	73.0–79.3	76.6–87.6	176	58.9–64.6	63.4–69.8	68.0–77.5
187	69.8–75.5	73.7–80.0	77.3–88.5	177	59.5–65.4	64.0–70.4	68.5–78.1
188	70.3–76.2	74.4–80.7	78.0–89.4	178	60.0–65.9	64.5–70.9	69.0–78.6
189	70.9–76.9	74.9–81.5	78.7–90.3	179	60.5–66.4	65.1–71.4	69.6–79.1
190	71.4–77.6	75.4–82.2	79.4–91.2	180	61.0–66.9	65.6–71.9	70.1–79.6
191	72.1–78.4	76.1–83.0	80.3–92.1	181	61.6–67.5	66.1–72.5	70.7–80.2
192	72.8–79.1	76.8–83.9	81.2–93.0	182	62.1–68.0	66.6–73.0	71.2–80.7
193	73.5–79.8	77.6–84.8	82.1–93.9	183	62.6–68.5	67.1–73.5	71.7–81.2

* Indoor clothing weighing 2.3 kg for men and 1.4 kg for women.
† Shoes with 2.5 cm heels.
Source of basic data: *Build Study (1979)* Society of Actuaries and Association of Life Insurance Medical Directors of America.
Copyright 1983 Metropolitan Life Insurance Company.

Company, 1983) or as the body mass index (BMI). The latter can be derived from the formula:

$$BMI = \frac{Weight\ (kg)}{Height^2\ (m^2)}$$

The average BMI for the general population is 20.

The use of these measures allows a clearer estimation of weight loss in a standardized way. This is especially true in those who have been previously obese (BMI greater than 27 or % MPMW greater than 120).

AETIOLOGY OF EATING DISORDERS

There is little doubt that the aetiology of eating disorders is multifactorial (Hsu, 1983). There is a large area of overlap between the putative factors involved in the aetiology of anorexia nervosa and bulimia nervosa and for this reason they can be considered together.

Sociocultural factors

The need to be thin is central to the psychopathology of eating disorders and this originates in part from the sociocultural pressures in Western society. Whilst the average weight of women has increased (Metropolitan Life Insurance Company, 1983), the current fashion is for thinness. Social pressures to achieve this thinness lead to social dieting which can herald either anorexia or bulimia nervosa. Contrasting pressures are present in the developing world where eating disorders are uncommon. Here the presence of body fat symbolizes affluence against a background of fear of starvation through poverty or natural disaster.

Genetic and family factors

Anorexia nervosa tends to run in families and a recent twin study (Holland et al, 1984) reported a higher concordance for anorexia nervosa in monozygotic compared with dizygotic twins, suggesting a genetic component.

Environmental factors within families have been shown to predispose to eating disorders. Parental discord, loss of a parent through death or divorce, and childhood sexual abuse are some of these factors. Within the family setting, secondary gains can powerfully maintain the eating disorder. The presence of such a 'sick' family member can restore stability to an otherwise disharmonious parental relationship as a new alliance is formed to fight the illness. Other gains from the adoption of the 'sick role' include the avoidance of adolescent anxieties such as leaving home (to college or by marriage), forming sexual relationships and sitting examinations.

Psychodynamic factors

Bruch (1973) stated that anorexia nervosa is a struggle for a self-respecting identity. Aspects of the development of individual identity and separation from parents are related to this issue. Adolescent females with poor self-esteem may seek to improve their self-worth by changing their external appearance, in particular focusing on being thin.

Physiological factors

It is difficult to separate the primary physiological changes of anorexia from the secondary effects of starvation. Russell (1983) suggested that a primary hypothalamic dysfunction may be present as indicated by the early loss of menstruation before weight loss in some patients. In addition, some patients continue to have hypothalamic dysfunction long after weight gain has occurred. However, other explanations seem more likely and will be discussed later.

Crisp (1977) suggests that anorexia nervosa is rooted in the psychobiological regression of the individual to a functionally prepubertal state, and can be regarded as phobic avoidance of adolescent/adult weight. Biological and psychological reversal of the maturational changes of puberty allow the avoidance of the adolescent fears and tasks described earlier.

Relationship to other mental illnesses

The eating disorders have been said to be related to depressive illness (Cantwell et al, 1977) both genetically and in terms of neurotransmitter changes. Although an arguable issue, the balance of evidence appears to be against such a link, at least at a simple level. At times, other mental disorders, including frank psychosis and confusional states, arise in patients with eating disorders, but these appear to be coincidental or related to the physical aspects of starvation or electrolyte disturbance. However, it does seem that bulimic behaviour in some individuals is related to a wider behavioural disorder, with stealing, substance abuse and self-harm. Individuals so affected are suffering from abnormalities of personality development and generally have a worse prognosis.

GYNAECOLOGICAL FEATURES OF EATING DISORDERS

Menstrual abnormalities

Menstrual abnormalities are the most likely reason for the referral of an eating disorder patient to a gynaecology clinic. By definition, all females with anorexia nervosa have primary or secondary amenorrhoea, whilst 40–95% of those with normal weight bulimia nervosa will have irregular menstruation. This must be compared with a rate for female college students of 2–5% for amenorrhoea and 11% for oligomenorrhoea (Bachman and Kemmann, 1982). Female psychiatric inpatients have amenorrhoea rate of 27% (Flint and Stewart, 1983). Pyle et al (1981) found 26 out of 34 bulimics to have had one episode of amenorrhoea of at least three months' duration, whilst only 10 out of the 34 had weight loss below 85% of the MPMW. Johnson et al (1983) found that 50.7% of bulimics had irregular menses. Fairburn and Cooper (1982, 1984b) in two separate studies of bulimics found irregular menses in 39.7% and 36.8%, and amenorrhoea in 6.9% and 21.1%, respectively. Of those with anorexia nervosa, 4% have primary amenorrhoea.

Weight loss appears to be a major factor in the amenorrhoea of eating disorders. Four out of five normal volunteers had amenorrhoea after a 12% weight loss (Fichter and Pirke, 1984), and 28% of ballet dancers (who need to maintain rigid low weight whilst exercising rigorously) have amenorrhoea (Garner and Garfinkel, 1980). The greater the weight loss in bulimia nervosa, the greater the risk of amenorrhoea. However, other factors are involved. In anorexia nervosa, 25% lose menses before weight loss (Hsu, 1983) and only 70% regain normal menstruation when weight is regained.

Emotional upset prior to the onset of weight loss may explain this early amenorrhoea. Sixty per cent of women interned in concentration camps had amenorrhoea preceding their weight loss. In bulimia nervosa there is a relationship between irregular menses and the nature of the abstinence–bulimia cycle.

Failure of gonadotrophin secretion is the immediate mechanism for amenorrhoea in eating disorders in which there is profound disruption of luteinizing hormone (LH) and to a lesser extent follicle-stimulating hormone (FSH) (Garfinkel and Garner, 1982; Copeland and Herzog, 1987). The release of these hormones is pulsed. In anorexia nervosa the pulsation pattern resembles that in prepuberty (absent pulsation) or early puberty (only sleep-related pulsations).

LH release is stimulated by gonadotrophin-releasing hormone (GnRH) from the hypothalamus, and the amount is dependent on the degree of GnRH release or the responsiveness of the pituitary. The disturbances of anorexia nervosa are greater in degree than in normal weight bulimia nervosa. Serum oestradiol levels greater than 120 pg/ml indicate the maturation of an ovarian follicle. These were found in 8 out of 15 normal weight bulimics. Levels in anorexia nervosa were found to be much lower. Marshall and Kelch (1979) showed that primary hypothalamic failure of GnRH production was occurring rather than loss of pituitary responsiveness by demonstrating restoration of menses with exogenous GnRH. The most likely cause of this hypothalamic disturbance is weight loss, but the roles of nutritional inadequacy, bulimic behaviour, psychological stress, intrinsic abnormality and exercise cannot be ignored.

Oestradiol feedback modulates GnRH secretion. At puberty positive feedback of oestradiol develops, whilst prior to puberty the feedback is exclusively negative. In anorexia nervosa there is a return to this prepubertal pattern and therefore there is decreased GnRH secretion. The positive feedback, lost in anorexia nervosa, is essential for the surge in LH levels which triggers ovulation. Hence amenorrhoea reflects the failure of central nervous system control of reproduction. A decrease in peripheral oestrogen levels may have a role in amenorrhoea via this positive feedback mechanism.

Hypercarotenaemia has been suggested as a contributory factor in the menstrual abnormality of anorexia nervosa. Between 38 and 76% of cases have frankly elevated levels of serum carotene. Hypercarotenaemia is also associated with amenorrhoea amongst vegetarians (Kemmann et al, 1983) and can be corrected by dietary change. Although sometimes dietary in origin, in anorexia nervosa there is also a slower metabolism of carotene. This occurs in hypothyroid states.

Functional hypothyroidism occurs in anorexia nervosa due to the alternative peripheral conversion of thyroxine to inactive reverse triiodothyronine (rT_3) (see later). There is also a decrease in triiodothyronine (T_3) in normal weight bulimics, possibly triggered by intermittent starvation. Low serum FSH levels are correlated with low T_3 levels in bulimia nervosa.

Endogenous opioid activity is increased and leads to a decrease in GnRH production. The receptor sites involved in this opioid effect can be studied by the administration of naloxone which inhibits μ-receptors strongly and δ-receptors weakly. Naloxone increased GnRH release and also the frequency of LH pulses in the late follicular and mid-luteal phases. (This effect is modified by ovarian steroid production as oestrogen must be present.) Naloxone raised the LH levels in 11 out of 25 anorectic patients (Baranowska et al, 1984). Amenorrhoea was present before weight loss in 9 out of these 11 and it was postulated that this was due to decreased oestrogen. Increased levels of CSF encephalins are found in those with anorexia nervosa. The above effects appear to depend on noradrenergic pathways being intact.

Noradrenergic activity in bulimia nervosa appears to be decreased, leading to decreased LH secretion (Copeland and Herzog, 1987). It is postulated that this decreased activity may be due to decreased food intake and may be reflected in decreased peripheral noradrenergic activity.

Prolactin levels are increased resulting from psychological stress and can lead to amenorrhoea through decreased GnRH release. This appears to involve opioid pathways, as above, as naloxone re-establishes menstruation. Prolactin activity may be increased as a result of increased serotoninergic activity and this ties in with similar increases during stress. Increases of serotonin may have some direct affect on LH release from the pituitary.

The hypothalamic–pituitary–adrenal axis is hyperfunctioning in anorexia and bulimia nervosa and this is reflected in the dexamethasone suppression test, which shows failure to suppress cortisol (Copeland and Herzog, 1987). CSF corticotrophin (CRH) is increased in anorexia nervosa. CRH has a central effect on decreasing GnRH release in experimental rats. Stress-induced decrease of GnRH release may be mediated by increased CRH levels. Increased cortisol levels also decrease GnRH.

Exercise leads to amenorrhoea due to decreased LH pulse frequency (via decreased GnRH) (Bullen et al, 1985). The mechanism is unclear. Feicht et al (1978) studied 54 female athletes of whom 19 had amenorrhoea without weight loss. Amenorrhoea most closely related to the percentage of body fat, and it may be the decreased ratio of fat to muscle which is the trigger for amenorrhoea in female athletes.

Osteopenia and vertebral compression fractures have been suggested as long-term complications of the hormonal state leading to amenorrhoea in eating disorders. However, although certainly involved, decreased oestrogen levels are not well correlated with these findings. The best correlation with osteopenia is decreased levels of dehydroepiandrosterone sulphate (a secretion of the adrenal gland with androgenic effects). The levels are decreased in anorexia nervosa and are possibly related to increased cortisol levels and poor nutrition. Amenorrhoea usually recovers with weight gain. When menses fail to return they can be stimulated by clomiphene (which blocks oestrogen receptors in the hypothalamus and gives a surge of GnRH leading to ovulation).

Ovarian changes ·

In anorexia nervosa and non-specific weight loss related to amenorrhoea, the ovaries have been studied using ultrasonography (Adams et al, 1985; Treasure et al, 1985). The ovarian volume is reduced in those with severe anorexia nervosa, but increases logarithmically with weight gain. When the BMI reached $17\,kg/m^2$, multiple small cysts were shown in the ovaries. Following further weight gain (to an average BMI of $19\,kg/m^2$), a dominant cyst appeared. These changes, including the multifollicular stage, resemble those of normal puberty. In the multifollicular stage, the ovaries are normal or slightly enlarged in size and filled with six or more cysts, 4–10 mm in diameter. Stroma is not increased, in contrast to ovaries in women with polycystic ovaries (Stein–Leventhal syndrome). In the management of infertility, an ultrasonographic appearance of cystic ovaries (multifollicular ovaries) should alert the clinician to the likelihood of undernutrition as the primary disorder in need of treatment.

Fertility and pregnancy

There is no evidence that fertility is abnormal after the restoration of weight and menses in those who have suffered eating disorders. Dally (1969) found that 50% of his patients had children after recovery. Although patients should be counselled to wait for recovery, Hart et al (1970) induced ovulation in three patients and conception and pregnancy occurred normally. Guidelines suggested for the use of clomiphene in those recovering from eating disorders are:

1.   That the patient has reached a weight greater than 90% of the MPMW.
2.   That eating and attitudes towards it have normalized.
3.   That the patients have maintained themselves satisfactorily in this state for one year.

There appear to be no additional problems for those with eating disorders taking oral contraceptive medication. However, patients with anorexia nervosa should be discouraged from taking this whilst ill as it is likely to induce withdrawal bleeding, disguising amenorrhoea and allowing denial of the illness.

Unlike those with anorexia nervosa, many with bulimia nervosa have normal fertility and conceive. Lacey and Smith (1987) studied the inter-action of bulimia nervosa and pregnancy in 20 women. Bulimic behaviour diminished sequentially in each of the trimesters and 75% had stopped by the third. Symptoms tended to return in the puerperium, and 50% were symptomatically more disturbed than before conception. However, 25% of the patients remained symptom-free at follow-up presumed cured. Although not statistically significant there were high rates of fetal abnor-mality (cleft lip and palate), multiple pregnancies and obstetric compli-cations (breech and caesarean sections). Fifteen per cent reported slimming their babies in the first year by restriction of food intake.

Primary amenorrhoea and delayed puberty

Although the age range for anorexia nervosa is generally regarded as 13 to 20 years with a peak of 17 or 18 years, and it is therefore a postpubertal illness, it has been recognized that there are younger patients who develop the illness before puberty. Tanner (1962) described normal puberty. The first stage of puberty is the development of breast buds, followed by the growth of pubic hair and the growth spurt. Menarche is a late occurrence. Starvation from any cause is known to arrest growth and development, but 'catch-up' usually occurs.

Russell (1985b) described 20 patients who had developed anorexia nervosa before menarche. The onsets of their illnesses were between 9 and 14 years, with a peak at 12 or 13 years. All had primary amenorrhoea. Of the 20, six had normal breast development, four partial development and ten had infantile (Tanner stage one) breasts. Eight out of 14 with under-developed breasts responded to weight gain with further breast develop-ment. Height was affected by the anorexia nervosa. Only two out of 20 had heights in the 50th percentile, and only seven had heights within the 2nd percentile. On refeeding and weight gain, menarche occurred in only four patients before 16 years and 13 patients still had amenorrhoea at 18 years. Four further patients began to menstruate between 18 and 25 years.

Hence, anorexia nervosa has a profound effect on the pubertal develop-ment of those girls unlucky enough to commence the illness prepubertally. The illness effectively suspends puberty. Hormonal patterns remain pre-pubertal, with negative feedback of peripheral oestrogen on the hypo-thalamus persisting, and positive feedback, necessary for ovulation, failing to develop. As a late feature of puberty, menarche is affected in some patients in whom breast development has progressed normally. When refeeding and weight gain occurs, patients may have to wait months or years for menarche to occur. These observations seem to concur with those of Frisch and McArthur (1974), who estimated that at the onset of menarche fat must contribute 17% of the body weight, and that it must be 23% for regular ovulation.

'Catch up' on recovery does not necessarily occur in respect of breast development. For those in whom breast development fails, hormone therapy with oestrogen and progesterone can have a beneficial effect.

OTHER ABNORMALITIES OF HYPOTHALAMIC FUNCTION IN EATING DISORDERS

The effects of eating disorders on the reproductive aspects of hypothalamic dysfunction have been discussed earlier. Eating disorders have effects on other hypothalamic–endocrine functions.

Growth hormone is increased in anorexia nervosa. Levels normalize with recovery, but seem to be related to the increased calorie intake, occurring before normal weight is reached.

Thyroxine levels in eating disorders are normal or marginally decreased. Levels of thyroid-binding globulin remain normal. Triiodothyronine (T_3) levels are decreased, while the reverse isomer of T_3, reverse T_3 (rT_3), is increased. This change is due to altered metabolism of thyroxine in the peripheral tissues, in which thyroxine is converted to rT_3 instead of T_3. The extent of this alteration is related to fasting and weight loss and is a compensatory mechanism in starvation states. Thyroid-stimulating hormone (TSH) production by the anterior pituitary is normal in spite of low T_3 levels, as negative feedback control is obscured by the presence of rT_3. At the same time rT_3 is metabolically inactive at the tissue level and the basal metabolic rate falls as part of a functional hypothyroid state. However, the TSH response to thyrotrophin-releasing hormone (TRH) is reported to be delayed and blunted. Such blunting was found by Gwirtsman et al (1983) to be present in eight out of ten bulimics.

Cortisol levels are raised in eating disorders. It is arguable as to whether this is secondary to psychological stress, to the physiological stress of low carbohydrate intake (in which increased cortisol levels serve to prevent hypoglycaemia) or to general hypothalamic dysfunction. The dexamethasone suppression test, which would usually show a suppression of cortisol levels for 24 hours in a normal subject, fails to suppress in many with eating disorders. Gwirtsman et al (1983) found that 12 out of 18 bulimics showed abnormal cortisol suppression in spite of normal weight.

Prolactin levels are essentially normal in eating disorders except for low nocturnal levels. However, the effects of psychological stress on prolactin can cause levels to be raised, adding to the reproductive abnormalities discussed earlier.

INVESTIGATIONS AND DIFFERENTIAL DIAGNOSIS

Anorexia nervosa

Anorexia nervosa is made more difficult to diagnose by the patient's reluctance to accept the diagnosis and intervention. This denial is sometimes shared by the relatives who would prefer to spare their patient a psychological diagnosis and continually look for physical causes. It is because of these factors, together with the obvious physical symptoms, that anorexia nervosa is often referred to medical or gynaecological outpatients. However, it must be said that anorexia nervosa is relatively straightforward to diagnose. It is arguable whether diagnostic tests, further to a full history and mental state examination, are required. Pursuing endless investigations may be damaging to the patient's prospects of recovery as it reinforces the sick role, encourages the perception of the illness as physical rather than psychological, and may delay diagnosis and appropriate treatment.

It is useful to check serum electrolytes and creatinine in those who are severely ill or when bulimic behaviour is suspected but not admitted by the patient. Often tests such as serum zinc, serum copper, EEG and CAT scan, together with endocrine investigations, may be abnormal, but since they are secondary findings they do not help with the primary diagnosis and probably should be reserved for those with complications. Ultrasonography of the ovaries may have a role in monitoring the patient's therapeutic responses and predicting target weight and the return of menses, but again is of little use in primary diagnosis.

The differential diagnosis of anorexia nervosa can be divided into psychological and physical diagnoses. A number of psychological disorders can lead to secondary anorexia and mimic anorexia nervosa. The commonest of these is undoubtedly depressive illness, in which biological symptoms of early morning wakening and loss of weight, appetite, concentration and menses overlap with those of anorexia nervosa. Reference to the typical psychopathology, with fear of weight gain and disturbed body image, usually allows the distinction to be made. Severe anxiety states accompanied by anorexia may also be mistaken for anorexia nervosa. One variety of anxiety, social phobia, which can involve the fear of eating in company, may be particularly relevant to the differential diagnosis. Bulimia nervosa must also be distinguished from anorexia nervosa, but as there is overlap between the two conditions, this can sometimes seem arbitrary.

Non-specific carcinoma and leukaemia are part of the physical differential diagnosis of anorexia nervosa. Gastrointestinal disorders such as Crohn's disease, ulcerative colitis and malabsorption (e.g. coeliac disease), chronic infections (e.g. tuberculosis) and infestations (e.g. strongyloidiases), neurological disorders with wasting, and endocrine disease such as Addison's disease, anterior pituitary disease and hyperthyroidism all need to be considered. Tumours affecting the hypothalamus and mid-brain nuclei are particularly difficult to differentiate on occasions.

Bulimia nervosa

Bulimia nervosa is similarly referred to physicians and gynaecologists through mistaken diagnosis. Frequently these patients are distressed by their loss of control of eating and actively seek medical help, therefore being forthcoming about the nature of their habits. Unfortunately some feel unable to confide in others about their symptoms owing to self-disgust. These patients may present with superficial symptomatology or complications and can be referred for inappropriate investigation of their vomiting, diarrhoea, amenorrhoea, oligomenorrhoea, infertility, hoarseness or metabolic disturbance. Further difficulties arise as their weight is often within the normal range.

As with anorexia nervosa, laboratory investigations are of limited diagnostic value. A full history and mental state examination, together with adequate knowledge of the nature of the disorder, is usually enough to make a clear diagnosis. Electrolyte and creatinine estimations may be of use in judging the frequency and severity of the bulimic behaviour, but not the underlying diagnosis. Complications may require further physical investigation and this can include regular dental inspection to diagnose early caries caused by acid regurgitation.

The differential diagnosis of bulimia nervosa overlaps with that of anorexia nervosa and obesity. Depression and anxiety may be diagnosed in these patients by mistake. Social phobias of eating with others may present as dysphagia, nausea, diarrhoea and vomiting associated with eating, but it is situational and can be distinguished from bulimia nervosa by a full history. Physical causes need to be considered, e.g. peptic ulceration, chronic infections, cholecystitis and Crohn's disease. Infertility and amenorrhoea in a normal weight bulimic may present particular diagnostic problems.

THE TREATMENT OF ANOREXIA NERVOSA

Treatment regimens for anorexia nervosa are as varied as the multitude of theoretical models by which the therapists work. Often the task of treating severely cachectic anorectic patients falls to the physician after they have collapsed or developed physical complications. The approach to treatment on a medical ward, though often modified by a liaison psychiatrist, concentrates on refeeding and physical health and is in contrast with the other extreme, i.e. the psychodynamic treatment of the anorectic outpatient, where physical symptoms and weight may be ignored. Between these two extremes is an abundance of varied strategies for dealing with the illness, which, it must be said, are not mutually exclusive.

Inpatient treatment

Inpatient regimens are traditionally regarded as the mainstay of treatment, especially in the initial stages of treatment of severe weight loss. There is a widely held view (which is not necessarily correct) that anorectic patients are unable to change their attitudes about their weight until they have increased their weight above a reasonable threshold. William Gull, who originally described anorexia nervosa in 1874, argued that 'the patients should be fed at regular intervals, and surrounded by persons who would have more control over them, relations and friends being generally the worse attendants'.

The decision whether to admit anorectic patients for refeeding hinges on a fundamental difference of approach between inpatient and outpatient regimens. The anorectic inpatients have the responsibility for their eating and weight removed from them, whilst treatment as an outpatient throws such responsibilities for eating back upon the patient. Whilst neither approach is more correct, it is important that the therapist be clear about the philosophy and strategy of treatment. The therapist needs also to be aware of the changes in the nature of treatment which occur as a patient changes from inpatient to outpatient status.

Once the decision to admit a patient has been made, many patients can be persuaded to accept voluntary admission by their therapists and families, and a large proportion of these patients will agree to stay in hospital for the duration of the treatment. However, a considerable proportion of patients will refuse admission or will discharge themselves as soon as any progress with refeeding has been made. It is arguable as to whether it is legitimate to use the 1983 Mental Health Act to compulsorily admit patients with this disorder. On rare occasions where the condition is clearly life threatening, and where the patient is unequivocally mentally ill, then such a course of action may be justified, but it must be remembered that a degree of co-operation from the patient is required, as there is no way of forcing a patient to eat against their will without sedating them heavily and resorting to nasogastric feeding. It also should be appreciated that the staff of the ward accepting an anorectic patient need to be well trained and supervised. The management of these patients can lead to strong emotions amongst the staff and can demoralize a ward.

The physiological basis of refeeding is the formula that weight gain is directly related to the consumption of calories in excess of daily energy requirements; 1 kg (2.2 lbs) will be gained as a result of a positive calorie balance of 7500 Calories. Patients are usually asked to eat a normal diet in the first week (though they may need to start with half-normal portions for the first few days) and then are given double portions thereafter, amounting to between 3000 and 5000 Calories per day. Energy expenditure is minimized by resting.

The usual methods of achieving these aims are behavioural strategies. Although these can be applied pragmatically, in the stricter regimens a contract is made with each of the patients in which they are expected to eat the diet that they are given and be weighed weekly. In the early stages 'privileges' are withdrawn and they are not allowed contact with relatives and friends, must wear night clothes and remain on bed rest. Prior to meals, patients are asked to empty their bladders and bowels, and are not allowed to leave their beds for one or two hours after each meal. In addition they are observed closely to avoid deceptions such as exercising and the hiding of food. The patients are given target weights to achieve, at which the privileges are returned (including getting up, dressing and time off the ward).

As an adjunct to the basic behavioural approach, pharmacological treatment can be used to stimulate appetite and reduce anxiety. Phenothiazines such as chlorpromazine and thioridazine sedate the anxious patient whilst at the same time causing increased appetite and weight gain. Cyproheptadine, a more specific appetite stimulant, can be used, as can low-dose insulin injections (which stimulate appetite by complex metabolic effects including hypoglycaemia). Tricyclic antidepressants such as dothiepin and amitriptyline can be used to treat anxiety and insomnia, and also have a mild effect in stimulating appetite. Pharmacological treatments are best used for symptomatic relief, especially during 'crisis' periods in the behavioural regimens. As the patient's weight increases they need further psychotherapeutic interventions for they become increasingly aware of the issues which have caused and perpetuated the illness. Unless patients can overcome these issues, which include fear of independence and the development of sexuality, they will remain at high risk of relapse on discharge. Individual, group and family therapies are all useful and can include elements of assertiveness training, art and expression therapy, relaxation and stress management. Early plans are required about eventual discharge, including consideration of whether independent living away from the family is necessary.

Outpatient treatment

In recent years more psychiatrists have been willing to persevere with outpatient treatments for low-weight anorectic patients. It is certainly the treatment of choice for milder illnesses. Although recovery of weight may take longer, outpatient therapy has the advantage of giving the patient responsibility, at an early stage, for their own eating and weight. The very fact that relatives and carers alike demonstrate such marked anxiety over those with anorexia nervosa allows the patients themselves to remain morbidly calm about their cachexia and to avoid taking self-responsibility. This perpetuates the illness through secondary gain. Central, therefore, to outpatient management is to push responsibility and anxiety back on to the patient. Relatives and others are asked to withdraw from their pattern of interference and emotionality. This requires much reassurance during family sessions.

Whilst rapid weight gain is expected during a hospital refeeding programme, a slower pace of weight gain is the aim in outpatients. If anorectic patients increase their weight rapidly, then panic ensues and they feel 'out of control'. Therefore it is better to aim for a modest gain of 0.5 kg per week or fortnight. Patients can normally be persuaded to tolerate this insidious rise in weight and gradually become desensitized to their fear of weighing more. In this approach the patients need to be motivated by logical and blunt argument about the deterioration of their health and its effect on their aspirations for the future. Therapists should not avoid discussing unpleasant realities such as the 5% mortality rate and the possibility of chronicity in this condition. Formal family therapy, or family sessions as an extension of individual therapy, is extremely useful. This is especially true for the younger patients who are living at home. On occasions other models of therapy, such as marital therapy (for the older, married patient) may be appropriate. Social intervention, possibly in the form of help with independent accommodation and support, may be crucial.

Usually normal menses (and fertility) return with weight gain and are one indication of full recovery. If the delay before starting cyclical menstruation is prolonged, then consideration may be given to ultrasonographic investigation (as described earlier). Restoration of menses may be encouraged by one or two courses of clomiphene (50–100 mg daily for seven days) or alternatively luteinizing hormone releasing hormone (LHRH) may have the same benefit.

THE TREATMENT OF BULIMIA NERVOSA

After initial despondency about the lack of effective therapies for bulimia nervosa, a consensus is growing amongst psychiatrists that cognitive–behavioural strategies hold the most promise. In addition, it may be that pharmacological treatments will also be shown to be useful in future studies.

Cognitive–behavioural treatment

Differing forms of cognitive–behavioural programmes have evolved at different centres. These programmes have a variety of elements which can be applied according to the nature of the individual's problems (such as current weight, presence of impulsive, depressive or obsessional features, and the amount of motivation). Central to the behavioural approach is the adoption of regular eating with the aim of controlling the chaotic alternating between binge eating and starvation. Patients are asked to decide on a realistic calorie intake, and then divide it between three regular meals per day. Various strategies can reinforce regular eating and the sense of control over food intake. Patients can be asked to limit eating to only one or two places, such as the dining room/kitchen table at home and the rest-room/canteen at work, and be told to always set a knife, fork, spoon, placemat and glass of water, whenever and whatever they are eating. Other activities whilst eating, such as reading or watching television, are expressly forbidden. These moves serve to enhance the awareness of eating. They increase the sense of control over eating and make the patient appreciate eating as an enjoyable act in its own right.

A diary of eating is another important strategy. The patients are asked to record what they eat, when, where and whether it is followed by vomiting or laxative abuse. In addition they are asked to record what activity, if any, they are doing at the time, to rate their hunger on a scale of one to ten, and to comment about their predominant thoughts and emotions associated with any bulimic behaviour. By recording such information, the patients may feel more in control of their eating, and binge eating may decrease. Useful insights may be gained into the emotions and events which precipitate their bulimic behaviour. Patients should be requested to produce a hierarchical list of foods which are either likely to trigger binges or which they are most likely to binge on. Using such lists, it is possible to avoid exposure to these trigger foods and to construct a safe, non-threatening diet. This will allow the consumption of a stable and regular diet, and eventually the trigger goods may be reintroduced gradually.

Contingency plans can help patients deal with bulimic urges as they occur. These are alternative plans of action which replace binge eating with other pleasurable or self-indulgent activities such as reading, exercise or socializing. By carrying out these activities it is possible to avoid the bulimic behaviour by delaying it till the urge has passed. Strategies in which the purchase of food or laxatives is avoided may also be developed. By not carrying money or avoiding shops (perhaps travelling home by an alternative route), the opportunity to buy can be decreased. When a co-therapist, such as a close friend, relative or husband, can be involved, then they can help with such strategies. Also, by being present during the patient's eating they can decrease the likelihood of bulimia and vomiting.

In conjunction with these behavioural approaches, cognitive strategies are helpful. Patients, with the aid of the therapist, identify dysfunctional thoughts and attitudes which underpin the eating disorder. Some of these thoughts may be identified through keeping a diary as described above. These thoughts and attitudes are then examined, and evidence for and against them is marshalled. Patients are encouraged to replace the dysfunctional thoughts and attitudes with alternatives and helpful ones. Although initially this process seems laborious to the patient, and needs therapist help, it will progress to being automatic with continued practice.

Pharmacological approaches, as yet, are generally unsatisfactory and unproven. Patients with a major degree of depression or anxiety associated with bulimia may be helped by an anxiolytic antidepressent such as dothiepin or lofepramine. Appetite suppressants such as fenfluramine may decrease appetite generally and decrease bulimic behaviour, but this effect is merely symptomatic and is used as a temporary respite whilst other treatments are applied. The new antidepressants which selectively inhibit serotonin re-uptake at central neuronal synapses (fluvoxamine and fluoxetine) may hold promise for the future, but this has not yet been confirmed by double-blind trials.

Psychotherapeutic approaches using one of a number of styles may be of real benefit to patients, especially those who fail to improve with cognitive–behavioural techniques. Such patients are likely to have psychological problems rooted in early relationships. As with the other treatments for bulimia nervosa, the critical factor in improvement is the patient's motivation, without which failure is likely.

THE PROGNOSIS OF ANOREXIA NERVOSA

In spite of the enormous concern which anorexia nervosa causes amongst relatives and carers, the mortality is relatively low at 5%, and the majority of this group are chronic patients who die through suicide rather than the metabolic consequences. Reviewing a number of studies it seems likely that at four to eight years follow-up, 50% of patients will have recovered completely, 25% will have minor residual problems and 25% will have severe chronic problems with low weights and psychological and social disability. Steinhausen and Glandville (1983) have reviewed studies indicating prognostic factors. Good prognostic indicators are early age of onset, probably before 18 years (though prepubertal cases may have a worse outcome), hysterical personality, a good parent–child relationship and a short duration. In addition, higher socioeconomic status, the ease of recovery of weight and from psychopathology, and the presence of only dietary restriction and excessive exercising appear to be good prognostic factors. Unfavourable outcomes may be predicted by the presence of self-induced vomiting, purgative abuse, bulimic behaviour, extreme weight loss, depressive and obsessional–compulsive symptomatology and chronicity. Premorbid developmental and clinical abnormalities of behaviour, old maternal age, higher rates of physical complications and acute body perception disturbances also indicate a poor prognosis. Similarly, high neuroticism scores, psychological tests suggestive of psychosis, masculine sex and married status also predict worse outcome.

THE PROGNOSIS OF BULIMIA NERVOSA

This has only been studied in respect of the short- and intermediate-term outcome of small numbers of patients treated by specific regimens in special centres. Lacey (1983) studied 30 patients treated with an integrated behavioural–psychodynamic regimen. All patients showed decreased frequency of bulimic behaviour and 24 out of 30 patients ceased bulimia by the end of therapy. At four-year follow-up, 28 patients attended and 20 of these were still free of bulimic behaviour and the remaining eight had occasional bulimia three or four times per year.

Lacey describes four types of bulimia with differing outcomes:

1. *Type One*—in which there is no previous history of anorexia nervosa, weight phobia or massive weight loss. It has a very good prognosis.
2. *Type Two*—in which the patient has a previous history of anorexia nervosa but has 'recovered' to a normal body weight. There is no fear of normal body weight expressed. Prognosis is not as good as Type One.
3. *Type Three*—in which the patients enter bulimia from massive obesity although weight is normal on presentation. The long-term prognosis is poor.
4. *Type Four*—the 'multi-impulse personality' group in which bulimic behaviour is associated with alcohol abuse, drug abuse, stealing, over-dosing, 'cutting' behaviour and sexual disinhibition. This group have a very stormy course and poor outcome and are perhaps fundamentally different from the other three groups.

REFERENCES

Adams J, Polson DW, Abdulwahid N et al (1985) Multifollicular ovaries: clinical and endocrine features and response to pulsatile gonadotrophin releasing hormone. *Lancet* ii: 1375–1378.
Bachmann GA & Kemmann E (1982) Prevalence of oligomenorrhea and amenorrhea in a college population. *American Journal of Obstetrics and Gynecology* **144**: 98–102.
Baranowska B, Roxbicka G, Jeske W et al (1984) The role of endogenous opiates in the mechanism of inhibited luteinizing hormone (LH) secretion in women with anorexia nervosa: the effect of naloxone on LH, follicle-stimulating hormone, prolactin, and beta-endorphin secretion. *Journal of Clinical Endocrinology and Metabolism* **59**: 412–416.
Bearn J & Robinson PH (1985) Binges, vomiting and guilt. *British Journal of Psychiatry* **146**: 214.
Bruch H (1973) *Eating Disorders*. New York: Basic Books.
Bullen BA, Skrinar GS, Beitium I et al (1985) Induction of menstrual disorders by strenuous exercise in untrained women. *New England Journal of Medicine* **312**: 1349–1353.
Button EJ & Whitehouse A (1981) Subclinical anorexia nervosa. *Psychological Medicine* **11**: 509–516.

Cantwell DP, Sturzenberger S, Burroughs J, Salkin B & Green JK (1977) Anorexia nervosa. An affective disorder? *Archives of General Psychiatry* **34:** 1087–1093.

Cooper PJ & Fairburn CG (1983) Binge-eating and self-induced vomiting in the community. *British Journal of Psychiatry* **142:** 139–144.

Copeland PM & Herzog DB (1987) Menstrual abnormalities. In Hudson JI & Pope HG (eds) *The Psychobiology of Bulimia*, pp 29–54. Washington: American Psychiatric Press.

Crisp AH (1977) Diagnosis and outcome of anorexia nervosa. *Proceedings of the Royal Society of Medicine* **70:** 464–470.

Crisp AH, Palmer RL & Kalucy RS (1976) How common is anorexia nervosa? A prevalence study. *British Journal of Psychiatry* **128:** 549–554.

Crisp AH, Hsu LKG, Harding B & Hartshorn J (1980) Clinical features of anorexia nervosa. *Journal of Psychosomatic Research* **24:** 179–191.

Dally P (1969) *Anorexia Nervosa*. New York: Grune and Stratton.

Fairburn CG & Cooper PJ (1982) Self-induced vomiting and bulimia nervosa: an undetected problem. *British Medical Journal* **284:** 1153–1155.

Fairburn CG & Cooper PJ (1984a) The clinical features of bulimia nervosa. *British Journal of Psychiatry* **144:** 238–246.

Fairburn CG & Cooper PJ (1984b) Binge-eating, self-induced vomiting and laxative abuse: a community study. *Psychological Medicine* **14:** 401–410.

Feicht CB, Johnson TS, Martin BJ, Sparks KE & Wagner WW (1978) Secondary amenorrhoea in athletes. *Lancet* **ii:** 1145–1146.

Fichter MM & Pirke KM (1984) Hypothalamic pituitary function in starving healthy subjects. In Pirke KM & Ploog D (eds) *The Psychobiology of Anorexia Nervosa*, pp 124–135. New York: Springer-Verlag.

Flint N & Stewart RB (1983) Amenorrhoea in psychiatric inpatients. *Archives of General Psychiatry* **40:** 589.

Frisch RE & McArthur JW (1974) Menstrual cycles: fatness as a determinant of minimum weight for height necessary for their maintenance or onset. *Science* **185:** 949–951.

Garfinkel PE & Garner DM (1982) *Anorexia Nervosa: A Multidimensional Perspective*. New York: Brunner Mazel.

Garner DM & Garfinkel PE (1980) Socio-cultural factors in the development of anorexia nervosa. *Psychological Medicine* **10:** 647–656.

Gwirtsman HE, Roy-Byrne P, Yager J et al (1983) Neuroendocrine abnormalities in bulimia. *American Journal of Psychiatry* **140:** 559–563.

Halmi KA, Falk JR & Schwartz E (1981) Binge-eating and vomiting: a survey of a college. *Psychological Medicine* **11:** 697–706.

Hart T, Kase N & Kimball CP (1970) Induction of ovulation and pregnancy in patients with anorexia nervosa. *American Journal of Obstetrics and Gynecology* **108:** 580–584.

Holden NL & Robinson PH (1988) Anorexia nervosa and bulimia nervosa in British Blacks. *British Journal of Psychiatry* **152:** 544–549.

Holland AJ, Hall A, Murray R, Russell GFM & Crisp AH (1984) Anorexia nervosa: a study of 34 twin pairs and one set of triplets. *British Journal of Psychiatry* **145:** 414–419.

Hsu LKG (1983) The aetiology of anorexia nervosa. *Psychological Medicine* **13:** 231–238.

Johnson CL, Suckey MK, Lewis LD et al (1983) A survey of 509 cases of self-reported bulimia. In Darby PL, Garfinkel PE, Garner DM et al (eds) *Anorexia Nervosa: Recent Developments in Research*, pp 159–172. New York: Alan R Liss.

Kemmann E, Pasquale SA & Skaf R (1983) Amenorrhea associated with carotenemia. *Journal of the American Medical Association* **249:** 926–929.

Kendell RE, Hall DJ, Hailey A & Babigian HM (1973) The epidemiology of anorexia nervosa. *Psychological Medicine* **3:** 200–203.

Lacey JH (1983) Bulimia nervosa, binge-eating and psychogenic vomiting: a controlled treatment study and long-term outcome. *British Medical Journal* **286:** 1609–1613.

Lacey JH & Smith G (1987) Bulimia nervosa: the impact of pregnancy on mother and baby. *British Journal of Psychiatry* **150:** 777–781.

Marshall JC & Kelch RP (1979) Low dose pulsatile gonadotrophin-releasing hormone in anorexia nervosa: a model of human pubertal development. *Journal of Clinical Endocrinology and Metabolism* **49:** 712–718.

Metropolitan Life Insurance Company (1983) *Statistical Bulletin of the Metropolitan Life Assurance Company* **64:** 2–9.

Pyle RL, Mitchell JE & Eckert ED (1981) Bulimia: a report of 34 cases. *Journal of Clinical Psychiatry* **42:** 60–64.

Pyle RL, Mitchell JE & Eckert ED (1983) The incidence of bulimia in three college populations. *International Journal of Eating Disorders* **2:** 75–85.

Russell GFM (1979) Bulimia nervosa. An ominous variant of anorexia nervosa. *Psychological Medicine* **9:** 429–448.

Russell GFM (1983) Anorexia nervosa and bulimia nervosa. In Russell GFM & Hersov LA (eds) *Handbook of Psychiatry 4. Neuroses and Personality Disorders*, pp 285–298. Cambridge: Cambridge University Press.

Russell GFM (1985a) The changing nature of anorexia nervosa: an introduction to the conference. *Journal of Psychiatric Research* **19:** 101–109.

Russell GFM (1985b) Premenarchal anorexia nervosa and its sequelae. *Journal of Psychiatric Research* **19:** 363–369.

Sheehan HL & Summers UK (1949) The syndrome of hypopituitarism. *Quarterly Journal of Medicine* **42:** 319.

Simmonds M (1914) Ueber embolische prozesse in der hypophysis. *Archives of Pathology and Anatomy* **217:** 226–239.

Steinhausen HC & Glandville K (1983) Follow-up studies of anorexia nervosa: a review of research findings. *Psychological Medicine* **13:** 239–249.

Tanner JM (1962) *Growth at Adolescence; With a General Consideration of the Effects of Hereditary and Environmental Factors upon Growth and Maturation from Birth to Maturity*, 2nd edn. Oxford: Blackwell Scientific.

Treasure JL, King EA, Gordon PAL, Wheeler M & Russell GFM (1985) Cystic ovaries: a phase of anorexia nervosa. *Lancet* **ii:** 1379–1382.

3

Psychological aspects of gynaecological surgery

MARGARET OATES
DENNIS GATH

This chapter concentrates on the psychological aspects of hysterectomy, with or without oophorectomy, and sterilization. These two procedures are amongst the commonest performed in gynaecology. They have acquired a reputation for causing psychiatric morbidity and psychological distress. This bad reputation was based, in part, on the assumption that the loss of the uterus and sterilization could be equated to castration, with an assumption of inevitable conflicts over femininity and sexuality, and in part on early research findings. The available modern evidence, from studies carried out over the past 15 years, would suggest that this reputation is largely unjustified and that hysterectomy and sterilization in particular are not causally related to psychiatric morbidity, nor indeed to medium- or long-term psychological distress. This is in marked contrast to both early and modern studies linking childbirth to an excess of serious psychiatric morbidity. However, even in the case of childbirth there is some controversy whether it is associated with an excess of minor psychiatric morbidity (see Chapters 8 and 9).

Nonetheless, the available evidence is that psychiatric morbidity in gynaecological patients is higher than in the general population and other areas of medicine. It is, therefore, important that the gynaecologist should be aware of the signs and symptoms of psychiatric disorder, in particular those of depressive illness, anxiety states and other common minor psychiatric disorders. A brief account of functional psychiatric disorders is given in Chapter 12, and a fuller account can be found in standard psychiatric textbooks (e.g. Gelder et al, 1983). It is necessary to be aware of the possibility of psychiatric disorder and to include questions on emotional well-being and the biological symptoms of psychiatric disorder during gynaecological assessment, for the following reasons:

1. A past history of psychiatric disorder is repeatedly mentioned throughout the literature on gynaecological surgery as the most important predictor of adverse psychiatric outcome following operation.
2. Whatever the gynaecological procedure and its indications, a disturbed mental state before operation predicts an adverse psychiatric outcome.
3. Psychiatric disorder, or long-standing psychosocial problems, may increase a patient's complaints and decrease her capacity to cope with

symptoms that might otherwise be tolerable. These factors may lead to an increased risk of referral to a gynaecologist and subsequently of surgery.

4. Undetected and untreated psychiatric problems may interfere with treatment and delay recovery from surgery.

5. The presence of a disturbed mental state at the time of assessment may lead to issues about the timing of gynaecological surgery. In some cases the appropriate treatment, if carried out before surgery, may lead to a reassessment of a patient's indications for surgery, even rendering it unnecessary. In other cases, particularly if the patient is suffering from a major psychiatric disorder, it may be necessary to treat the psychiatric condition first, as gynaecological surgery may lead to a deterioration of this condition. In other cases, the indications for gynaecological surgery may have to take priority over the psychiatric state and both conditions may need to be treated concurrently. In other circumstances, gynaecological surgery may lead to a resolution of the psychological distress. In all of these situations it may be necessary for the gynaecologist to collaborate closely with the patient's general practitioner or a psychiatrist who specializes in this field.

6. Although the most important factors predicting adverse psychiatric outcome are preoperative, a significant minority of women do become psychiatrically ill following these procedures, and it is important for the gynaecologist to be aware of the risk factors associated with this adverse outcome.

Psychiatric morbidity in gynaecological patients

Neurotic psychiatric disorder (excluding alcoholism) is more common in women than in men in a general practice setting. Amongst women in general practice there is an excess of psychiatric morbidity in those women complaining of premenstrual tension, menstrual problems (menorrhagia and dysmenorrhoea) and perimenopausal problems (hot flushes and sweating) (Gath et al, 1987), and an increased likelihood of referral to a gynaecologist when menstrual and psychiatric problems co-exist.

There has been a suggestion (Garter and Dean, 1989) that the excess of admissions of women may be accounted for by psychiatric disorders associated with childbirth. It is possible that the association of psychiatric morbidity with menstrual complaints may also contribute to the excess of psychiatric morbidity amongst women, particularly in general practice populations. It is, therefore, not surprising that psychiatric morbidity in gynaecological outpatient clinics is also high, higher than that in women in the general population and in general practice (Ballinger, 1975, 1977; Worsley et al, 1977) and higher than that in patients attending general medical and surgical clinics (which includes men and women). High levels of current and past psychiatric morbidity have also been noted in many studies of patients selected for hysterectomy (Martin et al, 1977; Gath et al, 1981a,b), and in early studies of patients referred for sterilization (Enoch and Jones, 1975).

With the exception of gynaecological emergencies, such as ectopic pregnancies, ruptured ovarian cysts or gynaecological neoplasms, the majority of gynaecological conditions present because of a subjective experience of quantitative variations in normal physiology (premenstrual and perimenopausal phenomena, and menstrual problems) or problems with fertility. It is, therefore, not unreasonable to assume that an emotional disorder could lead to an increased awareness of these problems and a decreased toleration of them, and lead in turn to referral and, once referred, to surgery. Some clinicians might feel that some of the symptoms themselves might be psychogenic. An alternative explanation, however, for this excess of psychiatric morbidity at all stages in the 'chain' leading to surgery could be that the gynaecological disorders themselves are distressing, and could lead to secondary emotional problems, particularly if the person is vulnerable by virtue of previous history or family history of psychiatric disorder. Thus it can be seen that the causal relationships between gynaecological disorder and psychiatric disorder are complex and that evidence can be found to support both these hypotheses.

HYSTERECTOMY

Psychiatric outcome

The bad reputation—results from early studies

Before the early 1970s, many studies in Great Britain and the United States reported high rates of psychiatric morbidity following hysterectomy compared with other women and those undergoing other surgical procedures. This led to an assumption on the part of the authors that hysterectomy was causally related to psychiatric disorder. This view has persisted, despite the fact that these older studies were mostly retrospective and did not use modern standardized psychiatric assessments, and the patients studied had a heterogenous mix of gynaecological conditions. These studies, even if controlled, could not validly assume a causal relationship between hysterectomy and psychiatric disorder. This can only be done by prospective studies which examine the psychiatric status before and after operation. One of the most influential of the retrospective studies was carried out in an Oxford general practice population by Richards (1973) and has become a standard reference work. This showed that 33% of women developed a depressive illness in the three years following hysterectomy, compared with only 7% of controls. Later, in 1974, he compared a group of patients who were hysterectomized with a similar sized group of other surgical patients who had had a variety of other operations ranging from cholecystectomy to thyroidectomy. In the second study he found that 73% of the hysterectomy patients became depressed as opposed to 29% of the other patients. He also found that the hysterectomy patients had a higher number of postoperative physical complaints than did the other patients. Despite its influence, the

study is also essentially flawed by being retrospective, having a heterogenous group of gynaecological conditions, and by not using standardized
psychiatric assessments and case definitions of depression. (A useful review
of the early literature on hysterectomy is given in Gath and Cooper, 1982.)

Reputation revised—results of modern studies

Since the 1970s there have been a number of prospective studies contributing to the overall view that hysterectomy does not lead to an increase in
psychiatric morbidity or other adverse sequelae, such as a deterioration in
sexual functioning or marital satisfaction, nor to higher levels of distress
than other surgical procedures (Martin et al, 1977, 1980; Meikle and Brody,
1977; Coppen et al, 1981; Gath et al, 1981a,b). Although the methodology
of these studies and their inclusion criteria differ somewhat, they all used a
prospective design and standardized measures of psychiatric status and
other variables. The patients were assessed at intervals preoperatively and
postoperatively. However, the results of the studies were divided in one
important respect. Two studies, one in Canada (Meikle and Brody, 1977)
and one in Great Britain (Coppen et al, 1981), suggested that the levels of
psychiatric morbidity before and after hysterectomy were not abnormally
high, whilst the other two studies, one in the USA (Martin et al, 1977, 1980)
and the other in Great Britain (Gath et al, 1981a,b), found high levels of
psychiatric morbidity before hysterectomy, and, whilst reduced, high levels
were still found after operation.

The Canadian study (Meikle and Brody, 1977) was a postal survey
comparing women undergoing hysterectomy, tubal ligation and cholecystectomy. These patients represented 75% of a consecutive series. They were
assessed during the week before surgery, and six weeks and three months
after surgery, using a standardized questionnaire on their emotional state
and levels of tension and anxiety. There was no evidence that removal of the
uterus led to greater disturbance than did the other two operations, and at
no time did the postoperative response reach abnormal levels.

The American study carried out in St Louis (Martin et al, 1977, 1980)
assessed women preoperatively and one year postoperatively using standardized psychiatric assessments. They found high levels of psychiatric diagnoses
both preoperatively (57%) and postoperatively (66%), the difference not
being significant. However, despite the fact that there was no significant
difference in the number of women receiving a psychiatric diagnosis before
and after a hysterectomy, there was a highly significant difference in the
number of women with pathological scores on a standardized assessment of
depression (14 women preoperatively and only 7 women postoperatively).
Virtually all the patients who received psychiatric treatment after operation
had received such treatment before. The authors of this study concluded that
the findings did not support the hypothesis that hysterectomy is followed by an
excess of psychiatric symptoms, but rather that patients had fewer symptoms
after the operation than before it.

The study in the United Kingdom (Coppen et al, 1981), designed to
examine the effects of oestrogen administered after hysterectomy, also drew

conclusions about the relationship between the operation and depression. The patients (including a group who did not have a hysterectomy) were assessed before the operation and at six-weekly intervals for up to three years following it, using standardized psychiatric assessments, the General Health Questionnaire (GHQ) and the Beck Depression Inventory. Following operation the mean scores on both the GHQ and the Depression Inventory improved significantly, leading the authors to conclude that there was a decrease in depression and psychiatric morbidity after hysterectomy.

The second study in the United Kingdom was in Oxford (Gath et al, 1981), where a consecutive series of 156 women undergoing hysterectomy for menorrhagia of benign origin (fibroids, endometriosis, dysfunctional uterine bleeding) were assessed at four weeks preoperatively and at six and eighteen months postoperatively. This prospective study of a largely unselected group (90% of a consecutive series) and a relatively homogenous sample (only benign conditions included) using standardized psychiatric assessments and measures of personality functioning and social assessments, as well as gathering sociodemographic information. The use of a standardized assessment, such as the Present State Examination (PSE), of known reliability and validity and which has been widely used in many other studies and in different populations, makes it possible to compare findings in relation to psychiatric morbidity with that found in other populations. By using levels of definition on the PSE index of definition, it is possible to define psychiatric cases of a certain severity. All the patients were interviewed at their interval assessments by trained female interviewers.

Using level 5 of the PSE index of definition, 58% of the patients were defined as cases before hysterectomy. Postoperatively, the numbers fell to 26% at six months and 29% at 18 months, both reductions being highly significant. The level of psychiatric morbidity was therefore halved after hysterectomy. It was also found that of the women who were non-cases preoperatively, only a small number (nine out of 66 patients) became cases following operation, contributing to less than 25% of all psychiatric morbidity in terms of PSE cases that were found at the 18-month follow-up. In contrast, 57% of the women who had been PSE cases before the hysterectomy had become non-cases by the time of the 18-month follow-up. The majority of the women who were psychiatric cases following operation had been psychiatric cases before the operation. This leads to the conclusion that hysterectomy seldom results in psychiatric morbidity and, indeed, for many women results in an improvement in their psychiatric functioning.

Psychosexual outcome

There have been a very large number of papers over the last 30 years examining the impact of hysterectomy on sexual functioning. These have given figures as high as 37% (Munday and Cox, 1967; Dennerstein et al, 1977) and as low as 6% (Jackson, 1979) of patients reporting a deterioration in sexual functioning following hysterectomy. The findings of some studies, that over a third of women experienced a deterioration in their sexual life, together with the widespread equation of hysterectomy with castration and belief on the part of the public that hysterectomy affects their sexual life, has led to the assumption that hysterectomy has a negative impact on sexual functioning in a significant number of women. Few, if any, of these studies were prospective and most used very variable and non-standardized ways of assessing sexual functioning. The negative interpretation of their results is misleading. The results of most of these studies, even the earliest ones, could be interpreted in an alternative and more positive way as showing that in the majority of women studied hysterectomy led to either no change or an improvement in their sexual functioning. Almost all of the studies show that the women whose sexual functioning deteriorated were outnumbered by those women whose sexual functioning improved.

However, only prospective studies can determine the impact of hysterectomy on sexual functioning. The study of Martin et al (1980), previously mentioned, found that in those women who had sexual partners, only four out of 34 reported a decrease in the frequency of sexual intercourse postoperatively, whilst 11 out of 34 reported an increase and 19 no change. Coppen et al (1981) found no change in the frequency and quality of sexual intercourse after hysterectomy, and Gath et al (1981a,b) found that 80% of the patients had recovered at least their preoperative level of sexual activity by four months post-operation. At six months and 18 months postoperatively the frequency of intercourse had increased in 56% of their patients, decreased in 17% and remained unchanged in 27%. The reported enjoyment of sexual intercourse was increased in 39%, reduced in 20% and unchanged in 41%.

In conclusion, therefore, the literature on psychosexual outcome after hysterectomy would indicate that for the majority of women their sexual functioning is either unchanged or indeed improved after hysterectomy. Prospective studies lead to the conclusion that hysterectomy does not cause in itself a deterioration in sexual functioning. However, all studies from the earliest to the most recent show that a significant minority of women do report decreases in sexual activity or enjoyment (perhaps up to 20%) following hysterectomy, and in clinical practice this is an important issue. Various factors have been implicated in predicting this risk. Psychiatric status as measured by the PSE, preoperatively and postoperatively, was significantly associated with low frequency and enjoyment of sexual intercourse in the study of Gath et al (1981b). Other factors which may be of importance in individual cases are preoperative satisfaction with marriage and preoperative sexual functioning. If satisfaction in these areas was low before operation, it is unlikely to be improved by the operation and may in fact deteriorate. However, there is no evidence from large well-designed prospective studies that this is true for populations of hysterectomized patients as a whole. Age might also be considered to be an important factor in determining sexual behaviour following hysterectomy (Amias, 1975). Many patients undergo hysterectomy at an age when there may be a natural reduction in sexual drive unrelated to the operation. For younger women whose hysterectomy interferes with their plans for reproduction there may be feelings of sadness and loss (grief) which may interfere with their libido and sexual performance. The attitudes and expectations of the women, and indeed of their partners, before the operation can also be important in determining sexual functioning afterwards. Pessimistic views may be received from the medical profession, from friends and family, and from the media. Amias (1975) stressed that many women are convinced that hysterectomy inevitably leads to cessation of sexual activity. Drellich and Bieber (1958) and Dennerstein et al (1977) both found an association between preoperative anxiety concerning a possible deteroration in sexual performance and postoperative deterioration of sexual relations, libido and an increase in dyspareunia; however, both these studies were limited by being retrospective and using different assessments of sexual functioning. Physical factors, such as the type of hysterectomy, the indications for it, accompanying oophorectomy and subsequent hormonal functioning (including the presence or absence of hormone replacement therapy) might also be implicated in postoperative sexual functioning. There is little evidence from the literature of a differential effect of abdominal as opposed to vaginal hysterectomy, and many studies report that patients have resumed at least their level of preoperative sexual functioning at between two and four months post-operation (Craig and Jackson, 1975; Coppen et al, 1981; Gath et al, 1981a,b). The effects of oophorectomy on sexual functioning of patients who are hysterectomized is difficult to assess, as most of the studies which included these patients were retrospective and used methods of assessment of sexual functioning which are difficult to compare. Also, many of the patients will have had some residual ovarian tissue left behind or may have been receiving oestrogen replacement therapy. Nonetheless, the consensus of opinion from these studies, which range over the past 40 years, would seem to be that patients who have a hysterectomy and oophorectomy are no more likely to have psychosexual disturbance after surgery than those undergoing hysterectomy with ovarian conservation (Munday and Cox, 1967; Gath et al, 1981a,b). However, it seems reasonable to suppose that if oophorectomy leads to problems with vaginal lubrication and consequent dyspareunia that this will have an adverse effect on sexual functioning; this might be ameliorated by the use of oestrogen replacement therapy.

Lastly, a woman's view of her own femininity following hysterectomy (and her husband's view of her in this way) might be thought to be important in determining her sexual feelings afterwards. This might be expected to effect particularly younger women, and there have been anecdotal reports of women feeling that they have lost youthfulness and attractiveness and feel hollow or empty following hysterectomy. This kind of concept is difficult to investigate in conventional medical research. However, in the study by Gath et al (1981a,b), patients were asked at their 18-month follow-up direct questions about their feelings of femininity and the great majority reported them as undiminished.

Factors relating to psychiatric outcome

Despite the fact that the evidence from studies discussed in this chapter is that hysterectomy does not in itself lead to psychiatric morbidity, nor does it have in general adverse psychological sequelae, it remains true that there is a high level of psychiatric morbidity in patients awaiting operation and a high level (if somewhat lower) of psychiatric morbidity for at least 18 months following the operation (Martin et al, 1980; Gath et al, 1981a,b). It is therefore, important for the gynaecologist to be aware of the risk factors that might be important in predicting adverse outcome and to take into account psychiatric factors when assessing patients for operation. Three groups of factors have been put forward as determining psychiatric outcome after hysterectomy: psychiatric, physical and demographic.

Psychiatric factors

Whatever the methodology, there has been a remarkable consistency in the findings of the hysterectomy literature of the past 40 years that a history of preoperative psychiatric disorder is one of the main determinants of post-operative psychiatric disorder. Two examples of this are the study of Richards in 1973, in an Oxford general practice, which found that a history of depression before hysterectomy greatly increased the risk of depression afterwards, and the study in Iowa, USA (Martin et al, 1980), which found that virtually all patients receiving psychiatric treatment after hysterectomy had received similar treatment before the operation. In addition to a history of a psychiatric disorder in a patient at any time before the operation, the patient's preoperative mental state is also important, even in the absence of such a history. In the Oxford Study of patients awaiting hysterectomy (Gath et al, 1981b), psychiatric outcome was significantly related to psychiatric status before operation, as measured by the PSE. Martin et al (1980) also found that patients receiving a psychiatric diagnosis before operation were more likely to receive one postoperatively.

Physical factors

Physical factors that might influence the psychiatric outcome of hyster-ectomy include the gynaecological condition indicating surgery (cancer, benign conditions such as fibroids, endometriosis and dysfunctional uterine bleeding), the presence or absence of any uterine pathology on histological examination of the uterus, the type of hysterectomy (vaginal or abdominal), associated procedures such as oophorectomy or pelvic clearance, and the hormonal status of women afterwards. It is difficult to draw firm conclusions from the literature on any of these points because the methodology of the relevant studies is so different that comparison between them is not always possible. In particular, many of the earlier retrospective studies included women with a mixture of gynaecological conditions resulting in hyster-ectomy, whereas many of the later prospective studies include women who suffer from benign conditions only, excluding those with cancer and those who might have had more radical surgery. Any adverse outcome to hyster-ectomy in this latter group of women might be contributed to, not only by the effects of hysterectomy, but also by concerns that they might have about their prognosis. The problem of uncertainty about the effect of physical factors on psychiatric outcome is further compounded by the wide variation in indications for hysterectomy, both across time and in different countries, most notably the USA. This is particularly relevant as a high proportion of hysterectomies are performed because of excessive menstruation which, if of benign origin, may either result from demonstrable pathology in the uterus, such as fibroids or endometriosis, or from dysfunctional uterine bleeding, which occurs in the absence of demonstrable organic pathology. In this country, up to 50% of patients undergoing hysterectomy are diagnosed as having dysfunctional uterine bleeding and it is probably this group of patients which accounts for the variation in different countries and amongst different gynaecologists, and it is also probable that it is amongst this group that preoperative psychological factors have their most important influence. Many studies, notably Barker (1968) and Richards (1973), have suggested that postoperative psychiatric morbidity was more frequent amongst patients without significant pelvic pathology or histopathology. These findings have led to the widely held belief, on the part of gynaecologists and psychiatrist, that post-hysterectomy depression is related to the absence of 'true' organic pathology. However, the more recent prospective Oxford study conducted by Gath et al (1981a,b) found no significant differences, at any stage of their enquiry, between patients with benign organic menorrhagia and dysfunctional menorrhagia in terms of their mental states, previous psychiatric histories, psychosexual adjustments, marital functioning or personality type. It has already been established by Chimbira et al (1980) and Ballinger (1977) that there is little correlation between the complaint of menorrhagia, usage of sanitary protection and the actual measurement of blood loss. It may be, therefore, that it is the subjective experience of excessive menstruation, with its consequent disability and embarrassment, that is more important than the actual amount of blood loss or the pathology causing it. As hysterectomy inevitably leads to the relief of menorrhagia, this may account for the absence of any correlation between psychiatric outcome and the different types of benign organic pathology.

Abdominal versus vaginal hysterectomy. Gath et al (1981a,b) found no evidence of a differential effect on psychiatric outcome from using abdominal or vaginal surgery. Apart from this study, there is little evidence in the literature that this issue has been raised, and it would be difficult to interpret the results of early studies, as there has been an increasing trend towards vaginal hysterectomy over the past 20 years.

Hysterectomy and oophorectomy. The majority of studies over the past 20 years that have compared psychiatric morbidity after hysterectomy alone with that after hysterectomy and oophorectomy have found no difference in psychiatric outcome. Barker's (1968) retrospective case note survey found that patients who had undergone both procedures were no more likely to be referred for psychiatric treatment than those women who had had hysterectomy alone. Similarly, Richards, (1973) retrospective general practice survey found that women who had undergone both procedures were no more likely to develop postoperative depression that those who had undergone hysterectomy alone. Despite the limitations of these and many other earlier studies, in that they were retrospective and used non-standardized ways of defining psychiatric outcome, their findings are consistent with those of two more recent prospective studies—Martin et al (1980) in the USA, and Gath et al (1981b) in Oxford. In the USA study, removal of the ovaries did not affect the prevalence of psychiatric morbidity after hysterectomy. In the Oxford study, there was no significant difference in the numbers of women who were psychiatric cases before operation between the hysterectomy alone group and the oophorectomized group, nor was there any significant difference in the number of cases 18 months postoperatively. In both groups the level of psychiatric morbidity was more than halved. Amongst those women who had both hysterectomy and oophorectomy, hormone replacement therapy made no difference in psychiatric outcome.

Radical surgery. There is no available evidence from the literature of the effects of more radical surgery, such as pelvic clearance, partial vaginectomy, vulvectomy or concurrent radiotherapy, on psychiatric outcome. However, as the majority of women undergoing such procedures are likely to be suffering from malignant conditions, and many will have experienced technical problems with sexual activity after operation, it would seem reasonable that these women may have additional psychological problems, at least in the short-term, and their psychological distress will be compounded by realistic fears for their prognosis.

Demographic factors

Age, marital status and satisfaction, parity and social class have all been implicated in hysterectomy literature as being determinants of psychiatric outcome. A number of studies have suggested that younger patients are particularly at risk of psychiatric disorder after hysterectomy (e.g. Richards, 1973; Martin et al, 1977). However, these findings have not been supported by the more recent Oxford study (Gath et al, 1981a,b), which showed that younger patients were not at increased risk of psychiatric disorder; if anything, those over the age of 40 were more at risk. However, these differences may be partly explained by the gynaecological conditions for which hysterectomy was indicated in the different studies. In the Gath et al (1981a,b) study, only women who had benign conditions were included. The indications for hysterectomy in young women who have not had any children, or have not completed their families, must be very different to the indications in women who have completed their reproduction. Inevitably these younger women will as a whole have much more serious pathology than older women, and may not be represented in large numbers in many studies. Despite the lack of evidence from large prospective studies that age is related to psychiatric outcome, in individual cases the youthfulness of the patient may present major psychological issues. This is particularly likely to be so if it renders the patient infertile against her wishes. In such cases the hysterectomy may be followed by a pronounced grief reaction and the patient may require opportunity to ventilate her feelings and considerable sympathy and support, perhaps even counselling, to adjust to her loss of fertility and her previous expectations.

Marital status. Not all patients who have hysterectomies are married or sexually active; many will be single or divorced. It might be expected that there should be a difference in psychiatric outcome between these groups of women, and also between women who are happily married and those who are not. Despite this, there are few references to marital status or satisfaction in the literature. Barker (1968) found that the incidence of psychiatric referral was greatly increased amongst divorced or separated women compared with those who were married. However, Gath et al (1981b) found no such association in their sample, nor did they find any association between disorder and the quality of marriage (which was assessed by means of a standardized schedule).

Parity. It has long been thought that childlessness and low parity might be associated with poor psychiatric outcome. Drellich and Beiber (1958) and Kaltreider et al (1979) both suggested that desire for more children was significantly associated with poor outcome. However, both these studies were retrospective with unrepresentative sampling and did not use standardized measures of psychiatric morbidity. Studies by Barker (1968), Richards (1973) and Gath et al (1981b) found no such association; in addition low parity was found to have no effect on psychiatric outcome. As in the issue of age being related to psychiatric outcome, childless women, or those who have not completed their families, may have been excluded from the Gath et al (1981a,b) study by virtue of the more serious indications for their hysterectomy. Women for whom hysterectomy represents an involuntary loss of fertility, who had wished to have more children, may have a pronounced grief reaction postoperatively and may experience additional psychological distress, or even a depressive illness, as they adjust to the loss of their fertility and their changed expectations of life.

Social class. The hysterectomy literature contains surprisingly few references to the effect of social class. Despite suggestions by Kaltreider et al (1979) that adverse psychological reactions were associated with low social class, neither Richards (1973) nor Gath et al (1981a,b) found any evidence for this.

Conclusions

The available evidence suggests that preoperative morbidity and a preoperative psychiatric history are more important determinants of the psychiatric and psychosexual outcome of hysterectomy than are physical or demographic factors.

Implications for the assessment for hysterectomy

1. Approximately half of all the patients a gynaecologist sees will have a psychiatric illness, and following hysterectomy approximately a quarter will be psychiatrically ill. The majority of those women who are psychiatrically ill following operation will have been ill before it, or will have a past history of such an illness.

2.   If the patient presenting to the gynaecologist is currently well and has no past history of psychiatric disturbance, it is probable that she will have no adverse psychiatric or psychosexual sequelae to the hysterectomy.

3.   If the patient is currently psychiatrically well, but reveals a past history of psychiatric disorder, then the gynaecologist and the general practitioner should be alert to the possibility of this women developing a depressive illness in the first 18 months following hysterectomy. The indications for hysterectomy should be sound and the risks of conservative management balanced against the risks of developing a depressive illness. Early diagnosis of such an illness, and its swift treatment, will reduce the distress and morbidity caused.

4.   If the patient·is currently psychiatrically unwell, and particularly if she also has a past psychiatric history, then a careful assessment of both her psychiatric state and the indications for hysterectomy will be necessary. If she suffers from a major psychiatric disorder, such as manic-depressive illness or schizophrenia, and the gynaecological condition is not life-threatening, then the hysterectomy should be delayed until the psychiatric disorder has been adequately treated. For benign gynaecological conditions, the indications for hysterectomy will then need to be reassessed. Such a patient will normally be receiving medication at the time of the hysterectomy. After consultation with an anaesthetist, it may be necessary to stop medication, such as tricyclic antidepressants, lithium carbonate or phenothiazines, for one or two days at the time of the operation. However, it is important that such medication is re-instigated as soon as possible, as stopping it may lead to a major deterioration in the woman's mental state and complicate her surgical management. On the rare occasion when a woman is receiving mono-amine oxidase inhibitors, it may be necessary to stop this medication for at least two weeks prior to the administration of an anaesthetic. If the gynaecological condition is life-threatening and the woman suffers from a major psychiatric disorder, it may be necessary to press ahead with the hysterectomy and, in close collaboration with a psychiatrist, treat both conditions concurrently.

5.   If the woman is suffering from a minor or neurotic psychiatric disorder, such as a mild depressive illness or states of emotional distress or anxiety, it is important to assess whether this condition is being caused by the gynaecological condition or, on the other hand, whether the woman's emotional state causes her to be distressed by gynaecological symptoms which would otherwise be tolerated. The distress, social embarrassment and interference with social and domestic functioning that can result from menorrhagia may be considerable and may be sufficient to account for states of emotional distress, particularly in women who are vulnerable by virtue of a previous psychiatric history or difficult life circumstances. In cases where the gynaecologist has doubts as to whether the emotional state is a primary or secondary phenom-enon, help should be sought from the patient's general practitioner or a psychiatrist specializing in this field, delaying the decision for hyster-ectomy until after a psychiatric assessment; when indicated, appro-

priate psychiatric treatment may lead to a reassessment of the need for hysterectomy.

6. All patients awaiting hysterectomy will benefit from clear explanation of their condition and the procedures that are likely to be faced. They will all benefit from the reassurance that their sexual functioning need not be affected by the hysterectomy and that most of them will experience an improvement in their general emotional and physical health. However, it is not uncommon for patients, in the first one or two weeks after hysterectomy, to feel tired, lethargic, emotionally turbulent and over-sensitive and occasionally weepy. This postoperative syndrome, not unlike the postpartum blues (although rather more severe and peaking on the second day after operation rather than on the fifth day after childbirth), has been described by a number of authors, including Iles et al (1989). Both patients and their carers need to be reassured about this occurrence and its essentially benign nature.

7. There will be, occasionally, individual patients whose hysterectomy is particularly personally significant or distressing. Such patients might be those prevented from having children or for whom their condition and operation results in disability or realistic fears for their prognosis. These patients will have valid extra needs of sympathy, support and continuity of care. The clinicians should be alert to the possibility of such patients developing distressing grief reactions following the operation, or developing a depressive illness. Appropriate care and counselling may ameliorate, or even prevent, such conditions arising.

STERILIZATION

Like hysterectomy, sterilization in women has acquired a reputation of leading to psychiatric problems and a deterioration in sexual functioning in some women. This reputation is based on the findings of many studies (e.g. Campanella and Wolff, 1975; Enoch and Jones, 1975) which showed high rates of psychiatric disorder and other problems after sterilization. It is also popularly supposed that these adverse affects are greater amongst women in non-Western countries (Lu and Chun, 1967, Hong Kong; Khorana and Vyas, 1975, India), which if it were true would have important implications for gynaecologists treating members of ethnic minority groups in this country. Even if these studies were not essentially flawed by being retro-spective, involving a mixture of medical and social reasons for sterilization and using non-standardized forms of assessment of outcome, it would still not be possible to relate these findings to modern day clinical practice, as sterilization has changed markedly in many important aspects over the past 20 years. The most dramatic change has been in its frequency of use. It has become an increasingly frequent and commonplace choice of contraception in women in all parts of the world who have completed their families. In England and Wales between 1961 and 1975, there was a 12-fold increase in female sterilization (Bledin et al, 1978) and there have been similar increases in other countries. There have also been marked changes in the sociodemographic characteristics of the women (age and class), their parity, preoperative physical condition, and whether or not the sterilization was carried out as a specific, or interval, procedure or in association with some other event, such as childbirth or abortion. Twenty years ago sterilization most commonly occurred amongst older women of lower social class who had had a large number of children and who were in poor gynaecological health, and it resulted from a medical suggestion rather than a request on the part of the patient. The sterilization was frequently carried out shortly after childbirth, abortion or some other gynaecological procedure. Nowadays, sterilization is a widely accepted form of contraception which is used amongst women of all ages and all social classes. Women undergoing sterilization are therefore more representative of the population as a whole. It usually takes place as the result of a direct request from the woman as an interval procedure, unrelated to either childbirth or other gynaecological events. The women have fewer children and are in better gynaecological health, medical reasons for sterilization being less common than previously. There have also been major changes in surgical technique, particularly in the last few years, with a trend towards laparoscopic surgery and more recently the introduction of clip sterilization with a consequent change in both the degree of tissue trauma involved and the view of sterilization, from being a permanent and irreversible procedure to being one which is at least potentially reversible. There have also been parallel changes in social attitudes towards sterilization amongst the general population. Once it was a secret, even shameful topic, now it is openly discussed and commonplace. It is, therefore, not surprising that most of the prospective studies carried out in the 1980s show, in marked contrast to the earlier studies (and in contrast to the modern studies on hysterectomy), that preoperatively patients awaiting sterilization differ little in their psychiatric and sociodemographic characteristics from the general population, and that postoperatively there is no evidence of adverse psychological sequelae. This is true not only of Western Europe, but also of many other countries, with the exception, perhaps, of India.

The psychiatric status of patients before sterilization

In contrast to the hysterectomy studies and some earlier studies on sterilization (Enoch and Jones, 1975), recent prospective studies, using standardized methods of psychiatric assessment, have suggested that the psychiatric morbidity in women awaiting sterilization is no higher than in the general population. In the Oxford study of interval sterilization, using the PSE (P. Cooper et al, 1982), 10% of the population were PSE cases (level 5 PSE index of definition), which is the same as in the general population. In the Dundee study (Smith, 1979) which used the GHQ, 25% of the population were probable cases, again no higher than in the general population. In a study performed in Nottingham as part of the World Health Organization (WHO) 1984 collaborative collective study, using six centres throughout the world (Bledin et al, 1985; J. Cooper et al, 1985), which also used the PSE, the rate of psychiatric disorder in the United Kingdom centre was no higher in women awaiting sterilization than that which would be expected in the general population. Whilst it would seem that, in the United Kingdom at least, the population awaiting sterilization is relatively ordinary in terms of its psychiatric status, this may not be necessarily true in all countries in the non-Western world (see below).

Adverse sequelae to sterilization

Four main types of adverse psychological outcome to sterilization have been described in the literature—psychiatric disturbance, psychosexual problems, regret, dissatisfaction and the wish for reversal, and menstrual problems. Because sterilization has changed so dramatically over the past 20 years in terms of its frequency, the surgical techniques used and the characteristics of the women themselves, only the results of modern studies will be discussed. The effect of sterilization on mental health and on psychosexual and menstrual functioning can only be ascertained by prospective studies using standardized assessments in these three areas. For both of these reasons the discussion of outcome will concentrate on the results of two studies. The first was carried out in Oxford by P. Cooper et al (1981, 1982), in which 200 women were interviewed before sterilization, and at six and 18 months postoperatively. Several standardized measures of their psychiatric status were used, including most importantly the PSE, and pre- and postoperative standardized assessment of psychosexual functioning, marital satisfaction, postoperative regret and menstrual disturbance, as well as general sociodemographic data. The second study was an international collaborative study conducted by the WHO involving six research centres in the United Kingdom (Nottingham), India (Agra and Chandigarh), Columbia (Cali), Nigeria (Ibadan) and the Philippines (Manila) (Bledin et al, 1985; J. Cooper et al, 1985). This study, which was slightly different in design to the Oxford study, excluded women with past histories of psychiatric disorder but included sterilization following childbirth. However, in common with the Oxford study, women were assessed preoperatively and at six months and one year postoperatively, using standardized assessments of mental health (the PSE), psychosexual functioning, menstrual disturbance, physical health and regret.

Psychiatric outcome

Most recent prospective studies reveal that sterilization is not followed by increased rates of psychiatric disorder. The Scottish study carried out in Dundee by Smith (Smith, 1979), using the GHQ, found that the number of probable cases fell from 25% preoperatively to 15% at one year postoperatively. The Oxford study (P. Cooper et al, 1981, 1982) found that the level of psychiatric morbidity fell from 10.5% preoperatively (at level 5 of the PSE index of definition) to 4.7% at six months and 9.3% at one year postoperatively. In this study of the outcome of interval sterilization, only 6.7% of those women who had been non-cases before operation became cases after. This rate of new cases was no different to that expected in the general population over the same period of time. In a report of the

Nottingham centre of the WHO collaborative study (J. Cooper et al, 1985), which included postpartum as well as interval sterilization and a control population for both groups, no significant differences were found between all four groups at one year postoperatively and, over time, in terms of their mean PSE scores. The numbers of PSE cases was at no time higher than in the Oxford study, or higher than that which would be expected in the general population. However, in the Nottingham study the percentage of cases at level 5 of the PSE index of definition in the postpartum patients and their controls was 8.7% preoperatively (higher than the interval sterilizations and their controls) and had risen to 13% in the postpartum sterilization groups, the control group remaining unchanged over this one-year period. However, the numbers of actual women involved was small and this difference did not reach statistical significance. It is important to note that the Oxford study did not include postpartum patients.

Psychosexual functioning

Early studies tended to report high rates of psychosexual disorder following sterilization, and more recent studies lower rates. The studies of outcome in the United Kingdom have tended to report, over time, lower rates of sexual disturbance than studies from non-Western countries. The Oxford study (P. Cooper et al, 1981, 1982) used standardized interviews to assess sexual functioning preoperatively and at six months and 18 months postoperatively. At 18 months the frequency of sexual intercourse had risen in 28% of the women, fallen in 26% and remained unchanged in 46%. Sexual enjoyment had risen in 22%, fallen in 6% and remained the same in 71%. Of the 11% of patients who are dissatisfied with their sexual life following operation, the majority had expressed dissatisfaction at the preoperative assessment. The Nottingham study also assessed sexual functioning in terms of frequency, enjoyment and satisfaction, before operation and at six months and one year following operation. They found a reported improvement in sexual relationship significantly more often in sterilized patients than controls at one year, and this difference was most significant for the interval sterilizations compared with their controls. Positive pleasure in sex was reported more commonly at one year than at the preoperative assessment for the sterilization subjects, in contrast to the controls who tended to express less satisfaction at one year than they had done at the initial assessment. Similar findings were reported from the other five international centres, and there was also a statistically significant trend towards the sterilization subjects reporting improved relationships with their husband in non-sexual areas. As the most frequent reason given by the subjects, in this international study, for requesting sterilization was that they had completed their family, it would appear that absence of the fear of becoming pregnant results in an improvement in these areas of women's lives.

Effects on menstruation

It is often taught that sterilization results in at least a temporary change in menstrual pattern, in terms of irregularity and menorrhagia. From the hysterectomy literature there is an established association between the complaint of menorrhagia and disturbance of emotional state, and also a lack of correlation between the experience of menorrhagia and the objective measurement of blood loss. It therefore seems distinctly possible that problems with menstruation following sterilization may be one manifestation of adverse psychological outcome. This issue is particularly important in view of reports of a higher rate of gynaecological referral and of hysterectomy after sterilization (Templeton and Cole, 1982; Cooper, 1983). Gynaecologists would have reason to be very concerned if sterilization led indirectly to an increased risk of further gynaecological surgery, no matter what benefits it appeared to confer on women in terms of improved psychosexual and psychiatric functioning. The study in Nottingham on the effects of menstruation on elective tubal sterilization, which was both prospective and controlled (part of the WHO collaborative project) (Bledin et al, 1985), used a complex system of assessing menstruation, including measurements of heaviness and duration of loss, reports of clots, premenstrual tension, interference with daily life and usage of pads and tampons. This study was carried out on equal numbers of postpartum and interval sterilizations and their controls. There were differences, many of which appear to be internally inconsistent, between many of these variables, but overall there was no significant difference in the patient's estimation of the heaviness, duration of loss and pain in all four groups at one year, but there was a significant increase of the complaint of premenstrual tension, the interference of menstruation with daily life and the usage of pads and tampons in the sterilization group as a whole compared with the control groups. There was also a significant increase in the overall subjective assessment of the women of menstruation as an adverse experience than in the controls. However, these differences were more marked at six months and less at one year. It is interesting that over this one-year period of time, one third of the control groups of women reported a deterioration in their menstruation, in terms of heaviness and loss of clots. In their complex analysis of these variables the authors feel that many of these changes could be accounted for by changes in contraceptive usage over the period of time studied, in particular the use of the intrauterine device by the non-sterilized control groups and the change from oral contraceptives to sterilization in the index groups. This view is also supported by the findings of Lieberman et al (1978) and P. Cooper (1981). These two studies, along with others, found that after sterilization the amount and duration of menstrual loss was increased in women who had used oral contraceptives preoperatively and decreased in those who had used an intrauterine device (it was unchanged in those who had used barrier methods). It remains unclear as to whether the type of sterilization procedure affects menstrual functioning.

Regret

Regret is a difficult concept to measure in research as it can include the active pursuit of an operation for reversal of sterilization, feelings of loss about the end of fertility and dissatisfaction over changes in menstruation. Results from early studies frequently commented on high rates of regret, using some if not all of these concepts. However, most, apart from the methodological limitations, result from studies done at a time when less than half of the patients studied were sterilized at their own request, the rest being sterilized for medical reasons. Two recent prospective studies of regret found low rates. Smith (1979) found that 3% of a Scottish sample were dissatisfied one year after sterilization. In an Oxford study, Cooper et al (1982) found that 10% expressed some regret 18 months after surgery (mostly because of menstrual problems and the desire for another child); this included 4% of patients wishing they had not had the operation, 3% considering a reversal, and only 1% who had actually explored this possibility with their general practitioner. In the Nottingham study (Cooper et al, 1985), out of 114 patients followed up one year after sterilization, only seven were definitely not 'glad' that they had been sterilized and only two would definitely have the sterilization reversed if it were possible. There is little evidence to suggest that preoperative marital disharmony is related to postoperative regret. However, Winston (1977), reporting on women requesting reversal of sterilization, found high rates of marital disruption and new partnerships since the operation.

Cultural factors

Many of the studies reporting high rates of adverse psychological sequelae were carried out in non-Western countries (Lu and Chun, 1967; Khorana and Vyas, 1975). It is, therefore, particularly interesting to consider the results of the WHO International Collaborative Study (1985) which assessed patients prospectively in six centres in five different countries. This allows for comparison of the psychological sequelae of sterilization between sterilized women and their controls, set against norms for psychiatric disorder in individual countries. Over 900 women undergoing elective sterilization were examined in this way, both before operation and six months and 12 months postoperatively. At initial examination the prevalence of clinically significant emotional disorder ranged from 1.6% to 14.6% in four of the six centres, and was highest in Cali, Columbia (25.5%) and zero in Ibadan, Nigeria. In all centres, except Agra, India, women applying for sterilization had a somewhat higher rate of mental health problems than control subjects at initial examination. At the six-month follow-up, the prevalence of emotional disorder was still within the same range and continued to be higher in Cali. At 12-month follow-up, again the range remained the same except in Chandigarh in India, where it had risen to 29.2%. There were no significant differences in the frequency of mental ill health between the sterilization subjects and their controls in any of the centres, nor were there any significant differences in the prevalence of mental ill health in relation to the timing of the sterilization, i.e. if it was interval, postpartum or post-abortion. Chandigarh in India was the only centre that showed a consistent increase in rates of psychological disorder over time. In these two centres with high rates—Cali in Columbia and Chandigarh in India—the high prevalence of psychiatric disorder was explained by the more frequent occurrence of high-risk factors in these patients, such as a family history of mental disorder, social stress, low educational status and antecedent and current emotional disorders.

Although it might be supposed that women belonging to religious groups who abhor the use of contraceptive (e.g. Roman Catholicism) might have more problems with psychological adjustment, and guilt in particular, after sterilization, there is no evidence from the literature that this is so.

Risk factors for adverse psychological sequelae

There are consistent risk factors that emerge from the recent prospective studies of the outcome of sterilization, both in the United Kingdom and in other countries. Preoperative PSE scores, preoperative psychiatric morbidity and a past history of psychiatric disorder are all related to higher PSE scores after operation, psychiatric illness after operation, poor psychosexual outcome, and some measures of menstrual abnormality. Although age, social class and parity have in the past been implicated in determining risk, no such evidence was found in either the Oxford studies or the WHO Collaborative Study. The only other risk factor that appears to emerge from modern literature is postpartum sterilization as opposed to interval sterilization. In the Nottingham study, postpartum patients did less well compared with interval patients in terms of their psychosexual adjustment afterwards, as measured by frequency and enjoyment, although 40% of all sterilized women reported an improvement in their general marital satisfaction. The only women who reported a deterioration, in the sense of adverse effects of sterilization on their marriage, were postpartum women. Significantly fewer of the postpartum women were glad to be sterilized than were the interval sterilized women, and there were also more psychiatric cases at level 5 of the PSE index of definition amongst the postpartum sterilizations than amongst the intervals. Regret was also associated with postpartum sterilizations in this study, the only patients having seriously considered reversal in the group being those who had had a postpartum sterilization.

Implications for gynaecological practice

1. The majority of women will experience no adverse psychological sequelae to sterilization. Indeed, a substantial number will report an improvement in their general health, their sexual functioning and their satisfaction with their marriage.
2. Although the evidence is conflicting, there is a suggestion that sterilization may be followed by menorrhagia and an increased risk of hysterectomy. This may be attributable to previous contraceptive use and the method of sterilization, but a contribution may be made by psychological causes. Further prospective controlled research needs to be done to assess further this risk.
3. As with hysterectomy, there is strong evidence to link preoperative

psychiatric status and a previous history of psychiatric illness to adverse outcome in terms of both psychiatric illness, deterioration in psychosexual functioning and regret. This underlines again the importance of assessing the patient's mental state and eliciting a past history of psychiatric disturbance when patients are initially seen with a request for sterilization. If currently unwell, these patients should be treated before the sterilization, and if they are well but have a past history of psychiatric disorder, then both the gynaecologist and the general practitioner should be alerted to the possibility of the woman developing a depressive illness in the year following sterilization.

4, The evidence of the early literature of adverse psychiatric sequelae of sterilization when so many were performed post-abortion or post-partum, and the evidence from more recent studies again suggesting a slightly worse outcome for women who are sterilized postpartum, should lead to the avoidance of sterilization following childbirth or an abortion when it is practicable to do so. Interval sterilization, as an admissions specific procedure, would appear to confer the least risk on the patients. The avoidance of postpartum and post-abortion sterilization would appear to be particularly important if the patient has a current or antecedent history of psychiatric disorder.

5. Extra care should be taken in the assessment of patients from ethnic minorities, particularly those from the Indian subcontinent.

REFERENCES

Amias AG (1975) Sexual life after gynaecological operations. *British Medical Journal* **ii:** 608–609.

Ballinger CB (1975) Psychiatric morbidity and the menopause: screening of general population sample. *British Medical Journal* **iii:** 344–346.

Ballinger CB (1977) Psychiatric morbidity and the menopause: survey of a gynaecological out-patient clinic. *British Journal of Psychiatry* **131:** 83–89.

Barker MG (1968) Psychiatric illness after hysterectomy. *British Medical Journal* **ii:** 91–99.

Bledin KD, Beral V & Ashley JSA (1978) Recent trends in sterilization in women. *Health Trends* **10:** 84–87.

Bledin KD, Cooper JE, Brice B & Mackensie S (1985) The effects on menstruation of elective tubal sterilization: a prospective controlled study. *Journal of Biosocial Science* **17:** 19–30.

Campanella R & Wolff JR (1975) Emotional reaction to sterilisation. *Obstetrics and Gynecology* **45:** 331–334.

Chimbira TH, Anderson ABM & Turnbull AC (1980) Relation between measured menstrual blood loss and patients' subjective assessment of loss, duration of bleeding, number of sanitary towels used, uterine weight, and endometrial surface area. *British Journal of Obstetrics and Gynaecology* **87:** 603–609.

Cooper JE, Bledin KD, Brice B & Mackensie S (1985) Effects of female sterilization: one year follow-up in a prospective controlled study of psychological and psychiatric outcome. *Journal of Psychosomatic Research* **29:** 13–22.

Cooper PJ (1981) Elective interval sterilization in women: a prospective study of psychiatric, menstrual and social sequelae. DPhil thesis, Oxford University.

Cooper P, Gath D, Fieldsend R & Rose N (1981) Psychological and physical outcome after the elective tubal sterilization. *Journal of Psychosomatic Research* **25:** 357–360.

Cooper P, Gath D, Rose N & Fieldsend R (1982) Psychological sequelae to elective sterilization in women: a prospective study. *British Medical Journal* **82:** 461–464.

Cooper PJ (1983) Risk of hysterectomy after sterilisation. *Lancet* **i:** 59.

Coppen A, Bishop M, Beard RJ, Barnard GJ & Collins WP (1981) Hysterectomy, hormones and behaviour: a prospective study. *Lancet* **i:** 126–128.

Craig GA & Jackson P (1975) Sexual life after vaginal hysterectomy. *British Medical Journal* **iii:** 97.

Dennerstein L, Wood C & Burrows GD (1977) Sexual response following hysterectomy and oophorectomy. *Obstetrics and Gynecology* **49:** 92–96.

Drellich MG & Bieber I (1958) The psychological importance of the uterus and its function. *Journal of Nervous and Mental Disease* **126:** 322–336.

Enoch MD & Jones K (1975) Sterilisation: a review of 98 sterilised women. *British Journal of Psychiatry* **127:** 583–587.

Gater R, Dean C & Morris J (1989) The contribution of child bearing to the sex difference in first admission rates for affective psychosis. *Psychological Medicine* **19:** 719–724.

Gath D & Cooper PJ (1982) Psychiatric aspects of hysterectomy and female sterilization. In Granville-Grossman K (ed.) *Recent Advances in Clinical Psychiatry 4*, pp 75–100. London: Churchill.

Gath D, Cooper P & Day A (1981a) Hysterectomy and psychiatric disorder: levels of psychiatric morbidity before and after hysterectomy. *British Journal of Psychiatry* **140:** 335–342.

Gath D, Cooper P, Bond A & Edmonds G (1981b) Hysterectomy and psychiatric disorder: demographic, psychiatric and physical factors in relation to psychiatric outcome. *British Journal of Psychiatry* **140:** 343–350.

Gath D, Osborn M, Bungay G et al (1987) Psychiatric disorder and gynaecological symptoms in middle aged women: a community survey. *British Medical Journal* **294:** 213–218.

Gelder M, Gath D & Mayou R (1983) *Oxford Textbook of Psychiatry*. London: Oxford University Press.

Iles S, Gath D & Kennerley H (1989) Maternity blues: comparison between post-operative women and post-natal women. *British Journal of Psychiatry* **155:** 363–373.

Jackson P (1979) Sexual adjustment to hysterectomy and the benefits of a pamphlet for patients. *New Zealand Medical Journal* **90:** 471–472.

Kaltreider NB, Wallace A & Horowitz MJ (1979) A field study of the stress response syndrome. *Journal of the American Medical Association* **242:** 1499–1503.

Kennerley H & Gath D (1986) Maternity blues reassessed. *Psychiatric Developments* **1:** 1–17.

Khorana AB & Vyas AA (1975) Psychological complications in women undergoing voluntary sterilisation by salpingectomy. *British Journal of Psychiatry* **127:** 67–70.

Lieberman BA, Belsey E, Gordon AG et al (1978) Menstrual patterns after laparoscopic sterilization using a spring-loaded clip. *British Journal of Obstetrics and Gynaecology* **85:** 376–380.

Lu T & Chun D (1967) A long-term follow-up study of 1055 cases of post-partum tubal ligations. *Journal of Obstetrics and Gynaecology of the British Commonwealth* **74:** 875–880.

Martin RL, Roberts WV, Clayton PJ et al (1977) Psychiatric illness and non-cancer hysterectomy. *Diseases of the Nervous System* **38:** 974–980.

Martin RL, Roberts WV & Clayton PJ (1980) Psychiatric status after hysterectomy—a one-year prospective follow-up. *Journal of the American Medical Association* **244:** 350–353.

Meikle S & Brody H (1977) An investigation into the psychological effects of hysterectomy. *Journal of Nervous and Mental Disease* **164:** 36–41.

Munday RN & Cox LW (1967) Hysterectomy for benign lesions. *Medical Journal of Australia* **17:** 759–763.

Richards DH (1973) Depression after hysterectomy. *Lancet* **ii:** 430–432.

Smith AHW (1979) Psychiatric aspects of sterilization: a prospective survey. *British Journal of Psychiatry* **135:** 304–309.

Templeton AA & Cole S (1982) Hysterectomy following sterilization. *British Journal of Obstetrics and Gynaecology* **89:** 845.

WHO Collaborative Prospective Study Report (1985) Mental health and female sterilization. A follow-up. *Journal of Biosocial Science* **17:** 1–18.

Winston RML (1977) Why 103 women asked for reversal of sterilisation. *British Medical Journal* **ii:** 305–307.

Worsley A, Walters WAW & Wood EC (1977) Screening of psychological disturbance amongst gynaecology patients. *Australian and New Zealand Journal of Obstetrics and Gynaecology* **17:** 214–219.

4

Infertility and assisted reproduction

TREVOR FRIEDMAN

The investigation and treatment of infertile couples can represent a major part of a modern gynaecologist's workload. The advent of new techniques such as in vitro fertilization (IVF) and gamete intra-fallopian transfer (GIFT), as well as technological advances in the monitoring of ovulation, have produced an increasing array of procedures for the treatment of fertility problems. The interest and research in this field is, no doubt, due to an understanding that the desire to have children is a central part of most people's adult life, and that the inability to do this results in great distress. There has been debate in the UK about the use of resources for the treatment of infertility, as the couple can be considered not to be suffering from illness. This raises philosophical and ethical questions as to whether a person's right to have children or the inability to do so is of such importance that it deserves the use of society's resources, which could be utilized in treating other medical conditions.

In the USA, private medical insurance has often not covered fertility treatment and legislation has been introduced in some states requiring insurance coverage of infertility procedures. Legislation, (the Family Building Act) has also been introduced in Congress to make this more widespread (Schroeder, 1988). A central point in deciding the importance of treating such people is whether the level of distress or illness caused by their inability to conceive is great enough that treatment should be given to relieve their mental suffering.

This chapter will present a review of the psychological aspects of infertility, and its implications for investigating and treating the infertile couple. A brief report of the prevalence and causes of infertility will be presented, followed by a consideration of the areas in which psychological factors must be considered. Firstly, there is the emotional response of men and women to childlessness or difficulty conceiving. Secondly, there is the response to investigation and treatment of such couples, both in those who are treatable and those couples who are not. Thirdly, it is possible that, in certain couples, psychological factors may play a causative role in the production or the perpetuation of the infertile state. These aspects will be considered in turn, followed by a consideration of some of the specific treatments used.

INFERTILITY

Prevalence

In discussing childlessness it is useful to define the terms to be used. *Primary infertility* refers to women who have never conceived, despite exposure to the chance of pregnancy, whilst *secondary infertility* refers to women who have previously conceived but then subsequently are unable to. Both these terms generally refer to a period greater than 12 months. Childlessness may also result from *pregnancy wastage*, in which conception occurs but there is no live birth due to spontaneous abortion or stillbirth.

Infertility is generally regarded as a common problem, although its exact prevalence has been difficult to quantify. Data has either been drawn from demographic studies or from studies of health services, which are then extrapolated to the community. In demographic studies the situation is complicated by trying to assess the cause of couples' lack of children. This may be caused by, in addition to those conditions already stated, child mortality or unproven fertility. There are women who are not at risk of conception due to contraception or due to absence of cohabitation.

In the USA, the National Center for Health Statistics found that only 2% of women who wed want to be childless. Worldwide studies by the World Health Organization have found there is a great variation in the prevalence of infertility, giving rates of primary infertility as low as 1.5% in Thailand and Korea and as high as 13% and 23% in urban areas of Columbia (Belsey and Ware, 1986). In the UK a study in Bristol (Hull et al, 1985) of 708 couples seen at an infertility clinic, an incidence rate of 1.2 couples per 1000 population was determined. This represents at least one couple in six needing specialist help at some time in their lives because of an average period of infertility of 2½ years.

Causes

The interpretation of research into the causes of infertility can depend on the particular interests of the specialist clinic, but of more importance have been the advances in investigation which have led to greater number of couples having a diagnosable cause for their infertility. Most studies report that primary infertility accounts for 55–75% and secondary infertility for 25–40% of referrals. In the study by Hull et al (1985) the causes of infertility and rates found were: ovulatory failure 21%, tubal damage 14%, endometriosis 6%, male factors 26% and coital factors 6%; the infertility was unexplained in 28% of couples. The significance of over a quarter of patients not having a diagnosable cause and its relation to psychological factors will be discussed later.

Conception rates after two years and treatments for this group range from 78% for amenorrhoea and 72% for unexplained infertility to 11% for failure of sperm penetration. The overall chance of pregnancy was 72%, but this still represents a major period of uncertainty and treatment for many couples, over a quarter of whom fail to conceive.

Psychological responses

The effects of infertility on couples, and on women in particular, have been described on a number of occasions (Daniluk et al, 1985). Although these vary to some extent there are common features to them, many of which are typical of the response to loss and subsequent grieving (Karahasonglu et al, 1972; Mahlstedt, 1985; Cabau and de Senarclens, 1986).

The features of the response are typical of those seen in real or potential loss, such as that seen following bereavement, although the content is obviously centred about the lack of pregnancy. It is typified by initial surprise and disbelief, because fecundity is generally taken for granted, although as we have seen difficulties are in fact, a common problem. The couple may respond by trying harder to conceive and there may be components of denial, with one or both partners responding to the difficulty by not considering or avoiding acceptance of the problem. This may explain the varying lengths of infertility before couples present for treatment. Couples may then feel that their inability to conceive is unjust and may respond with anger as they try to understand 'why me?'. They may be distressed by pregnant women or young babies, and find it hard to reconcile their jealousy for these people. The problem is frequently not discussed with family or friends, either because they feel ashamed about their problem, or because they do not want the extra pressure of others wanting to know if they have become pregnant, although this can lead to a further feeling of isolation. There is a general assumption in society that couples can have children and they may become distressed by others asking about their lack of children, and by assumptions that they do not want children and are acting selfishly. Couples may become increasingly preoccupied with becoming pregnant; the treatment and investigation of fertility, which entails careful noting of basal body temperature, timing of periods and sexual intercourse, exacerbates this.

The grief of infertility is unusual in that it involves loss of potential life. It is harder to accept and come to terms with the loss when there is always the hope that they may become pregnant, and the woman's periods may serve as reminders of their loss in a process referred to sometimes as 'monthly mourning'. Couples may feel guilty and in their search for a cause of their infertility may site premarital sex, contraception, abortion, venereal disease, masturbation, homosexuality and even sexual pleasure (Menning, 1980; Sandelowski and Pollock, 1986)!

There also appears to be a difference between sexes in their approach to infertility problems. Women more commonly appear distressed and talk of a greater need for children ('feeling broody'). Men seem less concerned, at least initially, and seem more fatalistic in their attitude to being able to have children. This does not seem to be a psychological defence against distress, but rather that men are less driven to have children than women. The women more commonly visit their doctor first about the problem of infertility and the male partners are involved later. This difference in attitudes has sometimes been mirrored in clinical practice with women being intensively investigated before their husbands have had sperm counts.

There is considerable distress following miscarriage (Friedman and Gath, 1989), and this is more common in those women who have previously miscarried, so that one month following miscarriage 80% are distressed enough to achieve a level of psychiatric caseness. The group of women who suffer from habitual abortion may need particular support to risk further pregnancies which may lead to the pain of miscarriage (see Chapter 5).

In addition to these features of grieving, infertility may be a cause of sexual difficulties. Sexual intercourse may become associated only with having children, leading to a decrease in satisfaction, and mid-cycle dysfunction has been reported in 10% of men receiving treatment (Drake and Grunert, 1979). These authors also found 11 out of 51 men having postcoital tests had equivocal tests and six of these were negative when repeated. The absence of sperm was due to long-standing impotence in one case, secondary impotence in two cases and ejaculatory failure in three cases.

Other workers have identified particular sexual problems in this group, Walker (1978) emphasizing the problems of 'sex on demand' in postcoital tests and the possibility of extramarital affairs and Elstein (1975) the loss of libido and inhibition of orgasm due to the preoccupation with becoming pregnant. McGrade and Tolor (1981) found 35% of couples had sexual problems during treatment and not surprisingly 25% had difficulty with the postcoital examination. Women rated their sexual and marital relationships as more affected than their partners.

Bernstein et al (1985) interviewed 70 patients attending an infertility clinic and assessed 21% as exhibiting mild distress and 3% moderate distress. Recently, Daniluk (1988) studied 43 primary infertile couples longitudinally as they progressed through the medical investigation of their infertility. Levels of psychological distress were measured, as were changes in the satisfaction with marital and sexual relationships. The couples were interviewed after their medical consultations at various stages, and this indicated that more distress was experienced by couples during the initial medical interview and at the time of diagnosis. Rather surprisingly none of the participants' levels of distress was high enough to reach the level of a positive diagnosis or psychiatric 'caseness', as one might expect given the normal rate amongst the general population, and this may be partly explained by the number of couples who withdrew from the study. A relationship was found between greater dissatisfaction with sexual relationships and the diagnosis of unexplained infertility, and the author suggests that an extensive sexual history and assessment may be particularly useful in identifying couples whose sexual relationships may be in difficulty.

Comparison of fertile and infertile couples

There have been a number of studies to try and discover if there are differences between fertile and infertile couples. There are two reasons for undertaking this type of research. Firstly, such research will highlight differences in the personality or psychological state that may have led to the infertility. This idea has as it's basis the theory of psychosomatics of

Alexander and others in the 1930s that particular personality types were predisposed to developing particular physical illnesses such as asthma, gastric ulcers, etc. Early papers in the field of infertility propose links between personality, early childhood experiences and the development of infertility, but this concept of organ specificity has now largely been discounted. Secondly, investigation may discover if being infertile leads couples to be different from their fertile contemporaries. Unfortunately, only a few studies have used standardized quantitative measures and there is always the methodological problem of selecting control or comparison groups.

Harrison et al (1986a) compared 'emotionality' in 22 couples with at least a three-year history of unexplained infertility with that in ten control fertile couples. They found a significant increase in some measures of anxiety in the infertile women, but no differences in their partners. There were no significant differences in measures of personality. They went on to show that autogenic training led to a reduction in anxiety as measured by the Spielberger State Trait Anxiety Inventory (Spielberger et al, 1970).

In a study by Mai et al (1972) of 50 infertile couples (not only with unexplained infertility) were compared with 50 fertile couples. The study found no difference demographically, and investigation of sexual function showed frequency was the same in both groups, although interestingly the women reported intercourse as having been more frequent than their partners in both groups. Sexual difficulties were reported in 22% of the infertile group as compared with 10% of the fertile controls, but this difference did not reach statistical significance. In an older study Seward et al (1965) compared 41 infertile women with a control group of multiparous mothers, using projective tests.

Recent research has tackled some of the methodological problems of studying the relationship between psychological factors and infertility by investigating these groups prospectively. Paulson et al (1988) compared 150 infertile women with a comparison group of 50 women. They measured personality, anxiety, depression, self-concept and a measure of internal/external locus of control. The most striking finding was the remarkable similarity of scores between the infertile and comparison groups. They concluded that significant emotional maladjustment was no more prominent in women coping with infertility than for the general population, and that these results cast doubt on the assumption that stress may be a causal factor in infertility. In reporting subjects felt to have emotional maladjustment they found no relationship with the diagnosis of unexplained infertility.

These studies have looked at the question of whether infertile couples differ from fertile couples. There is some suggestion that amongst infertile couples there are greater levels of distress and sexual dysfunction. The studies suffer, on the whole, from either failing to investigate or not using standardized measures of depression, anxiety, marital, sexual and social functioning. The retrospective design of most of the studies means that it is not possible to tell if the differences existed before investigation and treatment or if the differences are the result of the experience of this treatment.

Psychological infertility

The term 'psychological infertility' can refer to a number of conditions in which psychological factors have either been shown or speculated as having a major effect.

Sexual dysfunction

Problems involving sexual intercourse are common, and in the population survey by Kinsey et al (1948) a total and apparently permanent erectile impotence was reported by 1.3% of married men under the age of 35 and by 6.7% aged under 50. It is important to exclude medical conditions such as diabetes and peripheral vascular disease that can lead to this condition, as well as the side-effects of many drugs, the most important being anti-hypertensives (especially adrenoreceptor antagonists) and some major tranquillizers. Excessive alcohol use impairs sexual performance, and loss of libido and sexual performance is common in depressive illness.

In primary impotence the commonest psychological aetiology is through a combination of low sexual drive and anxiety about sexual performance. In the investigation of infertility it is difficult to assess the veracity of couples reporting the frequency of sexual intercourse and sexual dysfunction, but small numbers of patients with these difficulties are reported in many studies. There is probably an under-reporting of such problems and there have been reports of non-consummation in couples after periods of many years before seeking help (Burchadt and Catalan, 1982). Indeed, impotence is common in response to stressful situations and the figure of 22% of couples, previously noted, reporting dysfunction is not surprising.

Psychiatric illness

Infertility can also occur in response to recognized psychiatric illnesses, such as severe depressive illnesses, where menstrual disturbance occurs. This may sometimes be due to a loss of body weight due to a loss of appetite. In anorexia nervosa, weight loss and hypothalamic disturbance leads to amenorrhoea (see Chapter 2). The patient may be unaware of the cause or hide it from her physician. There is also evidence of menstrual disturbance in other psychiatric conditions such as schizophrenia. The pharmacological treatment with major tranquillizers leading to a rise in prolactin levels is probably the commonest cause of these disturbances.

Psychological factors and unexplained infertility

In considering the psychological aspects of infertility, of particular interest are those with idiopathic infertility. In the literature a number of terms are used to describe this group, e.g. 'unexplained', 'psychogenic' (Bos and Cleghorn, 1958; Stauber, 1972) or 'psycho-physiologic' (Seward et al, 1965; Mozley, 1976), but great care is needed in the precision with which these terms are used. In order to diagnose unexplained infertility, all the necessary investigations must have been completed, as Moghissi and Wallach (1983) examine in their review. This is not always true in many studies, and as advances occur in investigation, more of the cases of previously unexplained infertility may now be diagnosed as having some recognized pathology.

In those couples who have no recognized organic pathology, there is the theoretical possibility that the aetiology may be psychogenic. A number of studies have tried to examine the question of whether psychological factors are particularly important in those people with unexplained infertility, but the evidence described suffers frequently from the difficulties of retrospective analysis and the lack of quantitative measures of psychological factors. There is also the difficulty of detecting possible psychological effects amongst a group of subjects which may need to be very large because the psychological effect may be small and only affect a proportion of those couples with unexplained infertility. The decision also has to be made as to which psychological factors should be measured (depression, anxiety, etc) and how often, since to detect any effects the mental state of patients should probably be assessed frequently and, in particular, around the times of ovulation and implantation. These assessments may in themselves affect how people feel emotionally; this, and other methodological problems, illustrates the difficulty in designing a study to show an association between psychological factors and unexplained infertility.

The majority of women with unexplained infertility eventually conceive, so that in the study by Hull et al (1985) 56% at one year and 72% at two years were pregnant; moreover Harrison et al (1986a) notes that 46% of patients attending an infertility clinic conceived before starting active treatment. The reason for the delay in conception in these couples beyond that expected by chance is not known. It appears that in vitro fertilization in these couples may be as successful as for couples with tubal blockage (Wardle et al, 1985). A study of 500 couples attending an infertility clinic (Templeton and Penney, 1982) found an incidence of unexplained infertility of 23.5%. They compared patients with explained and unexplained infertility and found no difference in age, social class or coital frequency, and after nine years 34% of this group had still not conceived. In another retrospective study (Lenten et al, 1977) of 91 couples with unexplained infertility, 43% of the women conceived over eight years. Apart from small differences in the frequency of coitus, no differences were found between the two groups who did or did not conceive, in respect of demographic factors, menstrual history or contraceptive use. No psychological factors were investigated in these studies.

Dominici et al (1979) studied 31 couples with two years' unexplained infertility and compared them with fertile controls. At interview the sterile couples appeared more anxious and depressed but showed no difference on rating scales of anxiety or personality. The authors comment on great variability between couples and that tests on subgroups might have been more useful. The study obviously suffers from its retrospective nature but the authors conclude 'there are no significant or specific personality disorders in the sterile couples. In our opinion these disorders are not lacking but it is extremely difficult to bring them to light'.

Stress and unexplained infertility

The concept of stress has been suggested as being important in the aetiology of the infertility in those couples for whom no cause can be found. There appears to be a common sentiment amongst many workers in the field of infertility that this is important, despite the lack of any clear evidence to substantiate it, although stress seems more clearly implicated in cases of 'psychogenic' amenorrhoea following extreme dangers such as air raids, internment, etc. (Russell, 1972). Reports of conception in infertile couples following adoption, or on the cessation of treatment, have been seen as confirmatory evidence of the importance of stress. A number of studies looking at adopting in fertile couples have found low levels of conception of between 2 and 4% (Tyler et al, 1960; Aaronson et al, 1963; Sandler, 1965; Humphrey, 1971; Comninos et al, 1979), but they do not adequately specify the rate of conception amongst those couples with unexplained infertility. Rock et al (1965) compared 249 couples with unexplained infertility who adopted children with 113 similar non-adopting couples and found no evidence that it led to an increased rate of conception. The linkage between conception and relief of stress due to adoption or other factors appears to be due to retrospective attribution in which the low level of conception that occurs in these couples by chance is attributed to a recent life event. Thus it may be attributed to stopping investigations, stopping treatment, no longer 'trying' to get pregnant, considering or being accepted for adoption or finally successfully adopting a baby.

There remains the possibility that in a small number of couples psychological factors might have particular importance in the aetiology of their infertility. It may prove very difficult, other than in large prospective studies, to identify these few couples, as they will be lost amongst the majority of couples whose infertility does not have a psychological basis.

Neurophysiology of unexplained infertility

There have been a number of theories postulating how psychological factors might cause infertility; these include tubal spasm, limbic lobe effects on the hypothalamus, catecholamine effects on the reproductive tract and more recently by affecting prolactin function in ovulatory infertility (Harrison et al, 1979; Edelmann and Golombok, 1989). There continues to be much debate on the relationship between prolactin and stress (Delitalia et al, 1987). Harper et al (1985) in a study at an infertility clinic found a significant relationship between women's self-rated levels of anxiety and prolactin levels, and other studies have also reported similar correlations in different situations (Koninckx, 1978; Jeffcoate et al, 1986). In a recent study Friedman et al (1989) have found a relationship between anxiety and the change in prolactin level at different times in women attending an infertility clinic. However, other studies have failed to find any relationship between stressful situations and levels of prolactin (Nesse et al, 1980; Pearce et al, 1980).

O'Moore et al (1983) investigated 55 ovulatory infertile couples and found, by repeated prolactin estimation, that 39 of these women showed occasional spikes in their prolactin level, although these women were normo-prolactinaemic most of the time. These spikes of mild hyper-prolactinaemia (380–800 miu/l) were related to being stressed; they found higher anxiety rating scores in this group of patients than in women who did not show spikes in their prolactin secretion. They suggest that the inhibitory effect of prolactin may suppress pulsatile luteinizing hormone (LH) release and prevent the positive feedback of oestradiol on the LH surge. In this study they found that treatment with bromocriptine and clomiphene led to a significantly greater number of pregnancies than when treated with placebo, and suggested that drugs may provide more than just a beneficial placebo effect on those with high stress scores. This interesting finding, supported by similar findings from the same team (Harrison et al, 1981, 1986a,b), requires further investigation and validation. An earlier study (Wright et al, 1979) investigated the treatment of patients with unexplained infertility using bromocriptine or placebo. Bromocriptine produced a greater fall in prolactin levels than in the control group, but the rate of conception was the same for both groups. The study, however, did not include an investigation of psychological stress or of prolactin spiking.

There remains the possibility that for a proportion of patients with unexplained infertility their difficulties may indeed be explained in terms of their individual response to stress, leading to transient hyperprolactinaemia. If this result were corroborated it would require further elucidation of the mechanism causing transient secretion of prolactin, as well as suggesting the treatability of many couples for whom this had not been possible previously.

Management

In the treatment and investigation of infertility, couples are best served by the principles of good clinical practice. In particular this means explanation and information about the investigations and procedures upon which the couple are embarking, preferably by the same clinician throughout the treatment course.

The important question is whether or not infertility treatment, as opposed to treatment of other conditions, necessitates any special interest in the psychological well-being of the couple, and if so, whether this effects long-term outcome or satisfaction. It can be seen from a review of the literature that there is little to suggest, at the moment, that psychological factors play an important role in the aetiology of infertility, although sexual difficulties may be hidden from the clinician and detailed questioning may be necessary to elucidate the presence of problems in this area. It seems unlikely that psychological intervention would have an important effect on the rate of conception (unless evidence were produced that perhaps an anxiety reduction course had an effect on stress-induced transient hyperprolactin-aemia). The other reason for psychological intervention would be if great distress could be shown to occur from the investigation and treatment of infertility or long-term childlessness.

There has been relatively little research looking at the long-term effects of infertility, presumably due to the difficulty of identifying and studying a large group of infertile couples and of being able to assign their problems to their infertility. Monarch (1985) provides a review of the social impact of involuntary childlessness, and puts forward some evidence that it may lead to increased rates of divorce amongst couples as well as high levels of dissatisfaction with their lives. Owens and Read (1984) surveyed 387 members of the National Association for the Childless about their experience of subfertility testing and treatment. This is obviously a highly selected group but they found most couples satisfied with their treatment, although the treatment of male infertility attracted less satisfaction. Their dissatisfaction was most keenly felt about the amount of information they were provided with and the waiting times between appointments. The lowest degree of satisfaction was with the adequacy of provision dealing with emotional and psychological aspects. They also compared private with National Health Service treatment, and found the major differences were in the speed with which they were investigated rather than in the actual investigations and treatment.

The majority of couples consider undergoing investigation a stressful experience and that their difficulty with childlessness has been the most important area of their lives. In the study of 43 couples by Daniluk (1988), 97% felt there was a need for psychological services. They felt that provision of these services would be most helpful immediately following the diagnosis or a few weeks afterwards, but that it should be available at other times as well. Seventy-five per cent of the men would prefer to be seen as a couple, whilst only half the women felt this, more preferring to be seen individually. In this study, 54% of the men and 72% of the women said they would have used psychological assistance, but in practice the level of uptake may be lower. In a study by Paulson et al (1988), 27 of the 150 women (18%) actively sought counselling during investigation, and Bresnick and Taymor (1979) found only 62 out of 212 couples accepted counselling when offered. There does seem to be a general feeling that psychological intervention may be of importance and that there are a proportion of couples who would make use of such services. However, there has been little systematic study of the content of such counselling (Rosenfeld and Mitchell, 1979) and the outcome, both short- and long-term, of such intervention. Bresnick and Taymor (1979) found that counselling led to decreased levels of guilt, anger, frustration and isolation, that women were helped more than men, and that long-term treatment was better than short-term. The study was uncontrolled and in all studies of counselling it is important to offer a package that could be implemented realistically in an ordinary clinic, in terms of time and the level of expertise of the counsellors.

It has been shown, for example, that in other stressful situations associated with loss, such as stillbirth or perinatal death, counselling can appreciably shorten the period of distress, whilst enabling couples to come to terms with the situation. Psychological intervention in this group of patients should consist firstly of non-directive counselling to enable couples to explore their feelings towards their difficulties in becoming pregnant. This would allow them to explore the anger and frustration that they may be experiencing and which otherwise may become directed at themselves or their relationship. As investigations continue help may be needed with the stresses of particular tests, which may lead to an increase in sexual dissatisfaction, such as those performed postcoitally, and the couple may need to be helped to talk about this between themselves so that they do not lose enjoyment from their sexual relationship. If a diagnosis is made then this may lead to feelings of guilt by one partner and resentment from the other, and they can be helped to see that they are finding out the cause of the problems rather than assigning blame to one or other partner. Most clinics try to see the couple together rather than just investigating the woman first. Unexplained infertility may raise particular problems as the couples continue with follow-up in clinic, and perhaps treatment with drugs to promote their fertility, without ever understanding the cause of their problems. In this situation, as in others, people often paradoxically prefer to know a definite pathology rather than have it uncertain, even though this may have a worse prognosis in the long term.

Psychological intervention may also be necessary in the detection of formal psychiatric illness. It has yet to be shown whether or not there is an increased morbidity associated with infertility that might necessitate intervention. At the beginning of treatment one might expect increased rates of anxiety related to concerns about treatment, and that as the period of infertility increases there may be despondency leading to an increased rate of depressive illness.

There is little evidence to suggest that there is an increased long-term psychiatric morbidity, although this area has not been specifically researched. One could theorize that the failure to have children may lead to a lowering of self-esteem and increased incidence of negative thoughts about oneself. Beck's cognitive theory of depression would suggest that this way of thinking would place these couples at more risk of developing depressive illness in the future, and if this increased depressive illness were found (whether its basis was due to psychological cognitive processes or the social lack of children), it would strengthen the case for intervention during infertility investigation and treatment.

ASSISTED REPRODUCTION

Artificial insemination

In approximately one quarter of patients with infertility problems the condition will primarily be the result of male factors, and in such cases the only effective treatment may be artificial insemination (AI) using semen, either from the husband (AIH) or from an anonymous donor (AID). About 2500 births in the UK and 15000 births in the USA are achieved each year by artificial insemination.

Couples receiving investigations prior to treatment with AID share many of the experiences of couples undergoing infertility difficulties in general. The ability of otherwise childless couples to have children is undoubtedly of considerable benefit (David and Avidan, 1976), but the particular treatment, especially AID, may be highly stressful (Olshansky and Sammons, 1985). Couples may have particular difficulties in coming to terms with the diagnosis, husbands may feel guilty at their inability to provide children, and wives may feel guilty through 'not sharing their partner's reproductive failure' (Reading et al, 1982). These feelings of guilt and loss of self-esteem may contribute to transitory sexual dysfunction, with 10 out of 16 men reporting impotence lasting one to three months following the diagnosis, and only eight couples reporting no change in sexual pattern or mood (Berger, 1980). The use of donor semen may itself lead to difficulties because of conflicts with religious doctrine, anxieties about the donor, concerns about adultery, and other moral, legal and personal issues. A combination of these factors often leads to couples maintaining secrecy about their treatment and not informing the child of its origin (Snowden, 1985). This secrecy is often encouraged by nursing and medical staff.

We have already considered how psychological factors and stress may play a role in influencing fertility, and artificial insemination might be expected to accentuate any underlying problems. Artificial insemination may not be successful in causing pregnancy for many months, and indeed some couples may conceive years after beginning treatment. The cause of these delays is not always apparent. It might be hypothesized that in some women psychological factors affect the likelihood of conception and that it is when they are not overstressed that conception occurs.

At present no association between emotional state and conception in couples treated with artificial insemination has been found, but only a few studies have been conducted and they have had methodological limitations. Reading et al (1982) investigated 58 women prospectively for six months and found no differences in anxiety levels between women who conceived and those who did not. Interestingly, as has been noted by other workers in this field, the women themselves attributed the outcome of treatment to their psychological and emotional state at the time of insemination. Harrison et al (1981) detected no association between conception and anxiety in a small study. There are particular problems in studying this group of patients because, although their regular treatments would seem to make them appropriate for study, the problems of confidentiality and the reluctance of couples to be involved in the study tends to overshadow this (Carr et al, unpublished data).

Management

The ethical problems raised by AID and the need for consent by both partners to agree to insemination by a donor's sperm has meant that counselling is an inherent part of most treatment programmes. It is important that the legal and moral issues are discussed with the couple and that they receive information about the procedure.

There has been little research to investigate if other areas should be discussed with the couple or the best length of time for the couple to wait from diagnosis to treatment. The psychological support once treatment has started is often provided by the clinic nurse, who may not feel skilled for this task, and the husband who does not attend for treatment may be unable to obtain help. It may be that a form of denial from the husband about the treatment may be beneficial, but unfortunately this and other factors affecting long-term outcome are unknown. Some clinics set time limits for the length of treatment, whilst others leave it to the couple to decide when they should stop; it would be interesting to compare these two treatment approaches.

In vitro fertilization

Since the birth of the first baby using IVF in 1979, the use of such advanced technology has spread around the world. The success rate of such programmes overall is about 15% per IVF cycle and suggests that many couples are undergoing significant stress which may often not lead to ultimate childbirth. Investigation of the psychological aspects of IVF has followed the path of investigation of the psychological aspects of infertility in general. Many of the early papers lack methodological detail and do not use established measures of morbidity. Reviewing the literature it is possible, however, to give an overall assessment of the general findings of this research.

Investigators have studied couples attending for IVF to assess their personality and presence of psychological morbidity. Freeman et al (1985) studied 200 couples attending for pretreatment consultation. The most important finding from this and other studies is that the majority of couples show normal psychological profiles. As might be expected, half the women and 15% of the men reported that infertility was the most upsetting experience of their lives. In a recent study (Callan and Hennessey, 1989) women with explained and unexplained infertility on an IVF programme were compared with mothers and married women who were voluntarily childless. They were assessed with postal questionnaires and were found to report no difference in levels of self-esteem, psychological mood or contentment with their life. There was no evidence that infertile women were less happy with life. The results suggested that infertile women showed a strong need to be loved and that they perceive themselves as potentially good mothers. Infertile women generally disagreed that infertility had affected their marriages negatively, and indeed on scales of marital satisfaction infertile women rated better than mothers. A study in Hong Kong (Chan et al, 1989) found the psychological profile of women attending an IVF/GIFT programme as being similar to that of normal Chinese pregnant women. They were particularly interested in the amount of social support available to couples and that nearly half of the women were unwilling to disclose their treatment to other people.

It seems that for the majority of couples treatment with IVF is not associated with an increased level of psychiatric morbidity. Reading et al (1989) have shown in a study of 37 women that there is some distress that has features similar to grief associated with unsuccessful treatment during each cycle. They found no association between treatment outcome and psychological state. Harrison et al (1987), however, found a reduction in the quality of semen of men attending for IVF when compared with pretreatment levels. There was also a reduction in fertilization rates and they suggest that this change is due to the stress of the IVF programme.

It may be that the process of deciding to seek treatment with IVF is selective in choosing the most robust psychologically. There remains the possibility that in some couples where fertility is borderline, elevated stress levels may become of importance, as may be the case in unexplained infertility. There is a need for systematic prospective studies of IVF treatment using reliable measures of psychological status and correlating this with physiological measures. There remains the difficulty in finding useful comparison groups, although one may be most interested in comparing couples who are successfully treated and those who are not.

Management

The general principles outlined for the management of all infertile couples are obviously relevant to this group. There is good evidence that preparing people with information about their experiences enables them to deal with the experience better. Of particular importance are realistic expectations about the successful outcome of treatment. There has been concern at some clinics, despite having low success in achieving births, not differentiating clearly between rates of egg recovery and fertilization and the rates of eventual pregnancy, which are much lower.

There is a theoretical basis to suppose that women treated with IVF will suffer greater distress if they were to have a spontaneous abortion than other women, as they are more aware of the presence of a fetus within them (perhaps having seen it under the microscope), having early ultrasounds, as well as the obvious distress, after many problems, of having but yet losing a child.

SUMMARY

The inability to have children is a considerable cause of human distress. There is little evidence to suggest that the vast majority of infertile couples differ in their premorbid psychological make-up from their fertile contemporaries. There is understandable grief in response to their loss of the ability to have children and in vulnerable people this may be profound. There is little known of the long-term outcome of such couples, but it seems likely that for some it will be a devastating experience that will affect their life-time mental health. There are a large proportion of couples with unexplained infertility, but there is little evidence that this diagnosis is particularly associated with psychological factors, although research continues into possible links between stress and hormones that affect the reproductive system, such as prolactin.

Artificial insemination and IVF have particular problems, not only due to conception occurring out of normal sexual intercourse. In artificial insemination using donor sperm the problems of a genetically different father has similarities with the debate about egg donation for IVF. These technical procedures are undoubtedly stressful but generally, as for other treatments, if they are successful the rewards appear to outweigh any misgivings of the couples involved.

There is a need for further research as to whether psychological factors are causative in infertility as the absence of any link might indeed be reassuring to couples. We would also benefit from knowing the long-term outcome of couples for whom treatment is not successful.

REFERENCES

Aaronson HG & Glienke CF (1963) A study of the incidence of pregnancy following adoption. *Fertility and Sterility* **14**: 547–553.

Belsey MA & Ware H (1986) Epidemiological, social and psychosocial aspects of infertility. In Inster V & Lumenfeld B (eds) *Infertility: Male and Female*, pp 631–647. London: Churchill Livingstone.

Berger DM (1980) Couples reactions to male infertility and donor insemination. *American Journal of Psychiatry* **137**: 1047–1049.

Bernstein J, Potts N & Mattox JH (1985) Assessment of psychological dysfunction associated with infertility. *Journal of Obstetric, Gynecologic and Neonatal Nursing* **14(6)**: 63s–66s.

Bos C & Cleghorn RA (1958) Psychogenic sterility. *Fertility and Sterility* **9**: 84–98.

Bresnick E & Taymor ML (1979) The role of counselling in infertility. *Fertility and Sterility* **32**: 154–156.

Brooks JE, Herbert M, Walder CP et al (1986) Prolactin and stress: some endocrine correlates of pre-operative anxiety. *Clinical Endocrinology* **24**: 653–656.

Burchadt A & Catalan J (1982) Long standing unconsummated marriage. *British Journal of Family Planning* **8**: 22–25.

Cabau A & de Senarclens M (1986) Psychological aspects of infertility. In Inster V & Lumenfeld B (eds) *Infertility: Male and Female*, pp 648–672. London: Churchill Livingstone.

Callan VJ & Hennessey JF (1989) Psychological adjustment to infertility: a unique comparison of two groups of infertile women, mothers and women childless by choice. *Journal of Reproductive and Infant Psychology* (in press).

Chan YF, Tsoi MM, O'Hoy KM et al (1989) Psychosocial evaluation in an IVF/GIFT program in Hong Kong. *Journal of Reproductive and Infant Psychology* (in press).

Comnimos AC, Tsapaulis AD & Koussidou TI (1979) Conception after adoption. In Carenza L & Zichella L (eds) *Emotion and Reproduction*, pp 319–321. London: Academic Press.

Daniluk JC (1988) Infertility: intrapersonal and interpersonal impact. *Fertility and Sterility* **49**: 982–990.

Daniluk J, Leader A & Taylor PJ (1985) The psychological sequelae of infertility. The psychiatric implications of menstruation. In Gold N (ed.) *The Psychiatric Implications of Menstruation*, pp 77–85. Washington: American Psychiatric Press.

David A & Avidan D (1976) Artificial insemination by donor: clinical and psychological aspects. *Fertility and Sterility* **27**: 528–532.

Delitalia G, Tomasi P & Virdis R (1987) Hormone secretion during stress. Neuroendocrinology of stress. *Clinical Endocrinology and Metabolism* **1**: 391–414.

Dominici L, Coghi I, Pancheri P et al (1979) Psychosocial evaluation in couples with sterility without apparent cause. In Carenza L & Zichella L (eds) *Reproduction*, pp 261–271. London: Academic Press.

Drake TS & Grunert GM (1979) A cyclic pattern of sexual dysfunction in the infertility investigation. *Fertility and Sterility* **32**: 542–545.

Edelmann RJ & Golombok S (1989) Stress and reproductive failure. *Journal of Reproductive and Infant Psychology* (in press).

Elstein M (1975) Effect of infertility on psychosexual function. *British Medical Journal* **3**: 296–299.

Freeman EW, Boxer AS, Rickels K et al (1985) Psychological evaluation and support in a program of in vitro fertilization and embryo transfer. *Fertility and Sterility* **43:** 48–53.

Friedman T & Gath D (1989) Psychiatric effects of spontaneous abortion. *British Journal of Psychiatry* **155:** 810–814.

Friedman T, Carr EK & Jeffcoate WJ (1989) The relationship between prolactin and anxiety in women attending an infertility clinic. *Journal of Endocrinology* **123 (supplement):** 78.

Harper R, Lenton EA & Cook ID (1985) Prolactin and subjective reports of stress in women attending an infertility clinic. *Journal of Reproductive and Infant Psychology* **3:** 3–8.

Harrison KL, Callan VJ & Hennessey JF (1987) Stress and semen quality in an in vitro fertilization program. *Fertility and Sterility* **48:** 633–636.

Harrison RF, O'Moore RR & McSweeney J (1979) Stress, prolactin and infertility. *Lancet* 209.

Harrison RF, O'Moore AM & O'Moore RR (1981) Stress and artificial insemination. *Infertility* **4:** 303–311.

Harrison RF, O'Moore RR & O'Moore AM (1986a) Stress and fertility: some modalities of investigation and treatment in couples with unexplained infertility in Dublin. *International Journal of Fertility* **31(2):** 153–159.

Harrison RF, O'Moore AM, Mosurski K et al (1986b) Intermittent hyperprolactinaemia and the unexplained infertile couple: a placebo controlled study of combined clomiphene citrate bromocriptine therapy. *Fertility* **9:** 1–15.

Hull MGR, Glazener CMA, Kelly NJ et al (1985) Population study of causes, treatment and outcome of infertility. *British Medical Journal* **291:** 1693–1697.

Humphrey ME (1971) Childbirth following adoption. A myth revisited. In Morris N (ed.) *Psychosomatic Medicine in Obstetrics and Gynaecology*, pp 491–493. Basel: Karger.

Jeffcoate WJ, Lincoln NB, Selby C et al (1986) Correlation between anxiety and serum prolactin in humans. *Journal of Psychosomatic Research* **30:** 217–222.

Karahasonglu A, Barglow P & Growe G (1972) Psychological aspects of infertility. *Journal of Reproductive Medicine* **9:** 241–247.

Kinsey AC, Pomeroy WB & Martin CE (1948) *Sexual Behaviour in the Male*. Philadelphia: Saunders.

Koninckx P (1978) Stress hyperprolactinaemia in clinical practice. *Lancet* 273.

Lenton EA, Weston GA & Cooke LD (1977) Long term follow up of the apparently normal couple with a complaint of infertility. *Fertility and Sterility* **28:** 913–919.

McGrade SS & Tolor A (1981) The reaction to infertility and the infertility investigation: a comparison of the responses of men and women. *Infertility* **4:** 7–27.

Mahlstedt PP (1985) The psychological component of infertility. *Fertility and Sterility* **45:** 335–346.

Mai FM, Munday RN & Rump EE (1972) Psychiatric interview comparisons between infertile and fertile couples. *Psychosomatic Medicine* **34:** 431–440.

Menning BE (1980) The emotional needs of infertile couples. *Fertility and Sterility* **34:** 313.

Moghissi KS & Wallach EE (1983) Unexplained infertility. *Fertility and Sterility* **39:** 5–21.

Monarch J (1985) *The social impact of involuntary childlessness*. PhD thesis, Sheffield Polytechnic.

Mozley PD (1976) Psychophysiologic infertility: an overview. *Clinical Obstetrics and Gynaecology* **19(2):** 407–417.

Nesse NM, Curtis GC, Brown GM et al (1980) Anxiety induced by flooding therapy for phobias does not elicit prolactin secretory response. *Psychosomatic Medicine* **42:** 25–31.

Olshanky EF & Sammons LN (1985) Artificial insemination: an overview. *Journal of Obstetric, Gynecologic and Neonatal Nursing* **14(6):** 49s–54s.

O'Moore AM, O'Moore RR, Harrison RF et al (1983) Psychosomatic aspects in idiopathic infertility: effects of treatment with autogenic training. *Journal of Psychosomatic Research* **27:** 145–151.

Owens DJ & Read MW (1984) Patients' experiences with and assessment of subfertility testing and treatment. *Journal of Reproductive and Infant Psychology* **2:** 7–17.

Paulson JD, Haarman BS, Salerno RL et al (1988) An investigation of the relationship between emotional maladjustment and infertility. *Fertility and Sterility* **49:** 258–262.

Pearce JM, McGarrick G, Chamberlain GVP et al (1980) Lack of effect of interview and gynaecological examination on plasma levels of prolactin and cortisol. *British Journal of Obstetrics and Gynaecology* **87:** 366–369.

Reading AE, Sledmore CM & Cox DN (1982) A survey of patients attitudes towards artificial insemination by donor. *Journal of Psychosomatic Research* **26:** 429–433.

Reading AE, Chang LC & Kerin JF (1989) Psychological state and coping styles across an IVF treatment cycle. *Journal of Reproductive and Infant Psychology* (in press).

Rock J, Tietza C & McLaughlin HB (1965) Effect of adoption on infertility. *Fertility and Sterility* **16:** 302–305.

Rosenfeld DL & Mitchell E (1979) Treating the emotional aspects of infertility; counselling services in an infertility clinic. *American Journal of Obstetrics and Gynecology* **135:** 177–180.

Russell GFM (1972) Premenstrual tension and 'psychogenic' amenorrhoea: psycho-physical interactions. *Journal of Psychosomatic Research* **16:** 279–287.

Sandelowski M & Pollock C (1986) Women's experiences of infertility. *Journal of Nursing Scholarship* **4:** 140–144.

Sandler B (1965) Conception after adoption: a comparison of conception rates. *Fertility and Sterility* **16:** 3122–3123.

Schroeder P (1988) Infertility and the world outside. *Fertility and Sterility* **49:** 765–767.

Seward GH, Wagner PS, Heinrich JF et al (1965) The question of psychophysiologic infertility: some negative answers. *Psychosomatic Medicine* **27:** 533–545.

Siebel MM & Taymor ML (1982) Emotional aspects of infertility. *Fertility and Sterility* **37:** 137–145.

Snowden R (1985) The social implications of artificial reproduction. In Thompson E, Joyce DN & Newton SR (eds) *In-vitro Fertilisation and Donor Insemination*, pp 319–328. London: Royal College of Obstetricians and Gynaecologists.

Spielberger CD, Gorusch RL & Lushene RE (1970) *Manual for the State Trait Anxiety Inventory*. Palo Alto, California: Consulting Psychiatrists Press.

Stauber M (1971) The diagnosis of psychogenic sterility. In Morris N (ed.) *Psychosomatic Medicine in Obstetrics and Gynaecology*, pp 488–490. Basel: Karger.

Templeton AA & Penney GC (1982) The incidence, characteristics and prognosis of patients whose infertility is unexplained. *Fertility and Sterility* **37:** 175–182.

Tyler ET, Bonaparte J & Grant J (1960) Occurrence of pregnancy following adoption. *Fertility and Sterility* **11:** 581–587.

Utian WH, Goldfarb JM & Rosenthal MB (1983) Psychological aspects of infertility. In Dennerstein L & Burrows E (eds) *Handbook of Psychosomatic Obstetrics and Gynaecology*, pp 231–248. Amsterdam: Elsevier Biomedical Press.

Walker HE (1978) Sexual problems and infertility. *Psychosomatic Medicine* **19:** 477–484.

Wardle PG, Mitchell JD, McLaughlin EA et al (1985) Endometriosis and ovulatory disorder: reduced fertilisation in vitro compared with tubal and unexplained infertility. *Lancet* **ii:** 236–239.

Wright CS, Steele SJ & Jacobs HS (1979) Value of bromocriptine in unexplained primary infertility: a double-blind controlled trial. *British Medical Journal* **286:** 1037–1039.

5

The loss of early pregnancy

SUSAN ILES

In obstetrics little is taught about the emotional aspects of loss of early pregnancy. One reason may be the assumption that a woman cannot, and perhaps does not need to, mourn a baby that she has lost early in pregnancy and that emotional distress is not to be expected. Another reason is that many women are not followed up either by doctors or midwives after the loss of early pregnancy, so emotional distress often goes undetected. A further reason may be that there has been relatively little research, until recently, into the emotional sequelae of loss of early pregnancy.

Doctors are often ill-equipped to detect and manage the emotional sequelae of loss of early pregnancy. They will have been taught little about it, and they will have had little contact with women who have suffered loss of early pregnancy. Such women tend not to stay long in hospital, and students are often kept away from them.

There are important reasons why doctors should be trained in the detection, assessment and management of the emotional sequelae of loss of early pregnancy. Firstly, if doctors do not anticipate a woman's emotional distress, then they are unlikely to detect or assess it. Secondly, when doctors are uncertain as to how to manage emotional distress, they often cope by disregarding the patient's emotional symptoms altogether.

The aim of this chapter is to provide information about the emotional sequelae of loss of early pregnancy. The grief that occurs after any loss will be described. The emotional sequelae of loss of early pregnancy in three situations will be described: social termination of pregnancy, spontaneous abortion (miscarriage) and termination of pregnancy for fetal abnormality. Much of the information provided will be drawn from recent research. Attention will be paid not only to the recognition and treatment of emotional distress in these circumstances, but also to the identification of women who are particularly likely to experience severe emotional distress.

Grief

Grief is the normal response to loss—not only to the loss of a loved person known well to the bereaved and to others, but also to the loss of an early pregnancy and to losses of parts of the body, for example, a breast. The grief that follows the loss of a known, loved person shows a characteristic pattern which can also be recognized after other major losses, including the loss of an early pregnancy.

Typical grief has three well-recognized stages: (a) non-reaction, (b) full reaction, and (c) resolution.

Non-reaction. This initial stage of grief can last minutes, hours or days. The bereaved person appears free from distress and may act as if nothing has happened. He or she may describe a state of emotional numbness, or inability to react to the loss. This apparent lack of emotion can be misinterpreted as a sign of 'coping well'.

Full reaction. This second stage of grief can last for a variable number of weeks and perhaps several months; after this, the intensity gradually diminishes, although there may be exacerbations at significant times such as the anniversary of the death. The features of the full reaction fall into three categories: psychological, social and physical. Typical psychological features of grief include depressed mood, tearfulness, loss of interest in usual activities, guilt, anger (towards self, the family and the professionals), perceptual disturbances, and behavioural abnormalities such as constantly revisiting places associated with the deceased. Social features of grief include withdrawal from social contact and difficulties in relationships with other people. Both of these features can result in removal of opportunities for comfort. This social isolation can be compounded when the newly bereaved are avoided by those who either do not know what to say, or those who are embarrassed by displays of emotion. Common physical features of grief are the so-called 'pangs' of grief. These are bouts of autonomic disturbance, which include tightness in the throat, choking sensations, sighing and shortness of breath. There may also be headaches, blurred vision, fatigue and poor appetite.

Resolution. Once the pain of grief has been experienced and borne, and the reality of the loss accepted, the bereaved can begin to adjust to life without the lost person. There is no clear end to grief, and the deceased is not, of course, forgotten.

The normal grief described above is not a psychiatric illness and should not be treated as such. In particular, the use of drugs should be avoided. Normal grief is best managed with support and understanding. Grief becomes abnormal when the symptoms are either unusually prolonged or intense. For example, the initial stage of non-reaction may go on for weeks or even months. In other cases, features of the full grief reaction may be exaggerated in both timing and intensity.

Risk factors for developing an abnormal grief reaction can be categorized as follows: (a) features of the loss, e.g. a death that was unexpected, untimely or particularly horrifying, or circumstances where the body was not seen after death; (b) features of the relationship with the deceased, e.g. an ambivalent relationship; (c) features of the survivor, e.g. history of psychiatric illness, a special vulnerability to loss; (d) social features, e.g. poor social circumstances and lack of a confiding relationship (Parkes, 1985). Abnormal grief requires skilled psychological treatment. The aim of such treatment is first to restore and reinforce normal stages of mourning, and then to assist the bereaved in reorganizing their life; permission to stop grieving may need to be given.

A few bereaved people will develop a well-defined episode of psychiatric illness, usually a depressive disorder. These people are often those who have shown a previous tendency to become psychiatrically unwell following stressful life events. These episodes merit appropriate treatment in their own right while help is being given with mourning.

SOCIAL TERMINATION OF PREGNANCY

First trimester social termination of pregnancy

Facts and figures

The 1967 Abortion Act legalized termination of pregnancy on social grounds, i.e. if 'the continuance of the pregnancy would involve risk of injury to the physical or mental health of the pregnant woman or any existing children of her family, greater than if the pregnancy were terminated'. The Act goes on to state that in the determination of such risk '. . . account may be taken of the pregnant woman's actual and reasonably foreseeable environment'. For the purposes of this chapter, termination of pregnancy carried out under these grounds will be referred to as 'social termination'. Most terminations of pregnancy carried out in England, Wales and Scotland under the terms of the 1967 Abortion Act are these social terminations; less than 2% are carried out for other indications such as fetal abnormality or risk to the life of the mother.

Following the introduction of the 1967 Abortion Act, the annual number of legal abortions in England, Wales and Scotland rose rapidly in the late 1960s and early 1970s from 58 000 (1969) to 174 000 (1973) (Munday et al, 1989). It was against the background of this rising rate that concern was raised about 'the nature of the long-term physical and emotional sequelae of termination of pregnancy' (Editorial, 1973). The rate fell in the mid 1970s, but since then it has risen steadily every year to 184 000 in England, Wales and Scotland in 1987 (Munday et al, 1989).

Research on the psychiatric outcome of social termination of pregnancy

Many clinicians feel that there should be no adverse psychological sequelae when a woman has chosen to have an unwanted pregnancy terminated. Others would argue that termination of even an unwanted pregnancy is likely to result in significant emotional distress in the short-term for most women and for some women in the long-term also.

Recent research has gone some way towards ascertaining the psychological sequelae of social termination of pregnancy. Most social terminations are carried out in the first trimester of pregnancy (86% in 1987)

(Munday et al, 1989), so most research has been directed towards these early terminations.

The results of early studies on the psychiatric sequelae of termination of pregnancy varied widely. Some studies found high levels of psychiatric morbidity after termination, while others found little or none (reviewed by Simon and Senturia, 1966). However, the methods used in these studies make it difficult to draw firm conclusions from them. Common methodo-logical problems were poor sample selection, failure to assess psychiatric status before termination, retrospective design, short follow-up period and inadequate assessment of mental state (Simon and Senturia, 1966). Also, these early termination studies were carried out when psychiatric disorder was one of the few grounds for termination of pregnancy. Psychiatric outcome is likely to be poor in women who were psychiatrically disordered when termination was requested. Such a poor outcome might be less likely in the psychiatrically healthier women who are able to obtain termination under newer legislation.

The psychiatric outcome of social termination of pregnancy can be deduced only from prospective studies which use: (a) standardized methods to assess psychiatric outcome; (b) a large sample; (c) short- and long-term follow-up; and (d) interviews for assessment. Relatively few studies fulfilling these criteria have been carried out since the introduction of the 1967 Abortion Act.

These requirements are met by the study of Greer et al (1976), which began only after the 1967 Abortion Act came into force. In a prospective study, a large cohort of women (360) undergoing first trimester social termination of pregnancy were interviewed on three occasions: before termination, three months later, and 15 to 24 months later. Mental state was assessed by both standardized measures and subjective accounts. Follow-up at three months was good (91%), but only 60% (216) of the women could be traced for the final interview. An important finding was that very few of the women (14) had their first consultation for psychiatric disorder in the two years following social termination of pregnancy; most of these episodes were felt by the women to be unrelated to the termination. However, figures about psychiatric consultation may not provide a full picture of psychiatric morbidity. At three-month follow-up, there were significant improvements in the following areas: depression (as assessed at interview by the rating scale of Hamilton, 1967), 'sexual adjustment' and 'interpersonal adjustment'. Mean Hamilton scores indicated that depression was only mild before termination, and insignificant afterwards. We are not told about depressive symptoms at final follow-up. The proportion of women who experienced 'considerable' or 'moderate' guilt before termination (37%) fell significantly to 13% at three-month follow-up and further to 7% at final follow-up.

Greer et al (1976) conclude that early social termination of pregnancy carries only a minimal risk of 'untoward psychological and social sequelae up to two years afterwards'. They emphasize the significant improvement after termination in psychiatric symptomatology, guilt, interpersonal relation-ships and sexual adjustment. All the women in this study received 'brief counselling' (Beard et al, 1974) before their termination; this may have influenced outcome.

To what extent are the conclusions of Greer et al (1976) borne out by the results of other recent research? Lask (1975) found that psychiatric outcome was 'unfavourable' at six-month follow-up in as many as 32% of the sample of 50 women. Outcome was 'unfavourable' if the woman regretted the termination or was still experiencing moderate or severe guilt, or if mental symptoms had developed anew or had persisted since before the termination. By contrast, Ashton (1980) claimed that, although up to half the women undergoing social termination experienced a short-lived emotional disturbance (detectable at eight weeks after termination), the symptoms had resolved by eight months in most of them. However, since two thirds of those interviewed at eight weeks in this study were lost at final follow-up, it is difficult to draw firm conclusions about outcome. Belsey et al (1977) found that only 13% of a sample of over 300 women felt guilty three months after social termination of pregnancy.

Two other studies demonstrated psychological improvement after social termination. Before termination, Brody et al (1971) found high levels of depression, withdrawal and social unease on a personality profile; six weeks later, these symptoms were less intense, and after a year the symptom profile was close to 'normal'. McCance et al (1973) interviewed over 300 women before social termination and 18 months afterwards (82% follow-up rate). Whereas before termination, 61% of the unmarried and 40% of the married women showed severe depression on the Beck Depression Inventory (Beck et al, 1961), only 1.4% of the unmarried and 4% of the married women did so at follow-up. While one third reported (retrospectively) that they had experienced regrets at three months after termination, 80% were glad they had had the termination by 18 months, with severe regret being felt by only 5% at this stage.

Thus, there seems to be broad agreement that for the majority of women, mental state at varying intervals after termination of pregnancy appears to be better than it was immediately beforehand. In a recent review Olley (1985) concludes that 'recent research has not confirmed the earlier fears of frequent serious mental illness following induced abortion'. Nevertheless, most studies identify a variably sized group of women who do seem to experience significant psychological sequelae which are not always short lived.

Factors associated with poor psychiatric outcome after social termination

Is it possible to identify women who are particularly likely to experience adverse psychological sequelae after social termination of pregnancy? Lask (1975) identified the following predictors of unfavourable psychological outcome: past history of psychiatric illness, psychiatric illness at the time of the termination, ambivalence about the termination, desertion by the partner, multiparity, age group 21 to 30, and being foreign-born. Ashton (1980) identifies similar risk factors, e.g. past psychiatric history and ambivalence, together with a poor obstetric history and high neuroticism scores. He emphasized that poor psychological outcome was often related to the woman's environment since the termination rather than to the termination itself. Belsey et al (1977) identified two groups of variables predicting psychiatric outcome after termination: (a) the relationship with the partner, e.g. feelings towards the partner, sexual adjustment and perceived emotional support; and (b) ability to copy with daily stresses, e.g. previous psychiatric disorder, suicide attempts and work record.

Psychiatric illness after social termination of pregnancy

Although social termination results in adverse psychological sequelae for some vulnerable women, severe mental illness in such circumstances is rare. Brewer (1977) found that hospital admission for psychosis within three months of social termination of pregnancy was less common (0.3 per 1000 terminations) than admission for puerperal psychosis (1.7 per 1000 deliveries).

Second trimester social termination of pregnancy

Little is known of the psychiatric sequelae of social termination carried out in the second trimester of pregnancy. Brewer (1978) followed up 25 of a group of 40 women who had undergone social termination of pregnancy between the 20th and 24th week of pregnancy. None of the 25 reported severe psychiatric sequelae, but we do not know what happened to the 15 (37%) who either refused follow-up or who could not be traced. Kaltreider et al (1979) compared psychological outcome after mid-trimester termination in two groups of women: 30 who had had dilatation and evacuation (DE) and 30 who had had induced labour. Three weeks after termination, 24% of the women who had undergone induced labour felt guilty, whereas none of the DE group did so. The induced labour group also had higher levels of depression and anger than the DE group. The results of this study suggest that the procedure of induced labour which is frequently used for second trimester termination is likely to be a particular source of distress afterwards.

It is difficult to say whether second trimester social termination creates more psychological distress than first trimester termination, since women requesting late abortion may be 'an atypical group with many social and psychological problems' (Savage, 1985). Although some terminations are delayed into the second trimester for avoidable procedural reasons, women presenting late with requests for termination often show the following features: (a) extreme youth; (b) denial of the pregnancy; (c) ambivalence about continuing with the pregnancy; and (d) poor social support (Kaltreider et al, 1979). These are some of the very factors which predict poor outcome after first trimester termination. Thus any excess psychiatric morbidity in women undergoing second trimester termination might only reflect the increased vulnerability of the women who undergo such late terminations.

Psychiatric sequelae of refused abortion

A discussion of psychiatric sequelae of termination of pregnancy is incomplete unless attention is paid to the psychiatric sequelae of carrying an unwanted pregnancy to term. McCance et al (1973) compared psychiatric outcome in women who had undergone termination with those who had been refused one. At 18 months' follow-up, regret at having continued the pregnancy was more common than regret at having had the termination. However, the incidence of depression at follow-up was no greater in those who were refused termination than in those who had undergone it. By contrast, Brody et al (1971) found that women who had been refused termination remained psychologically disturbed after their child had been born compared with the improvement noted over the follow-up period in those who had undergone termination. However, women who experience psychological disturbance after carrying an unwanted pregnancy to term may be those who might have experienced psychological disturbance after termination.

When a woman's request for social termination is turned down, not only must the consequences for her mental state be considered, but also those for the child if it were to be born. One study showed that a third of a series of women who were refused abortion resented their babies one to three years later (Pare and Raven, 1970). The incidence of delinquency and psychiatric disturbance is increased in children born after abortion was refused compared with a matched control group (Forssman and Thuwe, 1966).

Recognition and management of psychiatric disorder after social termination of pregnancy

Whereas some women experience very little psychological disturbance after social termination of pregnancy, others suffer significant disturbance. With appropriate management the occurrence of such distress may be reduced and any distress that does occur may be recognized and treated.

The reduction of the likelihood of psychological disturbance

This may be achieved by careful assessment of any woman who requests a termination. The following information should be sought: (a) the circumstances leading up to the conception of the unwanted pregnancy; (b) any ambivalence about the request for termination; (c) the attitude of the baby's father and her family to the termination; (d) her present social circumstances, including relationships; (e) her present mental state and past psychiatric history; and (f) what she would do if termination was refused. Women with significant doubts about having a termination should be given the opportunity to discuss them, since ambivalence about termination increases the risk of psychiatric disorder afterwards (see above). In these circumstances, referral to a psychiatrist is sometimes helpful, since this provides an opportunity to discuss the situation away from the pressures of the gynaecology clinic. A single, unhurried consultation is often all that is necessary to help the woman resolve her ambivalence, whatever her final decision.

If the woman appears to be under pressure to have the termination from the baby's father or her family, it is important to help her decide what she herself wants to do. It may be helpful to involve the partner or family in this discussion.

Information gained at this assessment interview can be used to identify women who are particularly likely to experience psychiatric disturbance after a termination. Such women should not be refused termination, but identified as being likely to benefit from follow-up and psychological support after termination. Studies are needed to evaluate the benefit of such an approach in preventing psychiatric morbidity in vulnerable women after social termination of pregnancy.

The recognition and treatment of psychological distress

It must be clear that such distress can be recognized only if women are followed up after social termination of pregnancy. Both hospital doctors and general practitioners need to be aware that some women do suffer distressing emotional symptoms in the early weeks and months after termination, and possibly for longer. These women may present with physical rather than psychological complaints, but if the doctor is aware of the recent termination, sensitive enquiry should uncover any underlying emotional distress.

Psychological distress arising after termination of pregnancy is best managed in most cases by sympathetic counselling. Such distress may result from both the termination itself and the woman's circumstances since then. With regard to the termination, the woman needs to be allowed to express not only her grief at the loss of a pregnancy, but also any guilt and anger that she may feel. She may need to be encouraged to mourn for her fetus, since accepting the reality of the loss is part of the normal mourning process. With regard to her circumstances, difficulties in interpersonal relationships and life-style may need to be explored; practical help and advice may be needed, e.g. with housing. Attention should be given to contraception and to plans for future pregnancies. It is not uncommon for a woman to feel an intense need to become pregnant again soon after a termination, and the reasons for this need to be carefully explored. She may need to be helped to understand that while she is seeking to fill the emptiness she feels after the termination, the social difficulties and poor relationships that led her to request termination remain unchanged.

Serious psychiatric illness

Serious psychiatric illness after social termination of pregnancy is rare. However, women with past psychiatric histories of major psychiatric illness, e.g. manic-depressive disorder and schizophrenia, may be particularly liable to relapse following a potentially stressful life event such as termination of pregnancy. Care should be taken to detect the first signs of relapse in such women at follow-up, so that appropriate specialist help can be initiated.

Late psychiatric sequelae

The psychiatric sequelae of social termination of pregnancy may not become apparent for some years. Kumar and Robson (1978) found a highly significant association between antenatal depression and anxiety and a history of previous termination of pregnancy. Sometimes, it is only during a later planned pregnancy that the grief and guilt of an earlier termination are expressed, particularly if there are difficulties with the pregnancy; failure to bear a wanted child may be seen as a punishment. Women may not always volunteer a past history of termination, especially if their current partner is unaware of it. It is therefore important to enquire directly about previous terminations when taking an obstetric history; such information may be invaluable in understanding and managing unexplained emotional symptoms which arise during a pregnancy. Sometimes it may only be after childbirth years later than a woman faces the full implications of a previous termination. However, no association has been demonstrated between postnatal depression and previous social termination of pregnancy (Kumar and Robson, 1984; Watson et al, 1984).

SPONTANEOUS ABORTION

Up to 20% of all clinically diagnosed pregnancies end in spontaneous abortion or miscarriage before 20 weeks of pregnancy.

Too often, spontaneous abortion tends to be seen as normal or 'nature's way', and therefore unlikely to create much psychological distress (Roberts, 1989). It is often assumed that if the woman has not felt fetal movement and has experienced only minimal bodily changes of pregnancy, she is unlikely to have become attached to her pregnancy, and as many fetuses which abort spontaneously are abnormal in some way, the mother should feel relief rather than grief. Against the first assumption, it can be argued that many women already do think of the fetus as a real person by the end of the first trimester; this belief is reinforced by the increased use of ultrasound scans very early in pregnancy. Against the second assumption, a woman may find it of little comfort to be told that the miscarriage might have been a good thing when she has become attached to her pregnancy; she may also blame herself for having produced an imperfect fetus. A further reason for the belief that little psychological distress follows spontaneous abortion is that women are rarely followed up afterwards, either by the hospital or by their general practitioner. To summarize, emotional distress after spontaneous abortion tends not to be anticipated, and so goes largely undetected.

It has been suggested that women with certain personality characteristics are particularly susceptible to spontaneous abortion. Simon et al (1969) found that women who had had a spontaneous abortion were more likely to show sado-masochistic conflicts and rejection of a feminine biological role than women who had had therapeutic abortions. However, personality characteristics are difficult to identify and define, and it is hard to see how they could cause spontaneous abortion.

Most studies on psychiatric sequelae of spontaneous abortion are difficult to interpret; design is usually retrospective, samples are often small or atypical and standardized interview methods were not used to assess mental state.

Some sequelae of spontaneous abortion were described by Cain et al (1964). Although their sample of women was atypical in that it was restricted to psychiatric patients, they identified psychological factors which could be of general relevance after spontaneous abortion. Such factors included: (a) the need to reverse previous preparation for and adjustment to the pregnancy; (b) fears about damage to future child-bearing capacity; (c) a sense of failure; (d) a need to actively mourn a child that had become real, both as an immediate presence and as a source of fantasy about the future; (e) guilt at not only her own possible role in causing the miscarriage (e.g. by taking too much exercise or paying insufficient attention to diet), but also over past misdemeanours for which she may feel she is being punished (e.g. a previous induced abortion); and (f) anger directed towards her partner or her doctor, or both. Cain et al (1964) also emphasized the impact of spontaneous abortion on the woman's partner, who often has to deal with his wife's grief and his own disappointment, yet may find himself the target for her anger. Children are often bewildered by what has happened, and may blame either themselves or their mother for the loss of the pregnancy. They may show anger to their mother for having deprived them of a potential sibling.

Grief after spontaneous abortion in a more representative sample of women was described by Leppert and Pahlka (1984). Twenty-two out of 136 pregnant women in their practice (16.2%) who had spontaneously aborted were interviewed soon afterwards. The grief was judged to be as intense as that occurring after stillbirth or neonatal death, and its pattern was very similar to that found after death of an adult. It was not until three to four months after spontaneous abortion that the women's grief began to resolve. The authors point out that there are no well-established rituals for mourning early pregnancy; society tends not to recognize spontaneous abortion as a loss, thus creating a 'private and unshared burden'.

To what extent does the psychological impact of spontaneous abortion differ from that of induced abortion? In a retrospective study, Simon et al (1969) interviewed two groups of women, 32 who had experienced a spontaneous abortion 10 to 15 years before, and 46 others who had had a social termination over the same period. While most women (78%) felt little or no guilt after the spontaneous abortion, 22% did feel guilty for many months afterwards, as did 35% of those who had had a social termination. Forty per cent (13 out of 32) of the women described feeling 'depressed' after the spontaneous abortion; 8 of these 13 had a diagnosable psychiatric illness at the time of the research interview many years later. The spontaneous abortion group were felt to show less 'psychopathology' than the social termination group overall. However, the 'psychopathology' which did appear in the spontaneous abortion group tended to be closely related to the spontaneous abortion, whereas that seen in the termination group seemed to be part of chronic difficulties which existed beforehand. The results of this study must be interpreted with caution, since in any retrospective study recall of past events is influenced both by time and by the woman's mental state at the time of the interview.

Occasionally, grief becomes abnormal after spontaneous abortion. For example, Corney and Horton (1974) described the onset of irritable and explosive behaviour in a woman four months after a spontaneous abortion. At the time of the abortion, she had been unable to express her grief and had appeared outwardly cheerful. Her symptoms resolved after she had been helped to grieve for her loss.

A recent study in Oxford overcame the problems of method that made earlier studies difficult to interpret (Friedman and Gath, 1989). Standardized psychiatric measures were used to assess mental state after spontaneous abortion in 84% (67) of a consecutive series of women admitted to hospital for evacuation of the uterus after complete or threatened spontaneous abortion. The women were interviewed four weeks after the spontaneous abortion. The main finding in this study was that levels of psychiatric morbidity were high in the four weeks after spontaneous abortion. Forty-eight per cent of the women were psychiatric 'cases' on the Present State Examination of Wing et al (1974); rates of psychiatric 'case' status using this measure are only 10–12% in women in the general population, but as high as 95% amongst psychiatric patients. Many of the women described features of typical grief. For example, an initial emotional numbness was common, as was guilt. Several women felt their grief was similar to that experienced after family bereavement. Three had attempted to harm themselves, either by overdose or wrist cutting.

Factors influencing psychological outcome after spontaneous abortion

Psychological outcome after spontaneous abortion will be influenced by the meaning of the event to the individual woman and how others react to the event (Graves, 1987).

There are a number of areas in which a woman can experience a sense of loss. Not only has a baby been lost, but there also may be a sense of loss of self-esteem as a parent, and a feeling of failure as a woman. Status as a pregnant woman or mother-to-be has also been lost. There may also be fear of loss of capacity to bear further children. It is this sense of loss that leads to the expression of emotions such as fear, frustration, sadness, shame, self-blame, guilt, anger and projected blame after spontaneous abortion. The woman's loss is often unrecognized or poorly understood by others. The mother can be isolated by a conspiracy of silence, designed to protect not only her but also those caring for her. When people do speak out, reassurances such as 'it was for the best' or 'you can always have another one' will be seen by the mother as minimizing her loss; this will increase her sense of isolation.

Friedman and Gath (1989) have identified two groups of factors which are significantly associated with psychiatric morbidity after spontaneous abortion: (a) personal vulnerability factors, such as single status, past psychiatric history and the personality dimension of neuroticism; and (b) obstetric factors, such as previous spontaneous abortion and childlessness (where there is no history of spontaneous abortion). Hall et al (1987) suggest that the following factors may be predisposing factors for pathological grief after spontaneous abortion: obsessive personality disorder, past history of depressive reaction, previous loss of children, and ambivalent relationships with the partner or parents.

Management after spontaneous abortion

Guidelines for the management of spontaneous abortion have been given by Graves (1987). He explains the need to facilitate expression of grief, and to restore or reinforce the sense of self-worth which is often destroyed or damaged after spontaneous abortion. Important points for management after spontaneous abortion are summarized below.

1. Women who have suffered spontaneous abortion should not necessarily be nursed in isolation while they are in hospital; isolation and avoidance of such women may lower self-esteem further and inhibit expression of grief.
2. Women need to be helped to face the reality of their loss so as to be able to mourn effectively. Since it is rarely possible for a mother to confront reality by seeing the baby after a spontaneous abortion, the reality of the situation needs to be emphasized by providing detailed information about what has happened. This reality also needs to be explained to the woman's family.
3. Women are desperate to receive information about the likely cause of their spontaneous abortion. In particular, they need reassurance that they were unlikely to have been responsible for the loss of their pregnancy. Such reassurance reduces the likelihood of self-destructive guilt.
4. Women need someone to listen while they discuss their experience, and with whom to share their sense of guilt and failure after spontaneous abortion. The listener must be aware of the normal stages of grief so that, for example, hostility is recognized as part of normal grief and therefore not responded to by anger or by avoidance of the patient. Women often find it helpful to be told about the features of normal grief, so that they know what to expect. They may find it useful to read books in which the experiences of other women following spontaneous abortion are described, for example those by Oakley et al (1984) and Lachelin (1985).

Studies are needed to evaluate the role of intervention such as that described above in reducing psychiatric morbidity after spontaneous abortion.

Just as after social termination of pregnancy, there are good reasons why a woman should be advised to avoid becoming pregnant too soon after a spontaneous abortion. A new pregnancy may inhibit the completion of mourning for the last baby; this unresolved grief may present as unexplained psychiatric symptoms later during the pregnancy or after the next baby is born. However, many women feel so intense a need to become pregnant again that they ignore such advice. Whilst many of these women will go through their next pregnancy with few if any psychological problems, carers should be watchful for signs of unresolved grief. It is not uncommon for a woman to remain emotionally detached from a pregnancy occurring immediately after a lost pregnancy, so as to protect herself in case this pregnancy also fails. Such detachment needs to be detected and discussed with the woman. Finally, during the next pregnancy after a spontaneous abortion, the woman will require extra support and encouragement, and will benefit from frequent reassurance. It is worth noting that whether or not she becomes pregnant again immediately afterwards, a woman who has experienced spontaneous abortion may go through a depressive reaction at the time of the expected birth of the lost baby (Hayton, 1988).

TERMINATION FOR FETAL ABNORMALITY

Facts and figures

Clause 4 of the 1967 Abortion Act allows termination of pregnancy if there is 'substantial risk that if the child was born it would suffer from such physical or mental abnormalities as to be seriously handicapped'. In 1987, 1915 terminations for fetal abnormality were carried out on women resident in England and Wales (Office of Population Censuses and Surveys, 1988). Between 1973 and 1981, the proportion of abortions carried out under Clause 4 of the Act remained constant at 1–2% (Turnbull and MacKenzie, 1983). As techniques of antenatal diagnosis become increasingly sophisticated and more widely available, it might be predicted that the total number of pregnancies terminated for fetal abnormality would increase.

Psychological sequelae

Some clinicians might predict that women would be relieved and grateful to know that their baby had a potentially serious abnormality before it was too late to have the pregnancy terminated. Termination should protect the mother from either the distress of giving birth to a baby unlikely to survive long, or the difficulties of rearing a handicapped child. They might also argue that as some women deliberately opt for diagnostic tests such as amniocentesis, then they should experience no distress if the result of the test turns out to be abnormal. They would not expect emotional distress and would expect relief rather than grief to be the predominant emotion. As with loss of early pregnancy in other circumstances, there is relatively little contact with the medical profession in the early weeks after termination for fetal abnormality, so again, any emotional distress that is experienced tends to go by largely undetected.

There are many reasons why termination of pregnancy for fetal abnormality may have adverse psychological sequelae, and why relief is not the predominant emotion for most women:

1. Virtually all these pregnancies are wanted, although not necessarily

planned. Termination in these circumstances can mean that a woman 'has to reject her wanted child' (Statham, 1987).

2. The great majority of terminations for fetal abnormality are carried out in the second trimester of pregnancy; relatively few are carried out in the first trimester following early diagnosis from chorionic villus biopsy. There are at least two reasons why termination in the second trimester might create psychological difficulty. The first is that by the second trimester the woman looks and feels pregnant; the attachment to her baby that began in the first trimester will often have been consolidated by feeling fetal movement. People outside the immediate family will know of the pregnancy, creating a necessity to explain and perhaps justify what has happened to the pregnancy. This is in contrast to spontaneous or induced abortion, when relatively few people tend to know of the early pregnancy. The second reason concerns the nature of second trimester termination. Within NHS hospitals this usually take the form of induced labour, stimulated by prostaglandins or, less often, by hypertonic saline; surgical methods of termination in the second trimester are rare in the NHS. Thus, for most women, there are up to 24 hours—sometimes longer—of painful labour, ending with the birth of a recognizable fetus. The woman's active involvement in such a termination is likely to be a particular source of distress, as shown by Kaltreider et al (1979) (see above).

3. If the handicapped child would have survived, many mothers are going to feel guilty about choosing not to care for it. Even when the child would not have survived, some mothers still feel guilty at having taken the decision to end the baby's life rather than letting the baby die in its own time; such mothers may have been against abortion in other circumstances, for example, they may be Roman Catholics.

4. For some mothers, the psychological impact of the termination for fetal abnormality is increased when they find out that this abnormality may recur. Not only has that pregnancy been lost, but future pregnancies are threatened.

5. Mothers having termination for fetal abnormality are often in their late 30s or in their 40s, particularly those having terminations for chromosomal abnormality. At this age, conception is more difficult and the risk of spontaneous abortion is higher, so such women may doubt their ability to go through with another pregnancy. Also, some of these older mothers may have remarried, and the abnormal fetus may have been the first, often vital, child conceived within the new relationship.

6. As with spontaneous abortion, the conception of an abnormal fetus is likely to generate guilt, a sense of failure and a loss of self-esteem.

For these reasons, and perhaps others, it might be predicted that termination for fetal abnormality would have adverse psychological sequelae for at least some women. As Turnbull and MacKenzie (1983) say, 'second-trimester abortion (for fetal abnormality) can be a traumatic ordeal . . . with potential long-term psychological sequelae despite skilful and sympathetic care'.

Research on the psychiatric outcome of termination for fetal abnormality

Whereas much research has been carried out on the psychiatric sequelae of social termination, relatively little has been carried out on termination for fetal abnormality. Two early papers (Peck and Marcus, 1966; Pare and Raven, 1970) noted that poor psychiatric outcome is more likely after termination of a wanted pregnancy on 'organic grounds' (e.g. suspected fetal abnormality or risk to maternal health) than if the termination had been actively sought by the mother.

Blumberg et al (1975) interviewed 13 women just once at three months to three years after termination for fetal abnormality. Eleven of the 13 women said that they had been depressed after the termination; for two women, the distress was more severe than after a social termination and a stillbirth. Two possible sources for the guilt after such terminations were identified: first, the failure to produce a healthy child, and second, having made the decision to terminate the pregnancy.

Three subsequent small retrospective studies had findings which were remarkably similar to each other, namely that after termination for fetal abnormality, up to half of mothers are still experiencing significant emotional distress months or even years later (Donnai et al, 1981; Leschot et al, 1982; Jorgensen et al, 1985). In none of these studies were standardized measures used to assess mental state.

In a larger retrospective study by Lloyd and Laurence (1985), 48 women were interviewed on one occasion one to five years after termination for fetal abnormality. Thirty-six of the women (77%) recalled acute grief after the termination. Five of the six women who had also experienced stillbirth or neonatal death recalled similar grief. The grief after termination for fetal abnormality varied from 'mild tearfulness with sadness, lethargy and insomnia, to incapacitating grief with somatic symptoms'. Twenty-two of the women (46%) recalled still experiencing symptoms of anxiety and depression six months after termination for fetal abnormality; ten of them (21%) had received treatment for their symptoms. The women received very little support after termination for fetal abnormality. The authors suggest that the severity of the reaction after termination for fetal abnormality may be related to difficulties in mourning in these particular circumstances, for example the baby is often not seen, there is rarely a grave, and the mother's loss is often minimalized by others.

A current Oxford study (Iles, unpublished data) set out to examine psychiatric morbidity after termination for fetal abnormality in more detail. The aims of the study were to determine the frequency, diagnostic distribution, severity, duration and outcome of psychiatric disorders amongst women having termination for fetal abnormality, and to identify factors which would indicate women at high risk of developing psychiatric disorder. The design of the study was prospective and standardized measures were used to assess mental state; semi-structured interviewing was used so as to gain a detailed understanding of the experience of each woman. Seventy-one women were interviewed on three occasions in the year after termination for fetal abnormality: at one month, six months and 13 months afterwards. The main finding so far is that psychiatric morbidity in the first month is high. The proportion of women (39%) who were psychiatric 'cases' on the Present State Examination (see above) was four times higher than that found in the general population of women. Both the Present State Examination and other measures of mental state show that these women had levels of depression and anxiety comparable to that found in psychiatric inpatients and outpatients. Many of the women showed typical features of the grief that follows any bereavement, for example initial emotional numbness followed by sadness, anger, guilt and bodily symptoms.

From the interviews completed so far at six and 13 months, the findings show that the proportion of Present State Examination cases has fallen to general population levels. However, symptoms of anxiety and depression persist in a number of women who are not Present State Examination 'cases'. These symptoms are often associated with unresolved guilt over the termination, concern over the outcome of a new pregnancy, or failure to conceive another child.

Relatively little is known yet about factors which increase the risk of psychiatric disorder after termination for fetal abnormality. In the Oxford study, two groups of factors have so far been found to be associated with psychiatric morbidity one month after termination. Firstly, there are obstetric factors, such as whether or not the abnormality was life-threatening. Within the neural tube defect group, psychiatric outcome was poorer in women whose babies had spina bifida, and hence might have survived, than in mothers whose babies were anencephalic and hence unlikely to survive. A further obstetric factor was the duration of pregnancy at the time of the termination; psychiatric morbidity was higher for terminations carried out late in the second trimester. Secondly, there are personal vulnerability factors in the mother, such as a past history of psychiatric disorder and poor support from her partner at the time of the termination.

Management of termination for fetal abnormality

The research discussed above demonstrates that significant psychiatric morbidity does occur after termination for fetal abnormality. Management of women in this situation should have two aims: firstly, to minimize the likelihood of severe psychiatric disorder, and secondly, to recognize and treat psychiatric disorder when it does occur. Such management should begin before the diagnostic test is performed. It should be based on an understanding of the grief that follows any major loss (see above) and the information gained from detailed interviews of women after termination for fetal abnormality, such as those from the Oxford study.

The principles of management of termination for fetal abnormality are described below.

Before any specific antenatal diagnostic test, women should be told that they might be offered a termination if an abnormality were to be detected; their views on termination should be sought. Women who are against termination in any circumstances may decide not to have the test.

Women who are against termination but nonetheless request diagnostic testing should not be refused it. It may be valuable for such a woman to be able to prepare herself for the birth of a handicapped child, but she should be warned that a positive test result may lead her, quite unexpectedly, to consider termination. There is a particular dilemma over the use of routine ultrasound scans for, say, dating a pregnancy or checking on fetal growth. Should doctors withhold information about fetal abnormality from mothers who have stated themselves to be against termination in any circumstances, or should such mothers be advised to avoid ultrasound scans? The decision here can be taken only after consultation between the obstetrician and both parents. For a full description of the ethical aspects of prenatal diagnosis, the reader is referred to Crawfurd (1983) and Campbell (1984).

When diagnostic testing gives an abnormal result, care must be taken over how the news is broken. Ideally, both parents should be told together. If the abnormality has been detected in the laboratory, the information should not be given by letter or telephone but in person; a home visit by either the general practitioner or a member of the genetic or obstetric team is ideal. If the couple are recalled to the clinic to be given an abnormal result, they will be left suspecting that something is wrong whilst they await their appointment. If the abnormality is discovered during an ultrasound scan, the information should be given without delay; mothers soon become aware and distressed that staff are concerned about some aspect of the scan. It is often helpful to point out the abnormality on the scan to the parents; technical language should be avoided, and drawings may be helpful. The couple will then need some time alone to express their grief and to discuss what to do. These couples find it hard to return to the antenatal clinic to finish the consultation, and they should be seen away from the clinic, if possible.

The decision to terminate a pregnancy for fetal abnormality should not be made in haste nor should the parents feel under pressure to terminate the pregnancy. Some couples may have decided in advance to terminate a pregnancy in such circumstances, and their decision may be relatively easy. Others will not have considered the question, and may find it hard to decide. For all of them, initial information they were given about the abnormality may have registered poorly during the initial phase of shock and numbness that is so typical of grief. Information may need to be repeated, and perhaps supplemented with written information. It may be helpful if a paediatrician can talk to the couple about the prognosis for the child if it were to be born. Although it is not feasible to give the parents weeks to decide, they should not be forced to decide immediately about termination. They should be given time to discuss it between themselves and with the family, and perhaps with their general practitioner and, where appropriate, their priest. It should be stressed to them that while termination is an option, the hospital team is prepared to support them if they decide to go ahead and have the baby. Even when the prognosis is very poor, as for anencephaly, it may be better for some parents to mourn a child that has died in its own time after birth, rather than having to blame themselves for having taken its life.

Once a decision has been taken to terminate the pregnancy, care should be taken over the timing of the termination. Some women find it very distressing to wait several days for termination, particularly if they are feeling fetal movement. Others may request a few days' delay—either for domestic reasons or to give themselves time to be sure of their decision. These wishes should be accommodated wherever possible.

The termination itself should be handled sympathetically by staff who are experienced in dealing with mid-trimester terminations. A full explanation of the practical procedures involved should be given to the couple. Staff should make it clear that they know that this is the termination of a wanted pregnancy and not of an unwanted one. Analgesia should be adequate; women seem to cope less well with the pain of contractions when a happy outcome to the labour is not expected. The partner should be encouraged to stay with the woman; if this is impossible, the woman should not be left alone. It is particularly important that she should not be on her own when the baby is born. Staff may find themselves the targets of the anger which is such a common part of grief; this they should be prepared for, and accept.

It may be helpful for many women and their partners to see their baby after termination for fetal abnormality. After any death, seeing the body facilitates healthy mourning and minimizes the risk of abnormal grief (see above). The question of seeing the baby should be discussed with the couple well before the baby is born; otherwise, in the shock and distress of the birth, many couples may decide not to see the baby, a decision they may regret later. On the other hand, no couples should be forced to see the baby. The couple's expectations of what the baby will look like should be discussed with them before they see it. They are often afraid of it being a 'monster' and may need reassuring. The parents should be encouraged to hold the baby. Good quality photographs should be taken of the baby; memories fade even for parents who have seen the baby, while those who opted not to see the baby may request a photograph at a later date.

Some parents find it helpful to arrange a burial or cremation of their baby after termination for fetal abnormality. For such parents, the funeral signifies recognition that their child has existed and died, so is an important part of their mourning. Although death certificates are not provided in such circumstances, many undertakers are willing to arrange a funeral if they receive a note from a doctor explaining what has happened. Many hospitals have a bereavement welfare officer who will help with such arrangements. The parents should not be pressurized into arranging a funeral, but they should be made aware that it is possible. Whether or not there has been a funeral some parents choose to mark their baby's existence by planting a special shrub or tree in the garden; other parents may find it helpful to do the same.

After the termination, the woman and her partner should be warned what to expect, both physically and emotionally. Women are often unaware that they will experience physical changes similar to those that follow childbirth at term, e.g. lactation and vaginal bleeding. The symptoms of normal grief such as sadness, guilt and anger, should be explained to them. They should be warned to expect an exacerbation of their grief at both the expected date of full-term delivery and the anniversary of the termination. The general practitioner should be informed when the woman is discharged from hospital, and he or she should arrange to visit the mother soon afte discharge. Visits at home from a midwife and/or health visitor can be invaluable. Women should be encouraged to talk openly about their experience with their partner, family and friends; this helps others to acknowledge and share their grief. Many women say afterwards that it would have been helpful to have talked to someone who had gone through a similar experience, and to have received written information describing how they would feel. Both these needs can be met at least in some areas by the support group SATFA (Support for Termination for Fetal Abnormality).

The follow-up appointment at the hospital (usually at six weeks) needs to be handled with particular care. Mothers regard the visit as not so much an opportunity for a gynaecological check-up but as one for receiving information about the baby and, in particular, confirmation of the diagnosis. Couples find it distressing to return to the antenatal or postnatal clinic for this consultation, so this should ideally take place away from the clinic in the consultant's office. The couple should be seen by a doctor who was involved with the case, and all relevant information (e.g. post-mortem reports) should be at hand. The consultation should be unhurried, and the couple should be allowed to express their grief. They may need reassurance that they did not directly cause the abnormality. Genetic counselling should be offered. If there is any suspicion that the expression of grief by either partner is abnormal, referral for specialist help, for example to a psychiatrist, may be appropriate.

Couples should be warned that if they conceive another baby immediately, mourning for the baby that they have just lost may be impeded. Some couples do choose to delay the next pregnancy, while others conceive immediately. In the next pregnancy, many mothers deal with their anxieties about recurrence of the abnormality by detaching themselves from the new pregnancy until at least the time when the abnormality was diagnosed in the last pregnancy. After this, some mothers can relax and enjoy the new pregnancy; others remain anxious until the child is born, and need a lot of reassurance. If there is difficulty conceiving the next pregnancy, women become particularly distressed, as they now doubt their ability not only to have a normal baby but also to conceive.

CONCLUSION

Loss of early pregnancy through social termination, spontaneous abortion or termination for fetal abnormality results in typical grief for many women. For some of them, emotional distress is particularly severe. Recent research has identified risk factors which render some women particularly vulnerable to severe distress after early loss of pregnancy. Those caring for women during and after the loss of early pregnancy need to be aware that emotional disorder often follows, and they must be able to detect it. Management along the guidelines suggested in this chapter should do much to alleviate psychiatric disorder after loss of early pregnancy.

SUMMARY

It is often assumed that early loss of pregnancy is not followed by emotional distress. When such distress does occur, it often goes undetected. Early loss of pregnancy is frequently followed by typical grief such as that occurring after any bereavement.

Most recent studies have shown that although social termination of pregnancy in the first trimester has few adverse psychological sequelae for most women, there are vulnerable women who do experience significant emotional distress afterwards. Risk factors for poor psychological outcome include poor social support, past psychiatric history and ambivalence about the termination. The procedures used for second trimester terminations of pregnancy are likely to be a particular source of distress. Psychiatric disorder may also follow if termination is refused. Careful assessment of all women before social termination will identify vulnerable women who may benefit from counselling and support afterwards.

After spontaneous abortion or miscarriage, many women experience significant emotional distress, which persists for several months. Guilt and anger are common. Some women are particularly vulnerable to developing psychiatric disorder after spontaneous abortion, for example women with a past psychiatric history, poor social support, previous spontaneous abortion and personality traits such as neuroticism. Many women would benefit from follow-up and support afterwards; extra support and reassurance are often needed during the next pregnancy.

Termination for fetal abnormality is more likely to induce grief than relief for many women; these pregnancies are usually wanted, second trimester terminations are distressing, and there is often guilt at destroying a life and/or opting out of rearing a handicapped child. Recent research has demonstrated substantial levels of psychiatric morbidity after termination for fetal abnormality, particularly in those with a past psychiatric history, those with poor social support, and those who feel they have opted out of bearing a handicapped child. Women receive little support or follow-up after such terminations, yet many would benefit from it. Such women are in particular need of reassurance and support during a subsequent pregnancy.

REFERENCES

Ashton JR (1980) Psychosocial outcome of induced abortion. *British Journal of Obstetrics and Gynaecology* **87:** 1115–1122.

Beard RW, Belsey EM, Lal S, Lewis SC & Greer HS (1974) King's Termination Study II: contraceptive practice before and after outpatient termination of pregnancy. *British Medical Journal* **i:** 418–421.

Beck AT, Ward CH, Mendelson M, Mock JE & Erbaugh JK (1961) An inventory for measuring depression. *Archives of General Psychiatry* **4:** 561–571.

Belsey EM, Greer HS, Lal S, Lewis SC & Beard RW (1977) Predictive factors in emotional response to abortion. Kings Termination Study IV. *Social Science and Medicine* **11:** 71–82.

Blumberg B, Golbus MS & Hansen KH (1975) The psychological sequelae of abortion performed for a genetic indication. *American Journal of Obstetrics and Gynecology* **122:** 799–808.

Brewer C (1977) Incidence of post-abortion psychosis: a prospective study. *British Medical Journal* i: 476–477.

Brewer C (1978) Induced abortion after feeling foetal movements. Its cause and emotional consequences. *Journal of Biosocial Science* 10: 203–208.

Brody H, Meikle S & Gerritse R (1971) Therapeutic abortion: a prospective study I. *American Journal of Obstetrics and Gynecology* 109: 347–353.

Cain AC, Erickson ME, Fast I & Vaughan R (1964) Childrens' disturbed reaction to their mother's miscarriage. *Psychosomatic Medicine* 26: 58–66.

Campbell AV (1984) Ethical issues in prenatal diagnosis. *British Medical Journal* 288: 1633–1634.

Corney RT & Horton FT (1974) Pathological grief following spontaneous abortion. *American Journal of Psychiatry* 131: 825–827.

Crawfurd M d'A (1983) Ethical and legal aspects of early prenatal diagnosis. *British Medical Bulletin* 39: 310–314.

Donnai D, Charles N & Harris R (1981) Attitude of patients after 'genetic' termination of pregnancy. *British Medical Journal* 282: 621–622.

Editorial (1973) Facts about abortion. *British Medical Journal* ii: 438.

Forssman H & Thuwe I (1966) One hundred and twenty children born after application for therapeutic abortion refused. Their mental health, social adjustment and educational level up to the age of 21. *Acta Psychiatrica Scandinavica* 42: 71–88.

Friedman T & Gath D (1989) The psychiatric consequences of spontaneous abortion. *British Journal of Psychiatry* 155: 810–814.

Graves WL (1987) Psychological aspects of spontaneous abortion. In Bennet MJ & Edmonds DK (eds) *Spontaneous and Recurrent Abortion*, pp 214–235. London: Blackwell Scientific.

Greer HS, Lal S, Lewis SC, Belsey EM & Beard RW (1976) Psychosocial consequences of therapeutic abortion. Kings Termination Study III. *British Journal of Psychiatry* 128: 74–79.

Hall RCW, Beresford TP & Quinones JE (1987) Grief following spontaneous abortion. *Psychiatric Clinics of North America* 10: 405–420.

Hamilton M (1967) Development of a rating scale for primary depressive illness. *British Journal of Social and Clinical Psychology* 6: 278–296.

Hayton A (1988) Miscarriage and delayed depression. *Lancet* i: 834.

Jorgensen C, Uddenberg N & Ursing I (1985) Ultrasound diagnosis of fetal malformation in the second trimester: the psychological reactions of women. *Journal of Psychosomatic Obstetrics and Gynaecology* 4: 31–40.

Kaltreider NB, Goldsmith S & Margolis AJ (1979) The impact of midtrimester abortion techniques on patients and staff. *American Journal of Obstetrics and Gynecology* 135: 235–238.

Kumar R & Robson K (1978) Previous induced abortion and antenatal depression in primiparae: preliminary report of a survey of mental health in pregnancy. *Psychological Medicine* 8: 711–715.

Kumar R & Robson K (1984) A prospective study of emotional disorders in child-bearing women. *British Journal of Psychiatry* 144: 35–47.

Lachelin GC (1985) *Miscarriage: The Facts*. New York: Oxford University Press.

Lask B (1975) Short-term psychiatric sequelae of therapeutic termination of pregnancy. *British Journal of Psychiatry* 126: 173–177.

Leppert PC & Pahlka BS (1984) Grieving characteristics after spontaneous abortion: a management approach. *Obstetrics and Gynecology* 64: 119–122.

Leschot NJ, Verjaal M & Treffers PE (1982) Therapeutic abortion on genetic indications—a detailed follow-up study of 20 patients. *Journal of Psychosomatic Obstetrics and Gynaecology* 1: 47–56.

Lloyd J & Laurence KM (1985) Sequelae and support after termination of pregnancy for foetal abnormality. *British Medical Journal* 290: 907–909.

McCance C, Olley PC & Edward V (1973) Long-term psychiatric follow-up. In Horobin G (ed.) *Experience with Abortion*, pp 245–300. London: Cambridge University Press.

Munday D, Francom C & Savage W (1989) Twenty one years of legal abortion. *British Medical Journal* 298: 1231–1234.

Oakley A, McPherson A & Roberts H (1984) *Miscarriage*. London: Fontana.

Office of Population Censuses and Surveys (1988) *Abortion Statistics*. London: HMSO.

Olley PC (1985) Termination of pregnancy. In Priest RG (ed.) *Psychological Disorders in Obstetrics and Gynaecology*, pp 173–203. London: Butterworths.

Pare CMB & Raven H (1970) Follow-up of patients referred for termination of pregnancy. *Lancet* **i**: 635–638.

Parkes CM (1985) Bereavement. *British Journal of Psychiatry* **146**: 11–17.

Peck A & Marcus H (1966) Psychiatric sequelae of therapeutic interruption of pregnancy. *Journal of Nervous and Mental Disease* **143**: 417–425.

Roberts H (1989) A baby or the products of conception: lay and professional prospectives on miscarriage. In van Hall EV & Everaerd W (eds) *The Free Woman*, pp 426–432. Carnforth: Parthenon Publishing Group.

Savage W (1985) Requests for late termination of pregnancy: Tower Hamlets, 1983. *British Medical Journal* **290**: 621–623.

Simon NM & Senturia AG (1966) Psychiatric sequelae of abortion. *Archives of General Psychiatry* **15**: 378–389.

Simon NM, Rothman D, Goff JT & Senturia A (1969) Psychological factors related to spontaneous and therapeutic abortion. *American Journal of Obstetrics and Gynecology* **104**: 799–806.

Statham H (1987) Cold comfort. *The Guardian* March 24.

Turnbull AC & MacKenzie IZ (1983) Second trimester amniocentesis and termination of pregnancy. *British Medical Bulletin* **39**: 315–321.

Watson JP, Elliott SA, Rugg AJ & Brough DI (1984) Psychiatric disorder in pregnancy and the first postnatal year. *British Journal of Psychiatry* **144**: 453–462.

Wing JK, Cooper JE & Sartorius N (1974) *The Measurement and Classification of Psychiatric Symptoms*. London: Cambridge University Press.

6

Normal emotional changes in pregnancy and the puerperium

MARGARET OATES

Now that maternal death is rare and perinatal death uncommon, pregnant women not only expect that they and their infant should survive childbirth in good condition but also that the experience should be dignified and meaningful. Most women will only have two experiences of childbirth and it needs to be right. The way in which they are treated and the memories of their pregnancies will leave deep impressions for the rest of their life.

The concentration of lay and media attention on delivery and the critical experience of giving birth has tended to detract from the emotional importance of the whole one year of pregnancy and the puerperium. This is a time of extraordinary psychological and physiological change. The experiences and management of pregnancy and the puerperium are just as important and just as critical, perhaps even more so, to the successful adjustment to parenthood and to the physical and emotional well-being of mother and child.

These four trimesters (three of pregnancy, one of the puerperium) represent the greatest transition in a woman's lifetime. They are not only a period of emotional and behavioural change, but also of valid emotional needs and vulnerability. If these changes are not recognized and their needs not met, not only will clinicians have to deal with angry, dissatisfied consumers, but also their patients may at best not enjoy the experience and at worst may suffer from increased physical problems and an increased risk of emotional disorders, either mental illness or difficulties in adjusting to motherhood and relating to their babies.

Familiarity with the range of normal emotional and behavioural changes and the valid psychological needs of women will facilitate appropriate care and also enable a swifter diagnosis of those women who are ill.

It is also important to recognize those women who have special needs, by virtue of their background, their previous problems with reproduction or difficult pregnancies and to meet these special needs.

PREGNANCY AND THE PUERPERIUM AS A TRANSITIONAL PHASE OR TIME OF ADJUSTMENT

First-time pregnancy and childbirth, whether or not the result of conscious planning, is the most momentous change of a lifetime for women and probably for men as well. Nothing will ever be the same again. The nine months of pregnancy can be seen as the transition to parenthood and, together with the three months of the puerperium, as a period of adjustment to the new style of relationships. The relative freedom, independence and personal-centredness of the childless state, and the often intense intimacy of early marriage, becomes irreversibly altered over this period of time. There are now new responsibilities, new constraints and new pressures, and relationships have to expand to include children, with an inevitable dilution of the romantic priority between husband and wife. To add to this there will be a prolonged period of often unaccustomed emotional vulnerability, particularly in women. There are many different models of understanding of the changes and needs that take place during this period; two of the most useful are the psychoanalytical post-Freudian view of pregnancy and the puerperium as a developmental crisis and the socioanthropological view of the same period of time as a rite of passage.

The developmental crisis

Erikson (1950) describes in his essay 'The Eight Ages of Man' the development of the human personality as occurring in stages or milestones, each a developmental crisis. Many of these are associated with physical and physiological change. They begin with birth and end with death and each involves the acquisition of new skills and the transition from one role to a new role with new responsibilities. This is a maturing process; at the end of each developmental stage the person is older and wiser but passes through a phase of emotional turbulence, during which they have emotional needs which must be met and conflicts which must be overcome. During these phases of development there is potential for growth and maturation but the person is also vulnerable. Psychologically one has to walk before one is able to run, and these developmental phases have to be undertaken in the correct sequence; each has to be successfully overcome before the person is equipped to cope with the next.

According to this model, reproduction should take place after the developmental crises of adolescence ('identity versus role confusion') and of independent adult life ('intimacy versus isolation'). This is the phase during which human beings have to come to terms with the inherent conflict involved in being an independent adult who accepts responsibility for their own actions, emotions and achievements and yet, at the same time, is able to form intimate and trusting relationships with other adults, whose needs and attributes are compatible with their own.

Inevitably in the Western world, where the choice of partners is made by individuals, this phase may initially involve a few mistakes. It is only when this phase has been successfully overcome that the human being is ready to move on to the next phase—that involving conflict of 'generativity versus stagnation', during which the human being has the capacity to supply the needs of children, which, initially, requires unconditional loving. This involves loving a child merely because it exists, not because of its behaviour or its achievements, and taking physical and hedonistic pleasure in the existence of the child. This unconditional loving of a child, as opposed to the conditional loving of other adults, is a very mature ability and one which is probably not possible in earlier developmental phases.

Erikson's model allows us to see how difficult it is for human beings to undertake the tasks involved in reproduction 'out of phase'. For example, during the adolescent crisis, the essential tasks of struggling to emerge from childhood and to become an adult are incompatible with parenthood. During the early phase of the 'intimacy versus isolation' crisis of early adult life, the struggles to cope with both independence and intimate relationships are all-consuming and again ill-equip human beings to cope with the demands of very young children. Therefore this model of understanding reveals to us two groups of patients who have special vulnerabilities and special needs: a teenager who is pregnant, or the young adult who is pregnant early on in the relationship or perhaps committed to a relationship by virtue of the fact of pregnancy. According to this model the ideal time to reproduce would be after the establishment of a permanent relationship, when such conflicts had been largely resolved. The model also underlines the importance of earlier experiences in the preparation for parenthood, in particular the most fundamental and earliest developmental crisis, that of infancy, when the basic conflicts between 'trust and mistrust' have to be resolved. This can only be done when the infant is supplied with unconditional loving from its caretakers. Problems arising then, and during the later conflicts of toddlerhood and early childhood which again require secure and loving parenting, reveal for us another vulnerable group of pregnant patients—those who have had damaging experiences in childhood, particularly those of parental deprivation and multiple changes of caretaker, such as occur in unsatisfactory fostering situations.

The model also provides an understanding for the essential emotional turbulence and discomfort, the emotional vulnerability and the need for trusting and supportive relationships from family and friends. According to Erikson and to commonsense, these feelings are an essential part of a human lot and will be experienced whenever a human being is going through a time of major change.

Rite of passage

Erikson's understanding of human development was not only influenced by Freudian developmental psychology, but also by social anthropology from his study of other societies. Societal recognition in the form of ritual prescribed behaviour and the acknowledgement of the needs of the individual accompanies many developmental crises. The survival in Western urbanized society of such rituals may be vestigial or no longer easily recognized as such because they have been taken over by institutions or religions.

Such rituals have an important function in marking the individual going through a period of change (after which he will have a different role personally and in society). They usually involve ceremonies, distinctive dress, feasting and gatherings (e.g. christenings, weddings, funerals), the acceptance and even facilitation of emotional expression (e.g. the same examples), and more importantly the acknowledgement of the reality of the individual's emotional turbulence and distress and the need for social and emotional support for a prescribed period of time (e.g. the formal mourning period of Victorian society and orthodox Judaism). These are most easily seen surviving in Western society in funeral and mourning behaviour. In non-Western and non-urbanized societies, those life changes involving the rite of passage, or transition to a new and larger role within society, also involve the isolation of the individual temporarily and their education by elders (e.g. adolescent rites and childbirth rites).

Most societies, apart from Western urbanized societies, have well-prescribed and documented rituals surrounding childbirth. These usually involve appointed childbirth attendants, and protection and isolation of the new mother and her infant from her immediate society, but in the company of older and experienced women. She is usually given special foods and attentions for a prescribed length of time and there is often a ceremonial re-entry into society. These rituals can be seen to serve the function of protecting the mother/infant pair from infection and hazard, providing a base for the acquisition of skills and self-confidence, and helping and supporting her throughout this period of transition to parenthood. These rituals also acknowledge her valid dependency needs and give her status in her new role.

Although the reader may see some surviving vestiges of these rituals in pregnancy behaviour (e.g. the change of dress) and in obstetric practice (e.g. antenatal clinic attendance, the postnatal check at six weeks) and in other common practices (e.g. christenings), many other essential components of the childbirth rite of passage which are present in other societies have been lost in ours. Of these the most important are the acknowledgement of emotional and dependency needs, the need for con-tinuous social support, the need for an acknowledgement of the changed role within marriage, family and society, and the absence of increased status associated with motherhood. The Trinidadian anthropologist, Professor Fernando Henriques, has suggested that when the accepted expectations of society are at variance with common practice, problems ensue for both the individual and society. The accepted stance of our society is that motherhood is important, the family is the pivot of society, and that children are precious, vulnerable and cherished. For many women, the reality may rather seem as if motherhood detracts from their value as individuals; they may be seen as less reliable employees, motherhood is used as an argument for woman's non-progression in the professions, children are not welcomed in the workplace, restaurants, hotels or shops, and sometimes not even at family gatherings such as weddings. Children are valued if they are quiet and untroublesome, soundly asleep and absent from evening entertainment with friends. Mothers are readily blamed for all problems to do with children but rarely praised if things are going well.

Whereas there is little evidence to suggest that the rates of postnatal mental illness, both minor or major, are less in those societies which have well-prescribed rituals surrounding childbirth, it may be that the transition to parenthood is more satisfying and a little easier in those societies, and that some of the more valuable aspects of the childbirth ritual could protect against postnatal depression and problems with mother/child relationships. Those interested in maternal and infant welfare in the Western world could learn much from studying the practices in other societies.

WOMEN WITH SPECIAL NEEDS

Very young, single and unsupported mothers

Women and their partners who begin parenthood attempting the essential emotional tasks of this phase of their life when their overwhelming personal needs reflect upon an earlier stage of development present with inherent problems and special needs. Deprivation in early childhood, particularly relating to maternal deprivation and rejection, or lack of consistent and stable parenting, such as happens with multiple changes of caretaker, lead the pregnant mother to be emotionally vulnerable. Her own dependency needs and needs for mothering may conflict with her child's needs. It is important that these valid dependency needs are met in order that she should be able to meet the needs of her child. If close caring relationships are not available then professional care may go some way to ameliorate the situation. Continuity of care within the antenatal clinic, with special effort to make time available for information, reassurance and counselling, together with the involvement of social casework where necessary and perhaps, if available, the involvement of a voluntary agency which offers social support and befriending throughout pregnancy, are some measures that may impact upon both maternal and infant psychological and physical well-being (Sokol et al, 1980; Klaus, 1986). These women and their partners may be very young, attempting to escape from their backgrounds and provide a secure emotional base for themselves by early marriage and parenthood, or they may be single and unsupported.

Older mothers

Older mothers who have been married for a long time, may have successful careers and have consciously delayed child-bearing, or have perhaps had fertility problems, or a later marriage with an awareness that the 'biological clock is ticking on' may also have particular problems with their first pregnancy. They may find it difficult to cope with the system of antenatal care and the loss of autonomy and control, and may even appear threatening to staff because of their articulated needs for participation and information.

They may also have over-idealized expectations of pregnancy, labour, breast-feeding and their own coping abilities afterwards. They may be at high risk obstetrically and are vulnerable to disappointment, a sense of failure and guilt if their pregnancies and deliveries are more complicated than they expect. The changes that come about in a marriage that has been consolidated over a period of ten years or more, caused by the impact of a baby on well-established life-styles, may be more difficult than they are for most people. These women and their partners have a particular need for continuity of care, adequate time, information and explanation, and an awareness on the part of the staff of their special needs and circumstances. A sensitive understanding of the difficulties, challenges, satisfactions and advantages of combining career and motherhood, the importance of counselling aimed at realistic expectations and a spirit of co-operative participation should reduce difficulties and make these clients a rewarding group of women to work with.

Previous loss

This group of women includes those who have lost previous pregnancies through termination of pregnancy, miscarriage, fostering/adoption, the death of a baby during pregnancy, the neonatal period or infancy, or the death of a baby who was one of a multiple pregnancy. Their grief may not be properly resolved before conception, and they will inevitably have considerable anxiety that the same thing may happen again. The birth of this baby will inevitably reawaken the experience of the last pregnancy and any unfinished grieving or unresolved conflicts surrounding the previous loss. Obstetricians and midwives should be sensitive early in pregnancy to expressions of emotional distress and anxiety in this group, and allow time for ventilation of these feelings and where appropriate, refer to those who have special expertise in grief counselling. It is particularly important that this group of mothers should be helped before the arrival of the next baby (see Chapter 14).

Precious baby syndrome

In addition to the group of mothers just described, who have experienced loss of previous pregnancies, sometimes multiple loss, there are women who have conceived as a result of infertility programmes, including in vitro fertilization, and who have had particularly hazardous and difficult pregnancies, with high levels of medical attention, sometimes necessitating prolonged periods of admission during pregnancy, multiple investigations, and sustained doubts about the viability or health of the unborn child. Their pregnancies are not relaxed and enjoyable but anxious and highly medicalized, and there may be a prolonged disruption of their normal domestic and social functioning. This group of patients, and their families, have high valid needs of continuity of care, extra time being made available for explanation and reassurance, and the opportunity to ventilate their fears and anxieties. After nine months of high levels of attention and medical care, the birth of a healthy baby can produce a paradoxical let down and feeling of loss, and it is important that this level of care is continued beyond delivery for a while.

Investigative procedures

Many women in these special needs groups, but also less remarkable women as well, undergo investigative procedures such as chorionic villus sampling, amniocentesis, and other investigations and observations because of the suspicion of retarded intrauterine growth. Although these procedures have now become commonplace in obstetrics, they still have the capacity to produce high anxiety levels in patients. Because of the inevitable doubts on behalf of the woman about the viability of her pregnancy until a satisfactory result is obtained (amniocentesis in particular), they may emotionally put the pregnancy 'on hold'. It is therefore essential that sufficient time is made available, before such procedures, to explain exactly what is happening. Distress and anxiety should be acknowledged and validated and opportunity given to ventilate these feelings.

Emergency caesarean section

Women having an emergency caesarean section, often at the end of a period of time in labour, may experience a sense of failure and even anger and resentment at failing to deliver vaginally, particularly if this is their first pregnancy. It is important that such feelings are acknowledged and the opportunity given to ventilate them. It is also important to help the patient understand that not only has she had a baby but also a major abdominal operation, and that her need for rest and her recovery after delivery may be different to those women who have had a vaginal delivery. This understanding may help reduce any additional disappointments in the puerperium.

EMOTIONAL CHANGES DURING PREGNANCY AND THE PUERPERIUM

General

Pregnancy may have less effect on the psychological status of women than is commonly assumed and for most women it is a phase of positive mental health. It is certainly not the case that pregnancy induces a distinctive, particular psychological state in all women (Elliott, 1984). In contrast there is now well-documented evidence of marked changes in women's psychological status following delivery, particularly in the first two weeks—the phenomenon known as 'the blues'. However, although studies measuring orthodox aspects of personality, psychological and emotional functioning produce conflicting evidence of change in women's psychological status during pregnancy, this does not mean that 'nothing is happening'. Most women are aware of the enormity of the change that is about to befall them, and are aware that they are more prone to anxiety and worry and more emotional than they were before the pregnancy. There are inevitable feelings of responsibility, or apprehension, and a sense of embarking upon a voyage into the unknown, with consequent alterations in emotional and cognitive state that change as the pregnancy progresses.

First trimester

The woman is now in a state of 'being pregnant'. Her mood is related to either the joy or upset at being pregnant, and also very much related to how distressing she finds the common problems of fatigue and nausea. Tearfulness and irritability are quite common. For those women who have had a previous miscarriage or a threatened miscarriage in the current pregnancy, it may be a particularly anxious time. It is quite common for women not to 'trust' their pregnancies until they are well established, and to avoid informing other people or making preparations for the birth until they are convinced that the pregnancy is viable.

Second trimester

During this phase of the pregnancy the woman begins to 'expect a baby'. Fetal movements and her visible expansion makes the developing baby an increasing reality. It becomes personalized and many women name and talk to their fetuses and worry about them in a highly personalized way. In general, women feel both physically and emotionally well during this stage of their pregnancy. They have to rely upon professionals and their technology to tell them how their baby is progressing, as most of the complications of pregnancy are symptom-free in the mother. This inevitable reliance upon professionals can bring about a distressing feeling of a loss of personal control, or autonomy, compounded by busy and impersonal antenatal clinics, and rarely seeing the same doctor twice. All women are anxious and worried to a greater or lesser extent about the well-being of their developing fetus. It is important that they should receive adequate information as well as reassurance at all times, but particularly about the purpose and results of investigations no matter how routine they may be to the clinician ordering them. During this stage and continuing throughout the pregnancy and puerperium, women easily become guilty. They are likely to attribute any adverse event in their pregnancy to their own lifestyle, personal habits or emotional state.

Third trimester

During the third trimester, women's coping resources are relatively diminished and they will find it more difficult than normal to manage major upheavals in their family life and events such as moving house. During the last months of pregnancy the anxiety and apprehensions begin to subside. As the survival of the baby becomes assured, she becomes increasingly impatient with the pregnancy and wishes for delivery. Emotionally she slows down, with a tendency to withdraw socially, becoming increasingly pre-occupied with preparing for the baby, although she remains easily moved to tears. During this last month to two weeks, her concentration, recent memory and new learning ability decline slightly and difficulty in sleeping is common. This, together with day-dreaming, an increasing absorption in the forthcoming birth and physical discomfort, may lead to intellectual tasks becoming more difficult. This may be of importance if the woman has high expectations of working in intellectually very demanding positions right up to the point of delivery, or if she intends to undertake difficult tasks during maternity leave.

Libido

Sexual activity and enjoyment usually diminishes during pregnancy. Many men and women are apprehensive about intercourse in the first trimester of pregnancy for fear of miscarriage, and later in pregnancy sexual activity again tends to be avoided partly because it is physically uncomfortable, but often because 'it does not seem right'. However, in the mid-trimester, many couples do engage in some sexual activity. Sometimes a sudden increase in libido occurs towards the end of a pregnancy (see Chapter 7).

Delivery

Women's emotional experiences during childbirth are so varied that it is difficult to make generalized statements. However, no matter how well prepared the woman is, the experience of first delivery must always come as something of a shock. It can take place in the middle of the night, usually in the unfamiliar surroundings of a hospital, and in the company of profes-sionals who the woman will not have met before. No matter how well rehearsed in antenatal classes, the physical sensations of labour are powerful, uncomfortable and strange. All women will be in a high state of arousal and it is very common for women to feel depersonalized (as if it is happening to somebody else) or derealized (in that everything around them seems strange and unfamiliar). They may be successfully coping with the first stage of labour with the help of the exercises they have been taught, only to find the sudden transition from first to second stage produces alarming and unexpected sensations, frequently producing transient episodes of panic and fear of losing control. Unfamiliarity with procedures and the sensations of delivery, together with a fear of the unknown, can lead to high levels of distress in a woman in labour, which can interfere with her management and later with her memories of, and satisfaction with, the experience of childbirth. Of all the factors which impact upon this state, one of the most important would seem to be the continuous presence of a midwife during delivery. Despite the now almost universal practice of the woman's partner, or other relative, being present during delivery, the fear of being left alone during labour is as real as in the past and the continuous social support of a midwife reassuring and explaining is as important as it ever was (Klaus, 1986).

Immediately post-delivery

If all has gone well and a normal, good birth-weight baby has been produced which can be handed to the mother immediately, then the commonest immediate reaction is one of ecstasy and relief. However, any concern whatever for the baby, no matter how trivial, will be extremely alarming to the mother. Her perception of time will be altered so that attention to the infant that lasts only for a few seconds will appear to the mother to be lasting for hours. Those mothers whose infants require resuscitation or transfer to the neonatal unit will be extremely anxious and fearful, and should be given an opportunity to see their baby and handle it as soon as possible, as well as the appropriate reassurance and information about its welfare. Under normal circumstances, with the infant given to the mother as soon as it is born, there is a culture constant pattern of behaviour which involves the mother greeting the baby and engaging in eye-to-eye contact with her infant (Klaus et al, 1975). The baby at this stage is usually awake and relaxed. She begins to explore her baby, peripherally first, but then eventually will unwrap and examine its body. Towards the end of this process the baby may make sucking movements and the mother may indicate that she wishes to suckle her baby. A sensitive attendant will notice the clues and facilitate this process. However, it is important not to rush the mother or to force her to do something which she is not comfortable about. An opportunity to feed the baby after delivery is related to later satisfaction with the baby and ease of feeding. For those women who have decided not to breast-feed, the opportunity to bottle-feed their baby in the delivery suite should be offered (Ball, 1987). This phase, which lasts up to eight hours, is usually terminated by sleep on the part of both mother and infant. Although it is obviously an important and pleasurable time of mother/infant attachment, it is probably not crucial to the human being (Klaus and Kennell, 1982). The majority of mothers deprived of this experience, because of early neonatal separation, make perfectly good attachments to their babies at a later stage and develop close relationships with them. For a minority of women the immediate response to their newborn baby is one of flatness and an absence of emotion and even for an unfortunate few, one of active distaste. Sometimes this is the result of a long and distressing delivery, or the use of analgesia or anaesthetics. Most of these women will gradually settle over the next 24 to 48 hours, and only a very few will have a more prolonged difficulty in establishing a relationship with their newborn child.

The puerperium

Marked emotional changes take place during the puerperium. They occur in the majority of women, although there is a tremendous *variation* in how distressing the experience is. Because it takes between six and twelve weeks for a woman to return to her normal emotional state, the puerperium can justifiably be described as the fourth trimester.

The first three days

This is known as the latent period because functional mental illness very rarely occurs during this time. It is also known as the 'pinks' because the normal state is one of euphoria and optimistic excitement, accompanied by difficulty in sleeping and a feeling of restlessness, unless the woman is uncomfortable because of an operative delivery. There is a danger that she will not take adequate rest and may over-exert herself physically. This is particularly likely to happen with early discharges from hospital and a tendency to minimalize the physical impact of childbirth. Midwives in particular know the value of strong advice given to newly delivered women to rest for periods of time during the day in bed, and to avoid taking up the reins of domestic duties too soon.

Three to ten days—'the blues'

This phenomenon is well known to both the lay public and the medical profession, and is also known as the baby blues or the three-day blues. Reports on its frequency vary from 80% to 15%, according to the symptoms included in the syndrome and their severity. However, most women and clinicians feel that this condition is very common, probably normal, and occurs in the majority of women. Despite the fact that all women are informed about 'the blues' in antenatal classes, it can still come as a great surprise and, although it is a benign and self-limiting condition, its occurrence can still upset and distress the recently delivered woman. 'The blues' can occur at any time between the second and tenth postpartum day, but the commonest day of peak symptom production is day five. The symptoms vary in their intensity and number, but include feelings of anxiety, tearfulness, changeability in mood and emotional turbulence, difficulties in concentration and feeling forgetful and muddled. It is also common for women to feel restless, oversensitive and easily upset and to have difficulty relaxing and sometimes sleeping (Kennerley and Gath, 1986, 1989). During 'the blues' it is easy for small worries to be blown out of proportion and for women to feel temporarily incompetent and inadequate. The tearfulness and emotional lability associated with 'the blues' can be embarrassing. Frequently the emotional turbulence of 'the blues' is compounded by difficulties in establishing breast-feeding. 'The blues' is self-limiting, but the distress can be diminished by physical comfort and reassurance. The associated problems with feeding require supportive and patient expertise, to help the woman develop her own flexible routine and confidence and autonomy with her baby. Some mothers find this easier at home with the help of her community midwife and her family, whilst others prefer to stay in hospital. The length of postpartum stay in hospital should, whenever possible, be tailored to a woman's individual needs and expressed wishes.

One week to three months

During this phase the woman's emotional state gradually returns to normal.

For the majority of women this will be their first ever experience of a newborn child. Its behaviour will be mysterious, unpredictable and confusing. The baby will seem fragile, totally vulnerable and dependent. Most women are therefore easily moved to anxiety and even panic by minor changes in their baby's behaviour. They will worry and feel guilty that they are not doing all that they should. These worries will often be paradoxical—worrying one minute about over-feeding and the next about starving the baby, or worrying why the baby is crying and not sleeping and then finding themselves waking the baby up after it has been asleep for two hours to make sure that it is still alive.

The unfamiliarity of the task and the fear for the safety of the child will be compounded by a lack of sleep. Breast-feeding mothers will suffer from insomnia, i.e. not sleeping for longer than three or four hours at a stretch for anything up to six to eight weeks. They will therefore be tired and will at times experience feelings of great exhaustion which will diminish their normal coping resources.

Most women will experience during this time feelings of great joy and pleasure, sometimes almost frightening in intensity. They will also experience, if only fleetingly, less pleasant feelings. Feelings of anger and frustration and even resentment that no matter what they do the baby is still crying or does not love or appreciate them. These transient unpleasant feelings can be very frightening and can lead a woman to believe that she is deviant or even has the potential to harm her own child.

Some mothers become very distressed by having occasional intrusive vivid thoughts of some harm coming to their baby. These thoughts are obsessional, i.e. unwanted and recognized as being silly, but nonetheless difficult to resist and distressing. Other common obsessional phenomena also occur during the puerperium such as a need to check (often the baby) and feelings of doubt and uncertainty and an inability to make even minor decisions. It is not uncommon for recently delivered mothers to be unusually preoccupied with cleanliness and a routine that she can never quite keep up with. Most new mothers remain easily upset and vulnerable, oversensitive to criticism and easily losing a sense of proportion. They may be prone to occasional feelings of sadness, inadequacy and guilt, particularly when very tired, and may burst into tears for no apparent reason.

In the early weeks, most new mothers feel intensely possessive about their babies and may dislike other people handling them, even their own family members. They will feel very anxious if separated from their baby and will prefer to have the baby within their sight at all times. This intense possessiveness combined with emotional vulnerability and occasional feelings of inadequacy can easily slip into jealousy if other people, like mothers or husbands, appear to be more competent than they. Much is said about husbands feeling left out or jealous of their wife's close relationship with the baby. However, it is equally easy for a husband's new found delight in his offspring to be misunderstood by his emotionally fraught wife who feels jealous (and guilty) that the baby has taken her place in his affections.

For the first four to six weeks after childbirth it is very common for women to continue having difficulty in concentrating and to find intellectual tasks more difficult than usual. This is at least partly caused by sleep disturbance and results in a poor memory and difficulty in making decisions. Again this may be a problem if the woman has expectations of returning to high levels of intellectual functioning within a few weeks of childbirth.

It is common for women to remain preoccupied with thoughts and visual images of the delivery for some weeks after birth and to talk about it at length and in detail. If the experience was disappointing or traumatic the woman may feel angry and cheated and find these emotions very uncomfortable.

It comes as a surprise to many women to realize just how lonely and socially isolated they can feel when alone all day with a much longed for baby. No matter how well loved, babies are not substitutes for adult conversation and company. This loneliness may be particularly difficult for women who have been used to the companionship and intellectual stimulation of a busy career or who are far from their families.

Resolution

This takes place between six and twelve weeks of the birth and usually occurs at about the time the baby becomes more predictable and responsive, allowing some kind of routine and a return to sleeping at night. However, occasional feelings of ambivalence and a sense of loss about the life before the baby, together with tiredness, may continue for some time. Breast-feeding mothers are particularly vulnerable until weaning is introduced. Libido takes some time to return. Sexual activity is not usually resumed before three months postpartum, but a true interest in sexual activity may take considerably longer to return, often well into the second year of the baby's life (see Chapter 7).

SUMMARY

There is tremendous individual variation in the response to the inherent emotional, psychological and cognitive changes that take place during pregnancy and the puerperium, particularly in first-time mothers. Although the psychological changes, particularly in terms of emotional and behavioural changes, have probably been overstated in pregnancy, there are undoubtedly marked changes in such aspects of functioning following delivery. Women should be aware of these changes and be prepared for them, and obstetricians and midwives should incorporate them into their management of patients. All women have valid psychological needs during pregnancy and in the puerperium, and these must be met in order to ensure maternal and infant health and maximum satisfaction with the experience. Antenatal and postnatal care should not result in a struggle for power and control between patient and obstetrician. Emotional reassurance and support can only follow upon adequate information. The best antenatal care and management of delivery requires a spirit of mutual trust and active participation on the part of the patient in the decision-making process. There is ample evidence to support the theory that continuity of care and the continuous supporting role of the midwife, particularly during delivery, exerts a favourable outcome in mothers and children.

REFERENCES

Ball JA (1987) Factors surrounding the mothers' emotional well-being six weeks after the birth. In *Reactions to Motherhood*, pp 77–116. Cambridge: Cambridge University Press.

Elliott SA (1984) Pregnancy and after. In Rachman S (ed.) *Contributions to Medical Psychology*, vol. 3, pp 93–113. Oxford: Pergamon Press.

Erikson EH (1950) Eight ages of man. In *Childhood and Society*, pp 239–266. Penguin Books.

Kennerley H & Gath D (1986) Maternity blues reassessed. *Psychiatric Developments* 1: 1–17.

Kennerley H & Gath D (1989) Maternity blues I. *British Journal of Psychiatry* 155: 356–362.

Klaus MH (1986) *Social support during labour*. Paper presented at Third Biennial Meeting of the Marce Society, Motherhood and Mental Illness, Nottingham.

Klaus MH & Kennell JH (1982) *Parent–Infant Bonding*. St Louis: CV Mosby.

Klaus MH, Trause MA & Kennell JH (1975) Does human maternal behaviour after delivery show a characteristic pattern? *Ciba Foundation Symposium* 33: 69–85.

Sokol RJ, Woolf RB, Rosen MG et al (1980) Risk, antepartum care, and outcome. Impact of a maternity and infant care project. *Obstetrics and Gynecology* 56: 150–156.

7

Sexual behaviour in pregnancy, after childbirth and during breast-feeding

ELIZABETH M. ALDER

Sexual relationships go through many changes throughout marriage when couples adjust to age and changes in circumstances. The transition to parenthood can be thought of as a psychosocial crisis and many authors, both lay and academic, have described the birth of the first child as an event of major social and emotional significance (Cowan and Cowan, 1988). The birth of a new baby is a time for traditional celebration and may be the most significant event in a couple's lives.

Marital satisfaction and parenting

In spite of the attention and approval given by society to new parents, several studies report a decline in marital satisfaction when couples first become parents, and this continues to decline during the child-bearing years. Marital satisfaction may only begin to increase when the children leave home, which suggests that the presence of children has a negative impact. Cowan and Cowan (1988) question the basis for the findings of these studies which often fail to control for differences in the length of the relationship. A number of longitudinal studies report a significant decline in questionnaire ratings of marital satisfaction over time, but there is also continuity in the quality of new parents' marriages (Feldman and Nash, 1984), and the postnatal state of the marriage is closely related to the pre-pregnancy marital state. Awareness of the marital and sexual changes during the child-bearing years may help the clinician to understand the attitudes, emotions and behaviour of couples under their care.

Sexual behaviour during pregnancy and the puerperium

Sexual behaviour, particularly in the primiparous couple, must therefore be seen in the context of a transition to parenthood. Cultural influences on sexual behaviour are considerable at this time. Many societies operate a sexual taboo on sexual relationships during and following pregnancy. Murdock (1967) in an ethnographic survey of 166 societies tested the hypothesis that societies practising animal husbandry and consuming milk would have a shorter postpartum taboo than those not. Non-dairying societies had a postpartum taboo of an average ten months duration, compared with an average of only seven and a half months in dairying societies. In addition, the mean duration was found to be twice as long in polygynous societies as in monogamous societies.

Lactation has been regarded as a natural contraceptive method which allows births to be spaced out by as much as two years. Lactational amenorrhoea has undoubtedly contributed to birth spacing in developing countries, but the effect may be confounded by existing postpartum taboos. Saucier (1972) points out that a postpartum taboo must represent a severe deprivation for the mother and for the men in monogamous societies. He therefore suggests that there must be strong pressures for its maintenance. He assumes that women's sexual interest and desire remain unchanged in the post-partum period, although there is evidence that even in the absence of any traditional sexual taboo in Western society, there may be a decrease in sexual activity and desire.

Method of feeding

The reasons why women choose either to breast-feed or bottle-feed has attracted much attention. In the developing world the manufacturers of infant formula have had much criticism for their promotional methods (Palmer, 1988). While the decision to choose a particular method may not always be seen as the concern of the obstetrician, there may be considerable endocrine and psychosocial implications. In addition to the psychological and social factors which influence sexuality during pregnancy and the puerperium, there are also considerable physical and hormonal changes which are closely related to the method of infant feeding. In particular, the high levels of prolactin in lactating women suppress ovarian oestrogen production, with consequent changes in vaginal lubrication and atrophy of the vaginal epithelium.

It also seems likely that there are hormonal influences on female sexual behaviour (Bancroft, 1989), and it has been argued that there may be a biological basis for postpartum mood change (Stein, 1982). Some of these influences on sexuality during pregnancy and the first postnatal year will be explored in this chapter.

SEXUALITY DURING PREGNANCY

Kinsey et al (1953) offer no data on sexual activity during pregnancy, which is a surprising omission given that a high proportion of their sample were married with families. Psychoanalytic approaches have emphasized the process of pregnancy as a way of maintaining the mother's drive towards motherhood and they stress the importance of motherliness to the development of the child (Sarlin, 1963). This may be difficult to reconcile with the suggestion that mothers are also sexually active and may pose a 'Madonna versus Mistress' conflict for the male partner.

Masters and Johnson (1966) reported on sexual activity during pregnancy in a study based on six women observed in their laboratory and 101 women followed during pregnancy. The six pregnant women showed few differences apart from heightened arousal during the second trimester and a longer resolution phase. In the larger sample most primiparous women reported a decrease in sexual responsiveness and interest during the first trimester, although 57 out of 68 multiparous women reported no change. In the second trimester 82 out of 101 reported an increase in coital frequency and sexual desire, although this decreased in the third trimester.

The mid-trimester rise in sexual activity and interest has been widely quoted since the publication of Masters and Johnson's study. A number of recent studies have been considered in a comprehensive review by Reamy and White (1987). Many of these did not find a mid-trimester rise in sexual activity and interest, but instead reported a linear decline over successive trimesters. Kenny (1973) found in a retrospective study of 33 primiparous women that the majority reported no change in desire, frequency of sexual intercourse, enjoyment or orgasm in the first trimester compared with pre-pregnancy. Frequency, desire and enjoyment fell during the third trimester, although the number of orgasms remained the same, possibly because of the fall in frequency of sexual intercourse which would make it more likely that any one occasion would be orgasmic. In a prospective study, Falicov (1973) interviewed 33 primiparous women throughout pregnancy. Ratings of frequency of sexual activity, sexual desire and eroticism all declined as pregnancy proceeded. There was some increase during the second trimester, but all levels were still below pre-pregnancy levels. Solberg et al (1973) reported the results of a large study of 260 women who were interviewed on the second or third day following delivery, by male medical students, and Tolor and DiGrazia (1976) studied 216 women recruited by physicians in a cross-sectional design across the three trimesters of pregnancy. Both these studies found that there was a general decline in interest, activity and satisfaction as pregnancy progressed. The evidence from these early studies is somewhat conflicting, but it seems reasonable to assume that most women experience a significant decline in sexual activity towards the end of pregnancy for a variety of reasons.

Many of the studies so far described have methodological flaws, e.g. small unrepresentative samples, retrospective data, inadequate baseline data, the use of postal questionnaires and non-standard methods of assessment. It is interesting that these same methodological criticisms have also been made about early studies of postpartum mood change (reviewed by O'Hara and Zekoski, 1988). Changing patterns of sexual behaviour and awareness, in addition to changing advice from obstetricians, may make generalizations from the early studies to the present day difficult. In a large prospective study of a predominantly middle class sample in London, Robson et al (1981) recruited primiparous women early in pregnancy and followed them for up to a year after delivery. They found little overall change in frequency of sexual intercourse in the first trimester, but a significant reduction in the third trimester. Those women who reported deriving little or no pleasure from sex before pregnancy were much more likely to have stopped having intercourse in the first trimester. By the third trimester only 40% said that they found sex enjoyable. Similarly only 26% of the whole sample reported having orgasm during the third trimester. They also found that many subjects reported a higher rate of sexual intercourse during the month before they became pregnant and 95 of the 119 said that they had been actively trying to conceive. The month before conception may not be a useful baseline for subsequent comparisons.

Masturbation

Many of the early studies have concentrated on sexual intercourse and coital orgasm, but many women masturbate and the study by Solberg et al (1973) is one of the few which asked about frequency of masturbation. They found that 50–60% of women who had masturbated in the previous two years abstained during pregnancy. It is possible that women who experience orgasm through masturbation may not report this in response to questions only based on coitus.

Male sexual behaviour during pregnancy

Very little attention has been given to the changes in sexual activity and interest experienced by the future fathers. Christensen and Hertoft (1980) in a small prospective study followed 32 primiparas from six months' gestation to six months following delivery. Like other studies they found that the sexual desire of women decreased during pregnancy and this was also reported by some of the men. Twenty-two per cent reported no sexual desire or a decrease by the third trimester and 38% of couples reported problems of sexuality in the first and second trimesters. Often both partners were dissatisfied with the frequency of sexual activity, the woman because it was too often and the man because it was too seldom! The effect of the partner's pregnancy on the male may vary—some men finding their wives increasingly attractive, while others are fearful of 'hurting' or feeling that the intrauterine presence renders sex 'improper'.

Changes in sexual interests during pregnancy in either or both partners may be interpreted as rejection or loss of affection and open discussion is important to ameliorate such feelings.

SEXUAL BEHAVIOUR AND LATE PREGNANCY

Although there may be no traditional sexual taboos during pregnancy, many women (and their partners) may be afraid that sexual intercourse towards the end of pregnancy will harm their baby. In the study by Masters and Johnson (1966) many women had been advised by their physicians to avoid intercourse at some time during pregnancy, but only 21 out of 71 husbands stated that they understood, agreed with or honoured the prohibition. It has been thought that intercourse with or without orgasm could precipitate labour. In a fascinating study, Zlatnik and Burmeister (1982) studied the timing of the previous occasion of sexual intercourse before delivery in relation to a number of outcome variables. Four hundred and thirteen women were interviewed on the first or second postpartum day to verify their medical records. Two thirds of this sample of mainly married and multiparous women had had intercourse within seven days of delivery and 23% had experienced orgasm. The timing of the last occasion of sexual intercourse and orgasm was not related to marital status or parity. However, there was a trend for more orgasm to be reported with more years of formal education. There was more reported orgasm in the absence of intercourse and less intercourse without orgasm in patients with more formal education. No relationships were found between pregnancy complications and the time of the previous intercourse in relation to the length of gestation. The authors admit that differential over- or under-reporting relative to educational level could be one explanation, but suggest that a more likely explanation might lie in the sexual relationship of the couple. More highly educated women may be more likely to have an equal sexual relationship with their partners and be more willing to participate in sexual behaviour. It is interesting to speculate that with changing patterns of sexual relationships, the future trend may be for more couples to continue with sexual activity for longer during pregnancy.

Adverse consequences

Naeye (1979) found increased placental contamination in patients who had coitus once a week or more compared with those who had none. However, there may have been changes over time, or differences in the reliability of data collection. Two other studies found no evidence of higher incidence of orgasm in late pregnancy in women who delivered prematurely (Solberg et al, 1973; Rayburn and Wilson, 1980). Zlatnik and Burmeister (1982) conclude that intercourse, orgasm or both need not be interdicted in late pregnancy for the majority of obstetric patients. Sexual activity does result in uterine contractions and so restrictions might be considered in those for whom premature labour is a threat. It seems likely that the sexual desire of most women has already declined by the last few weeks of pregnancy, but for those who are still sexually active there seems little evidence to advise against it unless there are strong contraindications.

SEXUAL BEHAVIOUR IN THE FIRST POSTNATAL YEAR

The women in Masters and Johnson's (1966) study showed a wide range of sexual behaviour patterns. Some returned to pre-pregnancy levels within a few weeks, while others were still not sexually interested three months after delivery. The majority had resumed sexual intercourse by six to eight weeks after delivery. Two later studies reported an increase in sexual desire following childbirth. Kenny (1973) in a study of a sample of 33 women found that sexual desire increased in 30%, decreased in 11% and remained unchanged in 52%. Tolor and DiGrazia (1976) reported that at the six weeks postnatal check-up, 69% had had intercourse twice a week or more and 35%

more than four times a week. Of the total sample, 31% said they would prefer to have sexual intercourse more often.

The findings of Jacobsen et al (1967) contrast with these results. In this large Swedish study they reported a much slower return to sexual activity. Ten per cent had not resumed sexual intercourse by three months postpartum. Falicov (1973) found that two thirds of her small sample of 19 resumed sexual intercourse within two months of childbirth. Five women reported increased capacity for eroticism, but half the sexually active women reported reduced coital frequency. Reasons given included delay to post-partum check-up, tender episiotomy site, fatigue, lack of time and lack of inclination. A small prospective study (Lumley, 1978) used trained women interviewers to collect data from a sample of 26 women and 20 husbands. Half of the couples said they had less sexual intercourse at three months, although enjoyment of sex and sexual feelings were reported as being as great (61%) or greater (23%) than before pregnancy. Robson et al (1981) in their prospective study found that one third had resumed intercourse by the sixth week following delivery and nearly all by the twelfth week. However, at 12 weeks postpartum, 57% reported that their sexual desire was reduced compared with pre-pregnancy levels, 33% reported no change and 10% an increase. A more recent study by Grudzinkas and Atkinson (1984) found that 50% had resumed coitus by the time of interview at about six weeks.

Overall the more recent studies which were prospective and had large samples showed a reduction in sexual activity during pregnancy and a slow return to pre-pregnancy levels during the first postnatal year.

There is thus considerable variation in sexual behaviour in the puerperium judging from the results of these studies. The pattern of sexual behaviour may have changed over the last 20 years but so has some obstetric practice. Some women may be told or believe that they should not have sexual intercourse until after the first postnatal check-up, which is usually performed six weeks after delivery.

Factors influencing sexual behaviour

Perineal pain

Fear of physical harm has been reported in a number of studies (Kenny, 1973; Lumley, 1978; Hames, 1980; Grudzinkas and Atkinson, 1984), and soreness at the episiotomy site may be common. In a study by Reading (1982), 60 out of 68 patients reported dyspareunia at three months postpartum, and most attributed this to the midline episiotomy. Robson et al (1981) reported that 40% had soreness and dyspareunia at three months and this could give rise to secondary vaginismus.

Contraception

Fear of another pregnancy may deter couples from resuming intercourse, but surprisingly most of these studies did not ask about contraception (e.g.

Kenny, 1973; Falicov, 1973; Tolor and DiGrazia, 1976; Robson et al, 1981). Contraception is not considered in the major review of sexual behaviour in the puerperium by Reamy and White (1987).

Contraceptive use in the year following delivery was investigated in a study of 317 women who left hospital breast-feeding (Dewart P. and Alder E.M., unpublished data). Eighty-five per cent completed a questionnaire on feeding patterns and contraceptive use. Over half (56%) of the mothers were still breast-feeding at four months after delivery. Forty-four per cent used the progesterone pill while breastfeeding and 29% used sheaths (Table 1). Most women who used the combined pill before pregnancy used the progesterone pill while breast-feeding, and then returned to the combined pill after weaning. Lumley (1978) considered that fear of pregnancy was an unlikely contributory factor in deterring sexual intercourse because her patients were offered a choice of contraceptive methods at the postnatal visit and three quarters of those still reporting pain were using a 'reliable contraceptive', although details were not given. Women who bottle-feed their

Table 1. Contraception and breastfeeding ($n = 269$).

Method	While breastfeeding		While not breastfeeding	
	n	%	n	%
Progesterone only pill	124	46	22	8
Combined pill	0	0	118	44
Sheath	78	29	49	18
Diaphragm	13	5	24	9
Intrauterine device	11	4	24	9
Other	43	16	32	12

babies are likely to ovulate about six to eight weeks following delivery and therefore the choice of contraceptive method becomes more relevant. In our studies of primiparous lactating women, many reported little concern about the timing of the next pregnancy, because they were already committed to child-bearing.

Changes in body image

Changes in body image have also been suggested as a factor that could influence postpartum sexuality. Concerns about vaginal changes were reported by Falicov (1973), but she also suggested that for some women the period of pregnancy seemed to 'aid in shedding traces of one's timidity in relation to bodily functions'. One of our primiparous subjects described how the experience of obstetric care during pregnancy and delivery meant that she had 'no shame left'. There are variable changes in shape and size of breasts during pregnancy and lactation and this may concern some women or their partners (Masters and Johnson, 1966). Hughes (1984) found no difference in scores on a scale of satisfaction with body image between mothers who breast-fed for at least four weeks compared with those who bottle-fed.

Fatigue

Fatigue has been mentioned in very few studies. There are no studies which have looked directly at fatigue in relation to sexual behaviour and, like contraception, it is not considered as a variable by Reamy and White (1987). Many couples with new babies have their sleep disrupted during the night. We studied 25 women who kept records of feeding patterns and sexual behaviour for 24 weeks following delivery (Alder and Bancroft, 1983). Nineteen babies were breast-fed for at least six weeks. Nine still woke for night feeds at 24 weeks of age. These babies were fed more frequently than those whose babies were not waking, and their mothers took longer to resume intercourse. However, we do not know whether couples who wish to resume sexual activity are more likely to encourage their babies to sleep through the night or whether sleeping babies encourage the resumption of sexual activity. None of these babies slept regularly in the parents' bed and none of the women said they would be comfortable having sexual intercourse in the presence of the baby.

Reported fatigue and reduced sexual activity may be either a symptom or a cause of depressive mood in lactating woman and a close relationship between sleep patterns, mood state and sexual activity would be expected, although this has not been carefully investigated. It is interesting that the study by Lumley (1978), which used data from interviews by married parous women rather than male medical students, considered both contraception and fatigue as possible factors. The reasons most frequently given for avoidance or dislike of sexual intercourse in this study were pain and tenderness in the episiotomy scar, and fatigue.

Breast-feeding

Breast-feeding is very important in the understanding of sexual behaviour in the puerperium for a variety of reasons. Breast-feeding may stimulate sensual feelings in the mother and in the infant. Newton (1973) describes this as an essential part of the mother–infant bonding process and the importance of the nipple and oral satisfaction has been stressed by psychoanalysts (e.g. Sarlin, 1963). Breast-feeding may also have parallels with parturition and coitus (Newton, 1973). Newton (1973) suggests that there is a close relationship between lactation and coitus in terms of the uterine contractions and nipple erection which occur both during suckling and during sexual excitement. Both coitus and lactation are accompanied by breast and nipple play and during sexual stimulation there are comparable skin changes.

The research literature on the association of breast-feeding and sexual activity gives conflicting results. Many of the early studies so far described did not consider lactation as a variable and breast-feeding is rarely adequately defined. A description of a woman as breast-feeding may mean that she always breast-fed, she breast-fed on leaving hospital, she breast-fed with formula supplementation or that she also gave solid food. Breast-feeding can be on demand or to a schedule; it can mean one evening feed or eight times during the day or night. If the extent of breast-feeding is not defined it makes it very difficult to assess the impact on sexual behaviour. In the widely reported study by Masters and Johnson (1966), 24 women breast-fed for at least two months. All of these reported significantly higher levels of sexual tension compared with their non-pregnant state and expressed a desire for rapid return to sexual activity. There are difficulties in generalizing from this study. The extent of breast-feeding was not fully described, the sample may have been highly selected, and women who chose to breast-feed in 1966 may not be representative of those breast-feeding in the 1980s. However, the findings of this study have been widely incorporated into books of advice about breast-feeding which suggest that breast-feeding mothers will have more sexual interest than bottle-feeders (e.g. Stanway and Stanway, 1983). Kenny (1973) found that three quarters of the sample thought that breast-feeding had little effect on their sex lives, but several women reported less desire during the first few postnatal months and more desire later on. However, details of breast-feeding in terms of number of feeds, night waking and supplementation were not given. Negative changes while breast-feeding have also been reported (Baxter, 1974; Grudzinkas and Atkinson, 1984). Robson et al (1981) found no relationship between frequency of intercourse or enjoyment of sex and whether or not the mother was breast-feeding at 12, 26 or 52 weeks postpartum. Post and Singer (1983) comment that much research in this area is characterized by deficiences in both design and sampling techniques and conclusions are difficult to draw.

Breast sensitivity has been reported to increase around childbirth (Robinson and Short, 1977), but there have been no controlled prospective studies of changes in nipple sensitivity during successive months of lactation. Fondling and caressing of breasts during sexual foreplay was reported by the majority of couples in the Kinsey Report (Kinsey et al, 1953) and there seems no reason to suppose this to have changed. Sexual excitement can lead to the let-down reflex. In our research studies, some women described how tender nipples and the fear of leaking milk inhibited breast and nipple stimulation during sexual foreplay. Hames (1980) found that 20% of a sample of 42 lactating women experienced sexual inhibition associated with breast tenderness and fear of milk leakage, although 12% were more sexually aroused. Some husbands (19%) were more likely to report sexual enhancement because of increased breast size, but 60% reported no effect. Nipple problems are very common and pain from sore nipples can be excruciating (Drewett et al, 1987).

Masters and Johnson (1966) reported sexual arousal to plateau levels in lactating mothers while suckling, including three to orgasm. In our study of 23 lactating women (Alder et al, 1986), only three (15%) reported any sexual feelings, although the majority found breast-feeding pleasurable. Nearly all (85%) had experienced uterine contractions while suckling their babies. These women all kept detailed weekly diaries of their sexual behaviour and it is unlikely that they would have consciously concealed sexual feelings if they had occurred. There was no difference in ratings between mothers of male or female babies. None of the mothers reported the penile erections in male babies described by Newton (1973) and the question provoked much amusement.

There is one study which looked specifically at breast-feeding and sexual response (Kayner and Zagar, 1983). Their sample was made up of 121 lactating women who had attended a conference on breast-feeding. They completed a questionnaire (48% response rate) asking for demographic details, feeding patterns, sexual behaviour and menstrual history. Nearly half (48%) of the sample slept with the child in the bed where it was allowed to nurse at will. Forty-three lactating women who were amenorrhoeic were compared with 48 who were menstruating. Twenty-three per cent of amenorrhoeics said their sexual response was greater before pregnancy compared with only 9% of menstruating women. Sexual desire was no different, but more amenorrhoeic lactaters rated their pre-pregnancy sexual relations as preferable to their most recent sexual relations. Significantly more amenorrhoeic women reported vaginal dryness than menstruating women. The sample was highly selected but there is no reason to suppose that this would bias the reports of menstruating or non-menstruating women.

The evidence for a direct effect of breast-feeding on sexual behaviour is conflicting. There is no doubt that breast-feeding on demand can be very fatiguing. However, the intense satisfaction experienced by many mothers may increase feelings of well-being. The prolonged hypo-oestrogenized state may contribute to painful intercourse and mothers (and their partners) may not be prepared for this, causing potential problems.

Postnatal hormonal changes

Hormone changes begin from the moment of implantation and continue for as long as the woman lactates. Towards the end of pregnancy there is an increase in the secretion of prolactin from the anterior pituitary and a few weeks before delivery oestradiol levels rise and progesterone levels fall. When the progesterone levels fall after delivery, prolactin stimulates milk secretion from the mammary glands. The production of prolactin is maintained by the suckling of the infant and oxytocin release allows milk to be ejected. In the non-lactating woman there is no suckling stimulus and the prolactin levels decrease, leading to resumption of ovarian activity.

It is often suggested that hormones are the cause of emotional changes after childbirth, and there has been much controversy over the importance of the influence of hormones in changes in mental state (George and Sandler, 1988). The sudden fall in progesterone has been suggested as a cause of mood change (Dalton, 1980). This was not confirmed by Nott et al (1976), who found only weak correlations between mood and hormone variables and because of the large number of comparisons these could be due to chance. Neither Kuevi et al (1983) or Metz et al (1983) found any difference in progesterone levels in those with or without postpartum mood disturbance. The role of prolactin has been shown to be related to maternal behaviour in the rat and is also of interest because of its relationship with dopamine metabolism (see Chapter 10). Prolactin is sometimes called the stress hormone because it is very susceptible to external influences. Ambulation, suckling and even anxiety at having a blood sample taken can all elevate prolactin levels. In lactating women there is a surge of prolactin after each breast-feed, so blood samples must be taken at least two hours after the last breast-feed; however, in many studies the timing of the sample is not given (Nott et al, 1976; Kuevi, 1983). There are a number of studies that have failed to find the expected association between prolactin levels and behaviour (Mathew et al, 1979; Nesse et al, 1980; Alder et al, 1986). Women who breast-feed frequently have higher levels of prolactin than those who reduce their suckling time (Howie and McNeilly, 1982). However, frequent suckling may also mean that the mother feels very tired, and this may be more important than the effects of increased prolactin.

Although there has been considerable interest in the hormonal basis of postnatal mood change, there has been little research on the hormonal basis of sexual interest and behaviour. The raised prolactin levels in lactating women inhibit the negative feedback of oestrogen on the hypothalamus, and ovulation is then inhibited because of the loss of luteinizing hormone pulsatile secretion from the pituitary. Oestradiol production is then suppressed as long as the prolactin levels are maintained by frequent suckling. Reamy and White (1987) do not discuss the implications of oestrogen deprivation apart from suggesting the use of lubricants. There are many studies of sexual problems in the perimenopause related to oestrogen deficiency (Chakravati et al, 1979) and, as we have seen, the lactating amenorrhoeic woman is endocrinologically similar to the postmenopausal woman.

Breast-feeding and hormones

The physiological and behavioural correlates of lactation in relation to sexual activity and interest have been the focus of a number of research studies (Alder and Bancroft, 1983, 1988; Alder et al, 1986). We found indirect evidence of a relationship between breast-feeding and depression from a follow-up study of a group of 103 mothers who had been studied before and after delivery (Cox et al, 1982; Alder and Cox 1983). Eighty-nine (85%) responded to a postal questionnaire sent 18 months after delivery. Women who breast-fed fully for at least 12 weeks and who had not given solids or regular milk supplements were described as total breast-feeders and were compared with those who had breast-fed but had introduced solid food or supplements before 12 weeks (partial feeders). More total feeders than partial feeders reported depressive symptoms and this difference reached statistical significance for non-pill users. Overall the group least likely to have depressive symptoms were the most likely to have returned to normal endogenous ovarian cycles, i.e. non-pill-taking partial breast-feeders. The total breast-feeders, who would have had high prolactin levels and low oestrogen levels, were the most depressed. This study relied on retrospective data and we did not measure hormone status. There could also be psychosocial explanations for the difference between the different feeding groups.

In a more intensive and, of necessity, smaller study we measured hormone levels and mood change in a group of 25 primiparous women for six months after delivery (Alder et al, 1986). Mood changes were measured by visual analogue scales and showed no correlation with levels of prolactin, oestrogen, progesterone or the timing of ovarian activity. The women also kept detailed diaries of their sexual behaviour (Alder and Bancroft, 1983) and were interviewed at 12 and 24 weeks after delivery. Fourteen of the 19 breast-feeders reported a reduction in sexual interest at the 12 week interview and for five of them the reduction was severe. When the androgen levels of the non-pill-taking lactating women were measured, the five with severe loss of sexual interest had significantly lower levels of androstenedione and testosterone than those whose sexual interest was not severely reduced (Alder et al, 1986). This suggested that there was no simple hormonal relationship with mood change but that sexual interest might be related to androgen levels, and there is other evidence for this (Bancroft, 1986). If there is a relationship between hormones and changes in mood or sexuality then the relationship must be very complex. There may also be a tendency for some women with an external locus of control to attribute their emotional changes to hormone changes. We are investigating this in a current study of oestrogen replacement therapy.

Breast-feeding persistence

Rates of breast-feeding duration or persistence vary across cultures and across socioeconomic groups within a culture (Jelliffe, 1976). There have been numerous studies which have sought to identify the reasons why women choose to breast-feed or bottle-feed or, having begun to breast-feed, choose to give up. Post and Singer (1983) review some of the evidence for influences on breast-feeding, including psychodynamic factors, the influence of significant others, personality differences and attitudes, and postnatal support. While they were impressed with the amount of advice and information available for physicians, nurses and expectant mothers, they found the research evidence was relatively inconsistent. Evidence can be found for all the factors discussed by Post and Singer (1983), but it is often weak and subject to methodological problems. However, a few findings are consistently reported. In Western industrial societies socioeconomic status is closely linked to breast-feeding (Martin and Monk, 1982; Martin and White, 1988). Many studies which compare breast-fed and bottle-fed infants are con-founded by the influence of socioeconomic status; these issues are clearly reviewed by Sauls (1979). Key attitudes have been found concerning breast-feeding within American ethnic groups (Baranowski et al, 1986). They identified four attitudinal factors which they called benefits for the infant, social inconvenience, personal inconvenience and physical inconvenience–medical benefit to infant. Attitudes predicted behaviour most in Anglo-American mothers. Multivarate statistical techniques are needed to predict length of breast-feeding persistence, and Quandt (1985) identified feeding style and maternal education as predictors. The most recent report of feeding practice in the United Kingdom (Martin and White, 1988) found that 40% of breast-feeding mothers had discontinued by six weeks. Women who do not attempt to breast-feed or who give up soon after leaving hospital tend to be young, single, smokers and to be from lower socioeconomic groups. It has been suggested that it is not only the social or demographic variables or attitudes that influence breast-feeding duration, but also the practical problems which arise when faced with the realities of breast-feeding (Alder, 1989). For many young mothers the problems associated with being too shy to feed in public, frequent and unpredictible feeds, feeling tied to the house and general fatigue may outweigh the advantages of breast-feeding.

Breast-feeding persistence and sexual behaviour

It is possible that women who persist with breast-feeding may be different in their sexuality from those who bottle-feed from birth or who wean early. If this is so then it is not necessarily the different hormonal profiles that are important but the psychosocial characteristics of the women themselves. If, for instance, women who go on to breast-feed are more sexually active, more orgasmic or more interested in sex than those who go on to bottle-feed, then any postnatal differences such as those found by Masters and Johnson (1966) could be because of existing differences. If, on the other hand, we find that there are no antenatal differences or that they are in the opposite direction from postnatal differences, then we can look more closely for postnatal factors which could account for the differences. A prospective study was designed to answer this question (Alder and Bancroft, 1988). Ninety-one primiparous women were assessed early in pregnancy and again at three and six months postpartum. Women who persisted in exclusively breast-feeding were more likely to be from higher socioeconomic groups, which was an entirely predictable, previously reported finding (Martin and White, 1988). They were also more likely to report an episode of being 'happy' in the previous year, and scored lower on the neuroticism scale of the Eysenck Personality Inventory (EPI) (Eysenck and Eysenck, 1975). Neither of these two differences was associated with socioeconomic status, and none of these factors should have any adverse effects in the puerperium. None of the subscales of the Sexuality Experience Scale (Frenkin and Vennix, 1981) revealed any significant differences between mothers who either went on to breast-feed fully or to bottle-feed. At the postnatal follow-up at 12 weeks we found small but consistent differences between breast- and bottle-feeders. Breast-feeders were slower to resume sexual intercourse, they experienced more pain with intercourse and were more likely to report marked reduction of sexual interest and enjoyment compared with bottle-feeders. This negative relationship with breast-feeding confirms the findings of Kayner and Zagar (1983). The pain experienced during intercourse is likely to be related to the hypo-oestrogenized vagina, and anticipation of pain could inhibit sexual arousal.

Conclusions

We still do not understand the relative importance of social and endocrine factors in determining postnatal changes. The hormonal effect could be acting directly on the central nervous system or on the receptors (Deakin, 1988). There could also be peripheral effects resulting from changes in the vaginal epithelium. However, endocrine factors could be unimportant compared with the psychological and behavioural differences between breast- and bottle-feeders. Wright et al (1983) found that breast-fed babies were more likely to wake up in the night than bottle-fed babies, and this was independent of social class. The average age at which night feeding stopped was 10 weeks for bottle-fed babies and 16 weeks for breast-fed babies. Prolonged night waking could simply increase fatigue but it could also increase the worry that sexual activity might be interrupted. A higher proportion of breast-fed babies were still waking in the night at three years of age, so there could be long-term implications.

A further possibility is that breast-feeding women may somehow differ from bottle-feeding mothers in their relationship with their baby, but as we have seen there are enormous methodological problems in trying to disentangle the factors. The difficulty from the researcher's point of view is that babies cannot be allocated at random to be either breast- or bottle-fed. Although breast-fed babies can change at three months to become bottle-fed, bottle-fed babies cannot become breast-fed at three months, so a cross-over design is not possible. These methodological difficulties have made many studies difficult to interpret. Large samples and regression analyses are essential to understand the relationship of breast-feeding to mood, sexual behaviour or morbidity. Clinical experience often suggests that sexual problems first appear in the year following the birth of the first child. More knowledge and understanding of the changes in sexual behaviour in the puerperium might help to avoid these problems later in life.

SUMMARY

Sexual and marital relationships change throughout marriage and the transition to parenthood can be seen as a psychosocial crisis. Recent studies do not support the finding of Masters and Johnson (1966) that there is a mid-trimester rise in sexual responsiveness. Sexual behaviour decreases towards the end of pregnancy and a number of studies have found that in the majority of mothers there is only a slow return to pre-pregnancy levels in the first postnatal year. Some of the factors influencing the rate of return are discussed. Breast-feeding is important because of the hormonal changes it produces and it has been said to stimulate sexual feelings in both mother and baby. There is some evidence that breast-feeding has an adverse effect on sexuality in the first postnatal year. It is not clear whether this could be related to differences in hormone levels or differences in feeding behaviour. Fatigue and contraception have largely been ignored in studies of factors influencing postnatal sexual behaviour. Women who went on to breast-feed were found to be very similar on antenatal measures of sexual behaviour to those who went on to bottle-feed. The method of feeding is the major influence on the hormonal status, and the experience of painful intercourse reported by breast-feeding mothers may be related to low oestrogen levels. Breast-feeding persistence is influenced by both social and psychological factors and its effect on sexual behaviour is discussed.

REFERENCES

Alder E (1989) Why do not all mothers breastfeed? In van Hall EV & Everaerd W (eds) *The Free Woman. Women's Health in the 1990's*. Carnforth: Parthenon.

Alder E & Bancroft J (1983) Sexual behaviour of lactating women: a preliminary communication. *Journal of Reproductive and Infant Psychology* **1**: 47–52.

Alder E & Bancroft J (1988) The relationship between breastfeeding persistence, sexuality and mood in post partum women. *Psychological Medicine* **18**: 389–396.

Alder EM & Cox JL (1983) Breastfeeding and post natal depression. *Journal of Psychosomatic Research* **27**: 139–144.

Alder EM, Cook A, Davidson D, West C & Bancroft J (1986) Hormones, mood and sexuality in lactating women. *British Journal of Psychiatry* **148**: 74–79.

Bancroft J (1986) The role of hormones in female sexuality. In Dennerstein L & Fraser I (eds) *Hormones and Behaviour*, pp 551–560. Amsterdam: Elsevier.

Bancroft J (1989) *Human Sexuality and its Problems*, 2nd edn. Edinburgh: Churchill Livingstone.

Baranowski T, Rossin DK, Richardson JC, Brown JD & Bee DE (1986) Attitudes towards breastfeeding. *Journal of Developmental and Behavioral Paediatrics* **7**: 367–372.

Baxter S (1974) Labour and orgasm in Primiparae. *Journal of Psychosomatic Research* **18**: 209–216.

Christensen E & Hertoft P (1980) Sexual activity and attitude during pregnancy and the post partum period. In Forelo R & Pasini W (eds) *Medical Sexology*. PSG Publishing Company.

Cowan PA & Cowan CP (1988) Changes in marrige during the transition to parenthood: must we blame the baby? In Michaels GY & Goldberg WA (eds) *Transition to Parenthood*, pp 114–154. Cambridge: Cambridge University Press.

Cox JL, Connor V & Kendell RE (1982) Prospective study of the psychiatric disorders of childbirth. *British Journal of Psychiatry* **140**: 111–117.

Dalton K (1980) *Depression after Childbirth*, pp 357–364. Oxford: Oxford University Press.

Deakin JFW (1988) Relevance of hormone-CNS interactions to psychological changes in the puerperium. In Kumar R and Brockington IF (eds) *Motherhood and Mental Illness 2*, pp 113–132. London: Wright.

Drewett RF, Kahn H, Parkhurst S & Whiteley S (1987) Pain during breastfeeding: the first three months post partum. *Journal of Reproductive and Infant Psychology* **5**: 183–186.

Eysenck HJ & Eysenck SGB (1975) *Manual of the Eysenck Personality Inventory*. London: Hodder & Stoughton.

Falicov CJ (1973) Sexual adjustment during first pregnancy and post partum. *American Journal of Obstetrics and Gynecology* **117**: 991–1000.

Feldman SS & Nash SC (1984) The transition from expectancy to parenthood: impact of the first born child on men and women. *Sex Roles* **11**: 84–96.

Frenkin J & Vennix P (1981) *SES manual*. Amsterdam: Swets and Zeitlinger BV.

George A & Sandler M (1988) Endocrine and biochemical studies in puerperal disorders In Kumar R & Brockington IF (eds) *Motherhood and Mental Illness 2*, pp 78–112. London: Wright.

Goldberg W (1988) Perspectives on the transition to parenthood. In Michaels GY & Goldberg W (eds) *Transition to Parenthood*, pp 1–19. Cambridge: Cambridge University Press.

Grudzinkas JG & Atkinson L (1984) Sexual function during the puerperium. *Archives of Sexual Behavior* **13**: 85–91.

Hames CT (1980) Sexual needs and interests of postpartum couples. *JOGN Nursing* **9**: 313.

Howie PW & McNeilly AS (1982) Effect of breast-feeding patterns on human birth intervals. *Journal of Reproduction and Fertility* **65**: 545–557.

Hughes RB (1984) Satisfaction with one's body and success in breastfeeding. *Issues in Comprehensive Pediatric Nursing* **7**: 141–146.

Jacobson L, Kaij L & Nilsson A (1967) The course and outcome of the postpartum period from a gynaecological and general somatic standpoint. *Acta Obstetrica et Gynecologica Scandinavica* **46**: 183–203.

Jelliffe DB (1976) Community and sociopolitical considerations of breastfeeding. *Ciba Foundation Symposium* **45**: 231–255.

Kayner CE and Zagar JA (1983) Breast-feeding and sexual response *Journal of Family Practice* **17** (1): 69–73.

Kenny JA (1973) Sexuality of pregnant and breastfeeding women. *Archives of Sexual Behavior* **2:** 215–229.

Kinsey A, Pomeroy W, Martin C & Gebhard P (1953) *Sexual Behaviour in the Human Female.* Philadelphia: WB Saunders.

Kuevi V, Lawson R, Dixson AF et al (1983) Plasma amine and hormone changes in post partum blues. *Clinical Endocrinology* **19:** 39–46.

Lumley J (1978) *Australian and New Zealand Journal of Obstetrics and Gynaecology* **18:** 114–117.

Martin J & Monk J (1982) *Infant Feeding in the 80s.* London: HMSO.

Martin J & White A (1988) *Infant Feeding in 1985.* London: HMSO.

Masters WH & Johnson VE (1966) *Human Sexual Response.* Boston: Little, Brown.

Mathew RJ, Ho BT, Krakik P & Claghorn JL (1979) Anxiety and serum prolactin. *American Journal of Psychiatry* **136:** 1322–1326.

Metz A, Stump K, Cowan PJ, Elliott JM, Gelder MG & Grahame-Smith DG (1983) Changes in platelet alpha 2-adrenoceptor binding postpartum: possible relation to maternity blues. *Lancet* **i:** 495–498.

Murdock GP (1967) Post partum sex taboos. *Paedeuma* **13:** 143–147.

Naeye RL (1979) Coitus and associated amniotic fluid infections. *New England Journal of Medicine* **301:** 1198.

Nesse RM, Curtiss GC, Brown GM & Rubin RT (1980) Anxiety induced by flooding therapy for phobia does not elicit prolactin secretory response. *Psychosomatic Medicine* **42:** 25–31.

Newton N (1973) Interrelationships between sexual responsiveness, birth and breastfeeding. In Zubin J & Money J (eds) *Contemporary Sexual Behavior*, pp 77–98. Baltimore: John Hopkins University Press.

Nott PN, Franklin M, Armitage C & Gelder MG (1976) Hormonal changes and mood in the puerperium. *British Journal of Psychiatry* **122:** 431–433.

O'Hara MW & Zekoski EM (1988) Post partum depression: a comprehensive review. In Kumar R & Brockington IF (eds) *Motherhood and Mental Illness 2*, pp 17–63. London: Wright.

Palmer GK (1988) *The Politics of Breastfeeding.* London: Pandora Press.

Post RD & Singer R (1983) Psychological implications of breastfeeding for the mother. In Neville MC & Neifert MR (eds) *Lactation. Physiology, Nutrition and Breastfeeding*, pp 349–365. New York: Plenum Press.

Quandt S (1985) Ecological and behavioural predictors of exclusive breastfeeding duration. *Medical Anthropology* **9:** 139–151.

Rayburn WF & Wilson EA (1980) Coital activity and premature delivery. *American Journal of Obstetrics and Gynecology* **134:** 972.

Reading AE (1982) How women view post episiotomy pain. *British Medical Journal* **284:** 28.

Reamy KJ & White SE (1987) Sexuality in the puerperium: a review. *Archives of Sexual Behavior* **16:** 165–186.

Robinson JE & Short RV (1977) Changes in breast sensitivity at puberty, during the menstrual cycle and at parturition. *British Medical Journal* **1:** 1188–1191.

Robson KM, Brant HA & Kumar R (1981) Maternal sexuality during first pregnancy and after child birth. *British Journal of Obstetrics and Gynaecology* **88:** 882–889.

Sarlin CN (1963) Feminine identity. *Journal of the American Psychoanalytic Association* **11:** 790.

Saucier JF (1972) Correlates of the long post partum taboo: a cross cultural study. *Current Anthropology* **13:** 238–249.

Sauls HS (1979) Potential effect of demographic and other variables in studies comparing morbidity of breast-fed and bottle fed infants. *Pediatrics* **64:** 523–527.

Solberg DA, Butler J & Wagner N (1973) Sexual behavior in pregnancy. *New England Journal of Medicine* **288:** 1089–1103.

Stanway P & Stanway A (1983) *Breast is Best.* London: Pan.

Stein G (1982) The maternity blues. In Brockington IF & Kumar R (eds) *Motherhood and Mental Illness.* London: Academic Press.

Tolor A & DiGrazia PV (1976) Sexual attitudes and behavior patterns during and following pregnancy. *Archives of Sexual Behavior* **5:** 539–551.
Zlatnik F & Burmeister LF (1982) Reported sexual behavior in late pregnancy: selected associations. *Journal of Reproductive Medicine* **10:** 627–632.

8

Postpartum psychosis

R. KUMAR

Child-bearing is a time of repeated contact with health professionals, both antenatally and after delivery (see review by Hall and Chng, 1982). Improved standards of nutrition, better screening and general health care in pregnancy, and better obstetric and postnatal medical management are all factors behind the impressive 40-fold fall in maternal mortality rates over the past 50 years, and there has been a similar, but less steep, decline in infant mortality. There has, meanwhile, been no parallel reduction in the incidence of postpartum psychosis or, during the last 20 years since Pitt's (1968) classical study, in the incidence of postnatal depression. It would be reasonable therefore to argue that whatever improvements there have been in the general health of the population at large, in the standards of obstetric care, in general medical practice and in clinical psychiatry, they have made no impression on the incidence of mental illnesses related to childbirth.

There is, however, a framework in place and a mechanism in existence for attempting to achieve prevention and better early treatment of postnatal psychiatric disorders. The problem lies in articulating the pieces of the relevant machinery so that existing resources can be used to best effect. There can be few better opportunities for preventive medicine than the obstetric setting, given the repeated maternal antenatal contacts with medical and paramedical staff. Midwives and obstetricians can be persuaded of the importance of recognizing women at risk of puerperal mental illness, but they are likely soon to be disillusioned if their efforts are not followed by tangible improvements in the care of such mothers.

There is now ample evidence (see reviews in Brockington and Kumar, 1982; Inwood, 1985; Kumar and Brockington, 1988) that maternal mental illness during pregnancy and after delivery can exert severe adverse effects on the mother herself and on the rest of her family, especially on the newborn and developing child. These adverse effects are not limited to the mother's subsequent psychological and social adjustment or to the infant's cognitive and emotional development. Psychiatric illness can lead to increased obstetric complications with associated perinatal morbidity; for example, the ingestion of certain psychotropic drugs in pregnancy is linked with a greater risk of fetal malformation (see review by Brockington and Kumar, 1982) and non-prescribed substances such as alcohol and nicotine are also recognized as being a source of harm to the fetus. Inadequate nutrition, disorganized personal, domestic and social circumstances, and non- or late attendance for antenatal care are more likely to be seen in the presence of mental disturbance and can directly or indirectly contribute to ill health in the mother and in the baby. Not all mentally ill women are equally at risk and significant problems may arise only in a minority of cases, most often when a combination of adverse influences is at play. The nature of the mother's mental illness is also a major relevant factor.

Careful history-taking at booking-in clinics and effective liaison between obstetric staff and psychiatrists, as well as with the primary health care team and with social services in the community, can do much to prevent crises in labour and postnatal wards. Psychiatric emergencies will still occur despite such measures, because postpartum psychosis affects mainly first-time mothers, most of whom do not manifest obvious signs of vulnerability during pregnancy or during labour and delivery. If obstetric staff are generally sensitive to mothers' psychological well-being then it is likely that they will react quickly and appropriately to the signs of an impending psychotic illness in one of their clients.

The main part of this review will focus on postpartum psychosis, although there is, at present, no great difference in the therapeutic options when a woman becomes psychotic only after delivery as opposed to the case of a woman who has had past psychotic illnesses and who then becomes pregnant. Future research may reveal differences in aetiology and in response to treatments. Distinctions between 'pure' puerperal psychosis and illnesses that are coincident with child-bearing should therefore always be made, if possible. There are, of course, cases where women first have puerperal breakdowns and then subsequently develop non-puerperal psychotic illnesses. It may be necessary to classify subjects in a variety of ways depending upon the precise nature of the research questions that are being asked.

Childbirth is followed by three main types of psychological disturbance—the maternity blues, postnatal depression and postpartum psychosis. There is no special rationale behind the way the adjectives have been chosen and all three conditions could just as easily be qualified by any one of the descriptive terms. Indeed, a fourth term, 'puerperal', is often used inter-changeably with 'postpartum' in relation to psychosis; the puerperium is generally regarded as being of six weeks' duration but psychiatrists have borrowed the term from obstetrics and then used it to describe an associa-tion between events without, until recently, too much thought about its temporal limits (see discussions by Brockington et al, 1982; Kendell et al, 1987). Distinctions between the conditions are made easier if they have different names but the boundaries between the blues and postnatal depression and between severe depression and postpartum (depressive) psychosis are still empirical. There are many quite fundamental questions which still require answers. Are the qualifying adjectives which refer to child-bearing merely describing a coincidence of events or, at most, the setting in which the illness unfolds and by which it may be coloured, or is there some unique quality within these disorders, in their manifestations and causes, which specifically implicates childbirth and its attendant circum-stances as aetiological agents? Are the postnatal conditions themselves related to each other or are they separate entities, discontinuous in presentation and in origin? This review of postpartum psychosis is therefore preceded by brief discussions of the maternity blues and of postnatal depression.

Maternity blues

The maternity blues are transient emotional reactions, typically dysphoric, almost always evanescent, occurring towards the end of the first week postpartum. They occur in between 50 and 75% of mothers and because of this fact, and because of their mildness and transience, it is not appropriate to regard the blues as a disorder. Other points which may be extracted from Stein's (1982) comprehensive review are that the blues do not appear to be culture-bound, nor are they a function of hospitalization, they cannot be linked with any particular pattern of environmental stress and, as yet, no firm endocrine or metabolic basis has been identified. Nevertheless, the blues continue to be a subject for study mainly because of the possibility that meaningful correlations between biological and psychological events may permit extrapolations to more severe states, such as postpartum psychoses. This kind of strategy is reasonable provided that one remembers that the very high prevalence of the blues is bound to engender spurious coincidences with the rarer conditions. The search must be for subtypes which then can be shown to have predictive validity. There is not much point in simply sifting for associations which may lead to conclusions such as 'severe and persistent blues run into postnatal depression' or that 'irritability or tearfulness are prodromata of postpartum psychosis'. It would be surprising if such 'conclusions' were otherwise. No-one has yet picked out any particular psychological or metabolic 'blues' marker that predicts the later onset of a puerperal psychiatric disorder (see review by Campbell and Winokur, 1985).

Postnatal depression

Although the problems posed by postnatal depressive neurosis are obviously less acute and immediately less demanding than in the case of psychotic breakdowns, they merit at least as much attention and resource allocation. Postnatal depression is a hundred times more common than postpartum psychosis; several surveys have shown that 10–15% of women are clinically depressed in the first three months after delivery (see reviews by Kumar, 1982; O'Hara and Zekoski, 1988) and of them, only two or three out of every 100 are referred to psychiatrists (Nott, 1982). Of the remainder, about half remain undetected by family doctors (Kumar and Robson, 1984) or by health visitors (Briscoe, 1986), and most of those who are noted to be depressed are treated inappropriately with benzodiazepines or with subtherapeutic doses of antidepressants (Kumar and Robson, 1984). About a quarter of mothers who are depressed in the first three months postnatally are likely to go on to suffer with chronic severe depressions (Pitt, 1968; Kumar and Robson, 1984; Watson et al, 1984; Cooper et al, 1988). The extent to which there is a raised incidence of depression that is directly and specifically related to child-bearing is currently under discussion (Cooper et al, 1988; O'Hara and Zekoski, 1988), but this debate should not obscure the fact that whatever the combinations of causal factors, the number of new mothers who are depressed after childbirth is very large—a conservative annual estimate for the UK is 75 000 cases each year. There is good evidence that such depressions arise in circumstances of life stress, lack of social support and in the presence of marital conflict, factors which are themselves in turn likely to be exacerbated by maternal depression. The mothers, their families and especially their newborn infants must adapt to the debilitating impact of the depressive condition and there is emerging evidence of adverse effects of maternal postnatal depression on the cognitive development of the child (Cogill et al, 1986) as well as of links with later behavioural problems (Ghodsian et al, 1984; Wrate et al, 1985; Caplan et al, 1989).

How does child-bearing act as an aetiological agent? Brown and Harris (1978) and Paykel et al (1980) found that depression after childbirth was primarily a consequence of social and environmental adversity, childbirth bringing home to vulnerable women the hopelessness of their situation (see also Cox et al, 1989). Other evidence (reviewed by Kumar, 1982) indicates that there are factors which are specific to the child-bearing process which contribute to the onset of depression. There is, as yet, no sound evidence to support the suggestion (Dalton, 1980) that postnatal depression is a consequence of hormonal deficiency, specifically of progesterone (see Chapter 9 for a detailed discussion of the subject of postnatal depression).

POSTPARTUM PSYCHOSIS

A clinical entity?

Postpartum psychosis is the rarest and the most severe of the conditions considered here. But is it a clinical entity? The pendulum of medical (psychiatric) opinion has swung back and forth since the classic accounts of puerperal psychosis by Esquirol (1838) and subsequently by his pupil Marcé (1858). The debate and its background is admirably summarized by Hamilton (1962, 1982).

Postpartum, or puerperal, psychosis is not to be found in DSM-III nor in ICD-9—the two current versions of the major diagnostic and classification manuals of psychiatry. It goes without saying that postnatal depression also does not exist as a nosological entity but then, unlike puerperal psychosis, it never did. Many early authors from Esquirol and Marcé onwards were convinced of the importance of puerperal mental illness and their surveys showed that psychoses related to pregnancy, child-bearing and lactation accounted for between 3 and 10%, and sometimes more, of all female psychiatric admissions (Zilboorg, 1928; Osterman, 1963). Marcé (1858) had been struck by the variety of psychopathology in his puerperal subjects; they showed all the disturbances that could be found in other settings. This view was subsequently misrepresented as an argument against the idea of a clinical entity (see account by Hamilton, 1982). Kraepelin (1906) had put on record his opinion that puerperal psychoses had no specific characteristics which distinguished them from dementia praecox or from manic-depressive insanity and psychiatrists began to challenge the idea of a specific link. Ten years earlier, Crichton-Browne (1896) had asked if measles were to occur after childbirth would it be called 'puerperal measles'? This attractive argument ignored the fact that several surveys (reviewed by MacLeod, 1886) had already prepared the ground for this kind of question. If measles were indeed regularly found to occur in between one in 500 and one in a 1000 women soon after childbirth but not so frequently at other times, then the fact that parturient women had about a 20 times higher relative risk of contracting the disease would certainly be a most interesting subject for enquiry.

However, an influential paper by Strecker and Ebaugh (1926) attacked the concept of puerperal psychosis and American psychiatrists, with a few notable exceptions (Hamilton, 1962), swung behind this view. The condition disappeared from most American textbooks of psychiatry and obstetrics and DSM-I required the condition to be categorized under conditions unrelated to parturition (Hamilton, 1985). European psychiatrists were less volatile but nevertheless, gradually from ICD-7 through to ICD-9, they chipped away at the concept of puerperal psychosis as a clinical entity and eventually removed it. The two main reasons were that there were no clear distinguishing clinical features and no consensus about the time limits implied by the term puerperal, it having been taken to mean anything from six weeks to two years. Ignorance on two fronts, instead of leading on to better research, resulted in a denial of the possible existence of the condition. Psychiatry is still struggling with its diagnostic and classification systems and it makes curious reading to see that ICD-9 has more than a dozen different ways of categorizing paranoid symptoms and none for a condition which repeatedly and regularly necessitates mental hospital admission for child-bearing women (Kendell et al, 1987).

Campbell and Winokur (1985) list several reasons why there should be a separate diagnostic category for postpartum illness:

1. Research into these disorders is hindered because they are not recorded (e.g. Meltzer and Kumar, 1985).
2. It is premature to assume that the biological events surrounding parturition play no part as causal or predisposing factors—this forecloses the option that specific hormonal and other treatment strategies may emerge in time.
3. Maintenance of categories of postpartum illness may help to refine the understanding of affective disorders and reduce their heterogeneity.

Incidence

Over the years, by the crude criterion of admission to mental hospital, the rate of puerperal or postpartum psychosis has remained remarkably constant at about two per 1000 deliveries (Brockington et al, 1982; Inwood,

1985). Some psychotic mothers are not admitted to hospital and not all women who are admitted are psychotic. If more stringent clinical and temporal criteria are applied to cases of postpartum mental illness—i.e. the admission of a woman with definite psychotic symptoms and an onset within two weeks of delivery (e.g. Meltzer and Kumar, 1985)—the incidence rate may be corrected by approximately halving it. Expressed as 0.5–1.0 per 1000 deliveries this may seem inconsequential; set against an annual birth rate of more than half a million in England and Wales this means that each year about 500 women are affected with a severe mental illness which requires admission to hospital, the majority for the first time in their lives. About two thirds of the sufferers are first-time mothers and Kendell et al (1987) have estimated the relative risk for the occurrence of a psychotic breakdown for a primiparous woman in the first month after delivery is immensely higher than at any other time in her life—the relative risk being 35.

Onset, symptoms and course of illness

Onset

Most puerperal psychoses have an onset within the first two weeks of delivery (Brockington et al, 1982) and this includes practically every case where the syndrome is that of mania. The onset of severe depressive illnesses is spread over a longer time postpartum, but most cases of psychotic depressive illness—i.e. where there are delusions and/or hallucinations— also have an early onset (Meltzer and Kumar, 1985). Most classical descriptive accounts of puerperal psychosis (Hamilton, 1962) note that there is an initial 'lucid interval' of at least 48 hours following birth, during which the mother appears normal. The early signs of the illness are non-specific and include insomnia, agitation, perplexity and oddities and eccentricities of behaviour, which may be overlooked or dismissed as being 'maternity blues'. This phase of the illness may last for a few days before more easily identifiable signs of psychosis emerge. The significance of these early warning signs is often only recognized with hindsight, and information about this phase is usually gained retrospectively. However, in the cases where women are known to be at high risk of developing a puerperal psychosis (those with a past history of functional psychotic illness, either puerperal or non-puerperal), the observing clinician may well be aware of their signficance. By the time a psychiatrist is involved in the assessment and management of a mother with a postpartum psychosis, the illness has usually progressed to a point where her symptoms are causing mounting concern to her family and to those professionals who are looking after her. She is often found to be perplexed and frightened by what she is experiencing, as might anyone whose inner world is invaded by bizarre experiences and ideas over which there is no control and which seem to relate significantly with things that happen every day. She may be preoccupied with comments on the television which have taken on a special significance. She may feel that people appear to be whispering and plotting against her. She may have an inexplicable conviction that she is someone who is chosen, special and who has remarkable powers. Alternatively, she may be so convinced of her badness that she is afraid of infecting others with it, and that she, and even her baby, might be better off dead. It is not surprising, therefore, that in the early days of such an illness the mother is acutely disturbed, perplexed and confused. On careful testing it can be shown that such confusion is not that which is seen in toxic and organic states. The disorientation, if any, for time, place or person, tends to be patchy and inconsistent. Brockington et al (1981) have suggested that perplexity, non-organic confusion and bewilderment may be pathognomonic for puerperal psychoses. However, a direct comparison with non-puerperal acute psychotic states in their very early stages has yet to be made.

Symptomatology

Recent studies (Brockington et al, 1981; Dean and Kendell, 1981; Meltzer and Kumar, 1985; Kendell et al, 1987) using standardized and operational clinical criteria place postpartum psychoses within the spectrum of affective disorder. Pigeon-holing these conditions does not, however, do justice to their heterogeneity, lability and complexity. 'First-rank' symptoms of schizophrenia may be present intermittently and may be sufficient to result in categorization of the illness as schizo-affective. Many patients, however, remain in the group best described by the RDC (Spitzer et al, 1975) as 'unspecified functional psychosis'.

Course

Postpartum psychoses often have a stormy and fluctuating course but one of their most rewarding characteristics is the completeness of recovery in the great majority of women. There remains the distinct possibility of recurrence or relapse after a subsequent birth, estimated at 20–30%, and a raised life-time expectancy of recurrence outside child-bearing (Brockington et al, 1982). Women and their partners who contemplate extending their families after a first illness need to know about the risks of recurrence and, until there are ways of preventing relapse, the best strategy is support and preparedness should admission be needed (Kumar et al, 1983).

Onset of menstruation. This has been reported in some puerperal patients to be associated with psychotic relapse or exacerbation of symptoms (Brockington et al, 1988), but only systematic, prospective studies will tell us whether this is a chance finding or whether indeed the hormonal changes associated with menstruation in some way destabilize the process of recovery in some women. Neuroendocrine studies of recovering patients are complicated by the fact that most of them are still taking psychotropic drugs, which themselves have powerful effects on neurohormonal secretion. There have been occasional reports of women presenting with exacerbations of psychotic illness in synchrony with the menstrual cycle (Lingjaerde and Bredland, 1954; Gregory, 1957; Endo et al, 1978) and of more than expected symptoms of premenstrual syndrome in women with rapidly cycling bipolar manic-depressive illness (Price and DiMarzio, 1986). Putative neuroendocrine contributions to puerperal psychotic breakdown are currently under investigation and preliminary findings have been encouraging (see Chapter 10 and Wieck et al, 1989).

Aetiology

Almost all the relevant evidence about aetiology derives from epidemiological surveys and from a few studies of the genetics of these conditions. The data are all well summarized in reviews by Brockington et al (1982), Campbell and Winokur (1985) and in the major recent survey by Kendell et al (1987). The following factors stand out: psychotic breakdown is more common after first birth, in single mothers, slightly more common after caesarean section and there is evidence for a genetic loading. The morbidity risk for affective disorder in the relatives of women with only postpartum affective illness is raised and it is about the same in women with non-puerperal manic-depressive illness; the rates were about 33 per 1000 as compared with 1–2 per 1000 in the general population (Whalley et al, 1982). Most studies, except that of Thuwe (1974), also support Protheroe's (1969) observation that although postpartum probands show a family loading for psychiatric illness, there is no evidence for an increased risk of puerperal illness. There is also evidence that women with a history of bipolar manic-depressive illness are at greater risk of postpartum breakdown than are women with unipolar disorder. The links between the spectrum of post-partum affective psychoses and manic-depressive illness in general can be clarified by means of careful family studies of cohorts of women with either puerperal or non-puerperal onset of original illness and who have them-selves been followed up for several years so that rates of recurrence can be measured in relation to subsequent births or otherwise. Studies of twins (I. F. Brockington, personal communication) are also under way. It is striking also to note the factors which are *not* consistently found in association with postpartum psychotic breakdown—these include stillbirth, abortion, maternal age, gender of child, social class, environmental adversity and quality of the subject's own experiences of parenting. The link with single motherhood may reflect the fact that such women lacking the support of a spouse and additional family are more likely to be admitted. Most of the evidence which relates the onset of puerperal psychosis with psychological and social 'stress' factors has been derived from large scale epidemiological investigations (e.g. Paffenbarger, 1964; Kendell et al, 1987) and from studies of case notes (e.g. Dean and Kendell, 1981; Meltzer and Kumar, 1985). Much more detail and more rigour of method is required before it is possible meaningfully to test whether or not, or how, factors such as adverse life events, unsupportive relationships, high expressed emotion and obstetric stress play a significant part in puerperal psychiatric breakdown.

In summary, the blues, postnatal depression and postpartum psychosis do appear to be distinguishable from each other in their prevalence, mani-festations, outcome and aetiology. Systematic *prospective studies* are needed to test whether they do overlap in any way. Can one, for example, discern a 'malignant' pattern of psychological and behavioural responses a few days after delivery which then explodes into a florid psychotic state?

Admission to hospital

Delays in admission often occur because the early symptoms and signs of impending psychosis may be missed as a direct consequence of discontinuities in clinical supervision. The peak times of onset of these illnesses coincide with transition points in clinical care when mothers leave postnatal wards and when the family doctor and health visitor take over from obstetricians and midwives. Furthermore an awareness of the risks of mental illness is not uppermost in the minds of most obstetricians, midwives and general practitioners, that is until one of their clients experiences an acute and sometimes catastrophic psychotic breakdown. Even then, further delays ensue because of inadequate psychiatric liaison in this context and a lack of knowledge about the facilities that are available to avoid separation of mother and baby (Kumar et al, 1986; Appleby et al, 1988).

About a quarter of psychiatric admissions in the puerperium are cases where the mothers have a definite history of previous mental illness (Meltzer and Kumar, 1985; Kendell et al, 1987). Kendell et al (1987) in their Edinburgh study found that women with prior histories of manic-depressive psychosis (manic or circular) were at greatest risk of admission in the three months following childbirth (21.4%) and those with a history of depressive psychosis had a 13.3% rate of admission after childbirth. The rate of admission for schizophrenics was 3.4%, for women with prior histories of depressive neurosis it was 1.9%, and for all other diagnoses the rate of admission was 4.1%. Typically, manic-depressive patients are re-admitted because they suffer an acute puerperal relapse (Brockington et al, 1981; Dean and Kendell, 1981; Meltzer and Kumar, 1985) and the survey by Kendell et al (1987) shows that schizophrenic patients do not experience comparable rates of recurrence or exacerbation of their illnesses—only one of 22 schizophrenic women (having a total of 29 episodes of childbirth) was admitted during the period of the study. A review (unpublished) of consecutive admissions in two years (1987–1988) to the Mother and Baby Unit at the Bethlem Royal Hospital, on the other hand, shows that 12 out of 57 mothers admitted during a 22-month period had a definite history of schizophrenia. Thus in South London, the availability of a specialized mother and baby unit greatly increased the admission rate for schizophrenic women in contrast with Edinburgh, which did not have such a unit. The figures cannot, however, be directly compared because the Bethlem unit does not have a defined catchment area and it is not known how many schizophrenic mothers were *not* admitted to the unit during 1987–1988. Most of these admissions were not because the mother had experienced a flare-up of her illness, but rather to assess her motivation and competence to care safely for the newborn child, while at the same time meeting her own needs for treatment.

Admission under the Mental Health Act

It may sometimes occur, because of a profound disturbance of the mother's mental state, that she wishes to discharge herself from hospital or that she refuses to accept admission to a psychiatric unit when it is clearly in the interests of her own health and safety and in the best interests of the child for this to occur. Under such circumstances it is possible, using the Mental Health Act, to either detain a woman in hospital against her wishes or to effect an admission to a psychiatric hospital. The following sections of the Mental Health Act can be used:

Section 5(2). This is used only for a patient who is already in hospital and only when there is such an urgent necessity that the patient, suffering from a mental disorder, should be prevented from leaving the hospital and detained for her health and safety and the protection of others and it is not practicable to follow the normal procedures which would involve a delay which would prejudice the safety of the patient. Unless the psychiatric ward is within the same hospital and the same unit of management as the ward in which the patient is being detained, it is not possible to effect a transfer of a patient from a maternity ward to a psychiatric unit under this section.

Section 4. This should only be used when there is an urgent necessity that the patient should be admitted to a psychiatric unit and detained for assessment and in circumstances where the compliance with the normal procedure (Section 2) would involve undesirable delay. This section can be applied upon the medical recommendation of one registered medical practitioner (not necessarily a psychiatrist) and either the nearest relative or an approved social worker, who must have seen the patient within 24 hours of making the order. All parties must be in agreement. This section can be used to transfer a patient from a maternity unit to a psychiatric unit, or to admit the patient in an emergency from the community. It has a duration of 72 hours.

Section 2. This is the preferred section to use whenever possible and can be applied when the patient is thought to be suffering from a mental disorder of a nature which warrants the detention of the patient in hospital for assessment followed by treatment for at least a period and that the patient needs to be so detained in the interests of her own health and safety or that of other people (in this case her infant). This section of the Mental Health Act is applied on two medical recommendations, one doctor should be approved under Section 12(2) as having special experience in the diagnosis and treatment of mental disorder, the other doctor preferably being the patient's general practitioner. There must also be an application by either the nearest relative or an approved social worker, and all parties must have seen the patient within 14 days of the application and not more than five days apart. This section can last for up to 28 days and the patient has the right to appeal against her detention in hospital, after 14 days, to the Mental Health Review Tribunal.

Section 3. This order is for admission to a psychiatric hospital for treatment and Section 3 is normally applied if the patient is already known and the diagnosis clear. The grounds for admission should be that the patient is suffering from a mental illness of such a nature or degree that makes it appropriate for her to receive treatment in hospital, and that such treatment is necessary for her health and safety and for the protection of other people. It requires the medical recommendation of two registered medical practitioners, one of whom should be the patient's general practitioner and the other approved under Section 12(2), and either an application from either the nearest relative or an approved social worker. This section can last up to six months and can be extended by a further period of six months. The patient has a right of appeal to the Mental Health Review Tribunal.

It is good clinical practice to try, if at all possible, to obtain a psychiatric opinion and the emergency sections (Section 5 and Section 4) should only be used in a true emergency where any delay might be hazardous to the mother or infant. Section 2 respects the civil rights of the patient and allows for a careful assessment by both an approved and trained social worker and a psychiatrist. Its duration is usually long enough for the acute management of most puerperal conditions. It is also good clinical practice to always obtain close co-operation of the husband or partner and wherever possible of the family.

Treatment and the Mental Health Act

It is possible for a woman who is compulsorily detained to be so disturbed that she is also unwilling to accept treatment. It is possible under the Mental Health Act to prescribe emergency treatments without the patient's permission. Again, it is good clinical practice to obtain the consent of the relatives. However, if the woman is detained under Section 4 of the Mental Health Act, this order should first be converted to Section 3. Under Section 2 and under Section 3 of the Mental Health Act, certain forms of treatment, e.g. depot injections, electroconvulsive therapy, can only be carried out against the patient's will with the consent of the Mental Health Commission. The Mental Health Commissioners can be contacted by telephone at any time and a medical member of the Commission will visit the patient and, if in agreement after discussion with a responsible medical officer and other people, will authorize the treatment plan.

Mother and baby units

Britain is unique among Western countries in that, more often than not, babies are admitted with their mothers into psychiatric hospitals (Margison and Brockington, 1982). The rationale for joint admission of mother and baby is that despite severe mental and behavioural disorganization, separating a mother from her infant may have both short- and long-term adverse effects upon their relationship and upon the psychological development of the child. On the other hand, there is a small, but always worrying risk that a mother may harm or kill her child (D'Orban, 1979; Margison, 1982); there is also a concern about the possible undesirable impact on the developing infant of being with a severely disturbed mother. Finally, it may also be the case that placing a young baby in an institution where, inevitably, there are many 'caregivers' to help or 'take over' from the mother may of itself have some lasting influence on the child's development. There are, as yet, no reports of studies of child development or of parent–child relationships looking at the possible impact of early institutional care separately from the possible consequences of different kinds of maternal mental illness. There are also no reliable ways of predicting which infants are most likely to be 'at risk' of harm from their mothers, whether through impulse to harm or through neglect. Schizophrenic patients (Da Silva and Johnstone, 1981) and sometimes manic or psychotically depressed women (Margison, 1982) do rarely kill their children and clinical staff urgently need more sensitive indicators of potential risk.

Aside from the mother's mental condition *per se*, there are many other related factors which may affect her behaviour and her relationship with her infant—she may be heavily sedated by medication, she may have to discontinue breast-feeding, and access to her infant may be limited by staff because they are concerned about risk to the child or because of the nature of the facilities. Some hospitals encourage 'rooming-in', others have nurseries adjacent to the wards, and in others the child may be looked after in a paediatric ward at some distance from the mother (Kumar et al, 1986). Systematic studies of outcome have yet to be done which examine not only the impact of the mother's illness, but also the context in which this is managed.

Oates (1988) has recently described a pioneering clinical development in which an essentially hospital-based service has been extended out into the community. Domiciliary care of severely disturbed mothers has been shown to be a practicable, effective and preferable alternative to hospital admission. Intensive nursing care at home, backed up by quickly available medical intervention, produces quicker remission of the illness with easier rehabilitation of the recovering mother. In very severe cases, or if family support is lacking, admission of the mother and her baby into a hospital unit is still available.

Treatment

The duration of inpatient treatment may vary from a few days or weeks up to a year or more. The median stay for women with manic-depressive and schizo-affective disorders is about eight weeks (Meltzer and Kumar, 1985) and the treatments that are used are conventional drug therapy or electroconvulsive therapy (ECT). ECT is regarded by some clinicians as the treatment of choice, greatly shortening the illness and minimizing interference with breast-feeding (Protheroe, 1969; Sneddon and Kerry, 1985), but there have been no clinical trials to demonstrate conclusively that it is more efficacious. There is no sound evidence that treatment with hormones, such as oestrogen or progesterone, is effective, and research into possible neuroendocrine mechanisms in postpartum psychosis is virtually non-existent (see review by Campbell and Winokur, 1985). One reason for this lack is the difficulty in prospectively investigating a condition which occurs so relatively infrequently. Most of the work has focused on the blues and so far the results have been inconclusive. Dalton (1980) has described links with premenstrual symptoms and she suggests that progesterone therapy may be beneficial in the prevention of both puerperal disorders and the premenstrual syndrome, but her observations have not yet been verified by others.

A full account of the treatment of puerperal psychoses is given in Chapter 12.

FUTURE DEVELOPMENTS

Research into postnatal mental illness has recently emerged from a period in the doldrums. Prevention and early treatment of postnatal depression by counselling has been shown to be effective in the majority of cases (see Chapters 9 and 11) and it would be very helpful if there were reliable 'markers' to predict a good response to early pharmacotherapy in the small minority of mothers who go on to have chronic severe depressions. In a wider context, studies showing how depressed mother's interactions with their infants are impaired may lead to effective focused strategies for intervention (see Chapter 13). Postpartum psychosis remains as enigmatic a condition as it was when Hippocrates in 400 BC formulated the two main aetiological hypotheses implicating neuroendocrine dysfunction. Roughly translated into today's jargon these hypotheses entirely anticipate current ideas about possible disorders of the ovarian–pituitary–hypothalamic axis and about disorders which may emanate from or be reflected in the regulation of lactation. Uncovering possible endocrine contributions to the onset of illness will hopefully eventually lead to more specific treatments. Evaluation of different models of management is another urgent priority—is the outcome for mother, infant and others best when the mother and baby are admitted together, possibly with the additional option of home care, or is temporary separation better?

It should be possible to plan the deployment of services in a rational way, given knowledge of the constant incidence of postpartum psychosis. No comprehensive service can work without effective liaison between the different professional groups who are involved in normal child-bearing and those who may be called upon to deal with the mentally ill mother and her infant. The actual services will range from inpatient facilities, day attendance, outreach and domiciliary care, through to support and counselling by general practitioners and health visitors. In terms of cost and benefit is there not, for example, much to be said for devoting some resources to improving facilities for psychiatrically ill mothers even at the cost of less technology in obstetric suites or in neonatal intensive care units. These are medicopolitical decisions for health care planners to make and some of the data have been reviewed in this chapter. Mental health always receives low priority but perhaps a recognition of the special contribution of child-bearing to maternal psychopathology and to the repercussions this has in the next generation may lead to actual improvements in the allocation of resources.

REFERENCES

Appleby L, Fox H, Shaw M, Kumar R et al (1988) The psychiatrist in the obstetric unit: establishing a liaison service. *British Journal of Psychiatry* **154:** 510–515.

Briscoe M (1986) Identification of emotional problems in postpartum women by health visitors. *British Medical Journal* **292:** 1245–1247.

Brockington IF & Kumar R (1982) Drug addiction and psychotropic drug treatment during pregnancy and lactation. In Brockington IF & Kumar R (eds) *Motherhood and Mental Illness*, pp 239–255. London: Academic Press.

Brockington IF, Cernik KF, Schofield EM, Downing AR, Francis AF & Keelan C (1981) Puerperal psychosis. *Archives of General Psychiatry* **38:** 829–833.

Brockington IF, Winokur G & Dean C (1982) Puerperal psychosis. In Brockington IF & Kumar R (eds) *Motherhood and Mental Illness*, pp 37–69. London: Academic Press.

Brockington IF, Kelly A, Hall P & Deakin W (1988) Premenstrual relapse of puerperal psychosis. *Journal of Affective Disorders* **14:** 287–292.

Brown GW & Harris T (1978) *Social Origins of Depression.* London: Tavistock.

Campbell JL & Winokur G (1985) Postpartum affective disorders: selected biological aspects. In Inwood DG (ed.) *Postpartum Psychiatric Disorders*, pp 20–39. Washington: APA Press.

Caplan HC, Cogill SR, Alexandra H, Robson KM, Katz R & Kumar R (1989) The effect of maternal postnatal depression on the emotional development of the child. *British Journal of Psychiatry* **154:** 818–822.

Cogill S, Caplan HL, Alexandra H, Robson KM & Kumar R (1986) Impact of maternal postnatal depression on cognitive development of young children. *British Medical Journal* **292:** 1165–1167.

Cooper PJ, Campbell EA, Day A, Kennerley H & Bond A (1988) Non-psychotic psychiatric disorder after childbirth: a prospective study of prevalence, incidence, course and nature. *British Journal of Psychiatry* **152:** 799–806.

Cox JL, Paykel ES & Page ML (1989) *Childbirth as a Life Event.* Southampton: Duphar.

Crichton-Browne J (1896) Prevention and treatment of insanity of pregnancy and the puerperal period. *Lancet* **i:** 164–165.

Dalton K (1980) *Depression after Childbirth.* Oxford: Oxford University Press.

Da Silva L & Johnstone E (1981) A follow-up study of severe puerperal psychiatric illness. *British Journal of Psychiatry* **134:** 346–354.

Dean C & Kendell RE (1981) The symptomatology of puerperal illness. *British Journal of Psychiatry* **139:** 128–133.

D'Orban PT (1979) Women who kill their children. *British Journal of Psychiatry* **134:** 560–571.

Endo M, Daiguji M, Asano Y, Yamashita I & Takahashi S (1978) Periodic psychosis recurring in association with menstrual cycle. *Journal of Clinical Psychiatry* **39:** 456–466.

Esquirol E (1838) *Des Maladies Mentales.* Paris: J-B Baillière.

Ghodsian M, Zajicek E & Wolkind S (1984) A longitudinal study of maternal depression and child behaviour problems. *Journal of Child Psychology and Psychiatry and Allied Disciplines* **25:** 91–109.

Gregory RA (1957) The menstrual cycle and its disorders in psychiatric patients. *Journal of Psychosomatic Research* **2:** 199–224.

Hall M & Chng PK (1982) Antenatal care in practice. In Enkin M & Chalmers I (eds) *Effectiveness and Satisfaction in Antenatal Care*, pp 60–68. Lowenham: Spastics International Medical Publications.

Hamilton JA (1962) *Postpartum Psychiatric Problems.* St Louis: CV Mosby.

Hamilton JA (1982) The identity of postpartum psychosis. In Brockington IF & Kumar R (eds) *Motherhood and Mental Illness* pp 1–17. London: Academic Press.

Hamilton JA (1985) Guidelines for therapeutic management of postpartum disorders. In Inwood DG (ed.) *Postpartum Psychiatric Disorders*, pp 83–96. Washington: APA Press.

Inwood DG (ed.) (1985) *Postpartum Psychiatric Disorders.* Washington: APA Press.

Kendell RE, Chalmers JC & Platz C (1987) Epidemiology of puerperal psychosis. *British Journal of Psychiatry* **150:** 662–673.

Kraepelin E (1906) *Lectures on Clinical Psychiatry* (Revised and edited by Johnstone T). London: Baillière, Tindall and Cox.

Kumar R (1982) Neurotic disorders in childbearing women. In Brockington IF & Kumar R (eds) *Motherhood and Mental Illness*, pp 71–118. London: Academic Press.

Kumar R & Brockington IF (eds) (1988) *Motherhood and Mental Illness 2: Causes and Consequences*. London: Wright.

Kumar R & Robson KM (1984) A prospective study of emotional disorders in childbearing women. *British Journal of Psychiatry* **144:** 35–47.

Kumar R, Isaacs S & Meltzer E (1983) Recurrent post-partum psychosis: a model for prospective clinical investigation. *British Journal of Psychiatry* **142:** 618–620.

Kumar R, Meltzer ES, Hepplewhite R & Stevenson AD (1986) Admitting mentally ill mothers with their babies into psychiatric hospitals. *Bulletin of the Royal College of Psychiatrists* **10:** 169–172.

Lingjaerde P & Bredland R (1964) Hyperestrogenic cyclic psychosis. *Acta Psychiatrica Scandinavica* **29:** 355–364.

MacLeod MD (1886) An address on puerperal insanity. *British Medical Journal* **ii:** 239–242.

Marcé LV (1858) *Traite de la Folie des Femmes Enceintes, des Nouvelles Accouchees et des Nourrices*. Paris: J Baillière et fils.

Margison F (1982) The pathology of the mother–child relationship. In Brockington IF & Kumar R (eds) *Motherhood and Mental Illness*, pp 191–219. London: Academic Press.

Margison F & Brockington IF (1982) Psychiatric mother and baby unit. In Brockington IF & Kumar R (eds) *Motherhood and Mental Illness*, pp 223–237. London: Academic Press.

Meltzer ES & Kumar R (1985) Puerperal mental illness, clinical features and classification: a study of 142 mother and baby admissions. *British Journal of Psychiatry* **147:** 647–654.

Nott PN (1982) Psychiatric illness following childbirth in Southampton: a case register study. *Psychological Medicine* **12:** 557–561.

Oates M (1988) The development of an integrated community-oriented service for severe postnatal mental illness. In Kumar R & Brockington IF (eds) *Motherhood and Mental Illness 2: Causes and Consequences*, pp 133–158. London: Wright.

O'Hara M & Zekoski EM (1988) Postpartum depression: a comprehensive review. In Kumar R & Brockington IF (eds) *Motherhood and Mental Illness 2: Causes and Consequences*, pp 17–63. London: Wright.

Osterman E (1963) Les etats psychopathologiques du postpartum. *Encephale* **52:** 385–420.

Paffenbarger RS Jr (1964) Epidemiological aspects of postpartum mental illness. *British Journal of Prevention and Social Medicine* **18:** 189–195.

Paykel ES, Emms EM, Fletcher J & Rassaby ES (1980) Life events and social support in puerperal depression. *British Journal of Psychiatry* **136:** 339–346.

Pitt B (1968) Atypical depression following childbirth. *British Journal of Psychiatry* **114:** 1325–1335.

Price WA & DiMarzio L (1986) Premenstrual tension syndrome in rapid cycling bipolar affective disorder. *Journal of Clinical Psychiatry* **47:** 415–417.

Protheroe C (1969) Puerperal psychoses: a long term study 1927–1961. *British Journal of Psychiatry* **115:** 9–30.

Sneddon J & Kerry RJ (1985) The psychiatric mother and baby unit: a five year study. In Inwood DG (ed.) *Postpartum Psychiatric Disorders*, pp 98–110. Washington: APA Press.

Spitzer R, Endicott J & Robins E (1975) *Research Diagnostic Criteria for a Selected Group of Functional Disorders*. New York: Biometrics Research Division, NY State Psychiatric Institute.

Stein G (1982) The maternity blues. In Brockington IF & Kumar R (eds) *Motherhood and Mental Illness*, pp 119–154. London: Academic Press.

Strecker EA & Ebaugh FG (1926) Psychoses occurring during the puerperium. *Archives of Neurology and Psychiatry* **15:** 239–252.

Thuwe I (1974) Genetic factors in puerperal psychosis. *British Journal of Psychiatry* **125:** 378–385.

Watson JP, Elliott SA, Rugg JA & Brough DI (1984) Psychiatric disorder in pregnancy and the first postnatal year. *British Journal of Psychiatry* **144:** 453–462.

Whalley LJ, Roberts DF, Wentzel J & Wright AF (1982) Genetic factors in puerperal affective psychoses. *Acta Psychiatrica Scandinavica* **65:** 180–193.

Wieck A, Hirst AD, Kumar R, Checkley SA & Campbell IC (1989) Growth hormone secretion by human females in response to apomorphine challenge is markedly affected by menstrual cycle phase. *British Journal of Clinical Pharmacology* **27(5):** 700–701.

Wrate RM, Rooney AC, Thomas PF & Cox JL (1985) Postnatal depression and child development: a three year follow-up study. *British Journal of Psychiatry* **146:** 622–627.
Zilboorg G (1928) Malignant psychoses related to childbirth. *American Journal of Obstetrics
  and Gynecology* **15(2):** 145–158.

9

Postnatal depression: a serious and neglected postpartum complication

JOHN L. COX

Although most obstetricians are increasingly aware of the relevance of psychological considerations to the management of their patients, acquiring more specific knowledge of the psychiatric disorders which complicate childbearing is regarded as less important, or even as unnecessary altogether. The titles of recent papers published in the *British Journal of Obstetrics and Gynaecology*, and the lack of psychiatry in some postgraduate text books would indeed suggest that these disorders are not of particularly high priority. It is a purpose of this chapter, therefore, to describe the clinical aspects of postnatal depression which is one of the most serious complications of the puerperium and may affect at least 1 in 10 new mothers. I shall also attempt to answer some of the challenging and practical questions which are commonly asked by obstetricians about these disorders; questions which usually indicate clearly their reasons for scepticism about the relevance of this subject, and yet were asked because of the need to obtain lucid and practical answers to assist in the management of their disturbed patients.

What *is* postnatal depression? Is it 'just the blues'?

Marcé in 1858 was the first psychiatrist to describe in detail the puerperal psychoses which required treatment in hospital, although his teacher Esquirol (1845) had already observed that there were also many women with 'mild to moderate degrees' of psychiatric disorder who were treated at home and never recorded in hospital statistics. Despite this shrewd observation, most papers published until 20 years ago were descriptions of the postnatal psychoses which were treated in a mental hospital. For example, Menzies (1893) in one of these earlier papers gives detailed clinical descriptions of women whose paranoid delusions involved their husbands and the medical staff, and who also believed that their babies were an 'animal or elephant'. Interestingly, he also observed that women with the later onset 'lactational' psychoses had a 'quiet form' of depression, perhaps similar to postnatal depression of the present time, which only rarely is treated in hospital; more commonly such depressed women are to be found untreated at home and miserably failing to cope with household tasks.

One other conceptual difficulty is that the diagnosis 'postnatal depression' is not included in international classifications of mental illness and could be construed therefore to 'not exist'. However, puerperal psychoses do now appear in the new tenth edition of the International Classification of Disease (ICD), but *only* as a category to be used if criteria for other psychiatric diagnoses are not fulfilled. It is therefore regrettable that ICD-10 will not assist the routine classification of women with a specific postnatal mental illness, an anomaly which has occurred because these classifications do not take into account causal considerations and ignore the pragmatic criterion of 'popular usage'. The diagnostic terms postnatal depression and puerperal psychoses, however, do not necessarily imply a causal association between childbirth and depression, but indicate a temporal relationship.

The criteria for the diagnosis 'postnatal depression' used by most health professionals and used in this chapter include a morbid and persistent depressed mood, usually commencing six to twelve weeks after delivery, although at six weeks the mood is particularly labile so that making a *firm* diagnosis at the postnatal clinic can be particularly difficult. The mother with a postnatal depression is suffering from a 'non-psychotic depression' and does not usually experience persistent delusions (false beliefs) or have hallucinations, which are characteristic of a major depressive psychosis. Indeed, many women with postnatal depression do not at first sight appear to be unwell at all. Such depression is, however, definitely distinct from 'postnatal blues', which are restricted to the transitory weepiness, irritability and anxiety of the first two weeks after delivery.

Mothers recount their depression in a variety of ways but usually describe accurately the distress caused by their symptoms and generally recognize that they are not their usual selves. The following descriptions were provided by women who took part in our study of counselling in the management of postnatal depression, and were documented by Jennifer Holden (unpublished data).

> 'I have never felt like that in my life before. Nobody could speak to me because I would burst into tears at the least thing. I took an extreme dislike to everybody in this world except my baby. I wanted everybody to go away, I was interested in nothing.'

> 'It was terrible. It was like someone else taking over. I wasn't the same person any more. I didn't recognize myself. It wasn't me, that was what I kept saying. It wasn't me.'

> 'It was absolutely ghastly. It felt as if there was a physical weight inside that was dragging me down. I was pulling it around all the time; everything was an effort.'

Another woman described her depression in the following way:

> '. . . I enjoyed my pregnancy and I enjoyed having him, it was the greatest thing I have ever experienced until I came home. And then I thought, God, I don't want you . . . I have been sad before and I have been unhappy, but never like after I had Thomas, to the point where I just didn't want to live any more.'

Another woman described her depression as though something had got a hold of her which she knew was serious and required medical help. Indeed, for most such women postnatal depression is clearly recalled several years later and we found that for at least a half of these depressed women the disorder lasted for a year, and sometimes merged into a second postnatal depression following a subsequent pregnancy (Cox et al, 1984). It is clear, therefore, that this disorder is *not* a trivial illness, and is clearly distinct from the postnatal blues and the postnatal psychosis (which has an earlier onset— usually within three weeks of childbirth).

An understanding of how such depression may present to health professionals, which is described in the following sections, also underlines that this disorder cannot readily be dismissed by managers or consultants as the 'worried well'. Indeed, there is substantial evidence that such depression can cause havoc to a marriage, disrupt bonding to the baby, have an enduring negative effect on the attitude towards a subsequent pregnancy and may even influence adversely the development of the baby (see Chapter 13). Such depression could also initiate behavioural disturbance in an older sibling (see Kumar and Brockington, 1988). Postnatal depression, because of its severity and distress as well as its prolonged duration if untreated, is a major psychiatric disorder which may lead to suicide or rarely to threatened or completed physical child abuse.

How can postnatal depression be recognized?

The recognition of this disorder in clinical practice is more straightforward than might be expected, provided the doctor or other health professional worker knows what symptoms to look for. Most health professionals can readily be taught how to make this diagnosis, and a provisional diagnosis can usually be made after an interview which has not lasted more than 45 minutes.

The obstetrician, midwife, health visitor or general practitioner may be alerted to the possibility that a mother is depressed by observing one or more of the following:

1. A complaint of feeling low, worried, fatigued or having severe sleep difficulties.
2. Constant complaints of somatic symptoms such as headaches, abdominal pain or breast tenderness without an adequate physical cause.
3. An expressed fear that the doctor or health visitor will be excessively critical of her mothering ability, and may even be considering taking away her baby.
4. Excessive concern about a healthy baby and pre-occupation with minimal feeding difficulties. The mother is continuously over-solicitous and always responds immediately to the baby's demands.
5. Unexpected failure to attend a postnatal clinic.
6. 'Failure to thrive' of the baby.

Confirmation of the diagnosis

Once a mother is thought to be 'possibly depressed' or is regarded as a 'problem patient', then specific enquiry should be made as to the presence or absence of the following psychiatric symptoms:

1. Depressed mood. Almost all women will acknowledge when they feel down, sad, depressed, low-spirited or 'blue'. The question 'how do you feel in your spirits in these days?' will usually elicit this crucial information. The obstetrician can then determine the extent to which this depressed mood is a break with the normal mood state, and establish how long the mood has lasted, and how distressing it is. A depressed mood which has lasted for at least four weeks and which is accompanied by other symptoms of depression would confirm the diagnosis.

2. Excessive anxiety. Although being anxious (fearful, worried) can occur in the absence of a depressed mood, if anxiety *is* present it should be regarded as co-existing with depression unless shown *not* to be so. The best clinical rule of thumb is to assume that any mother who is anxious is also depressed.

3. Lack of interest and pleasure in doing things. Snaith et al (1978) regards such 'anhedonia' as a hallmark of depression. The lack of interest may show itself through an unusual disinterest in cooking, reading, or in maintaining or resuming sexual relations. Libido is often non-existent.

4. Early morning wakening, when not caused by a noisy baby or restless partner, is also a characteristic of depression, and when consistently present and prolonged is especially typical of the depressed phase of manic-depressive illness. Initial insomnia when the mother is kept awake by rounds of worrying thoughts or by an exaggerated need to listen to any sound from her baby may be another sign of a depressive illness.

5. Ideas of not coping, self-blame and guilt.

It can be seen that the clinical skills required to determine the presence or absence of these symptoms of depression are not particularly complex and usually are acquired during undergraduate or postgraduate teaching or from a post-qualifying refresher course such as those organized for midwives.

Is depression more common after childbirth than in non-child-bearing women?

There is little doubt that mental illness severe enough to require treatment in a psychiatric unit is substantially more common after childbirth than at other times. Kendell et al (1981) have found this increased risk to be as high as 16-fold. Pitt (1968) believed that a non-psychotic non-hospitalized depression following childbirth was also more common than in non-child-bearing women. The preliminary results of our North Staffordshire controlled study of postnatal depression being carried out by Dr Declan Murray, Mrs Gay Chapman and myself show a trend towards higher rates of serious depressive illness at 6 months postpartum compared with non-child-bearing controls. The non-puerperal controls in this study are being obtained from general practice lists and individually matched with the index group for age, marital status and number of children. This study to an extent has overcome some of the methodological problems of other controlled studies. Thus, although O'Hara (1989) found no significant differences in the frequency of depres sion in his controlled study, he acknowledged some limitations of the study design; some women, for example, dropped out from the study during its progress and there was the possibility that the controls were selected for good psychological health and were familiar with the research hypothesis. There may have been a marked practice effect of giving repeated measures of psychiatric morbidity over a period of time which could explain the reduction in levels of psychiatric morbidity in the control and index groups. It was also pointed out by Brown (1989) that the index groups may not have been selected for psychological health and that the controls who were acquaintances of the index subjects may have been closer to a random sample of the population as a whole. In addition, if the measures of psychiatric morbidity had continued until six months postpartum rather than completed at nine weeks, then it is possible that the differences found at nine weeks in the proportion of women who were depressed (10.4% index, 7.8% controls) which failed to reach statistical significance would have become so at this later period. Nevertheless, O'Hara did conclude that the impact of postnatal depression was substantially different from depression occurring at other times, and he underlined that marital adjustment was certainly markedly deteriorated in the index group. In another study of maternal depression by Cooper et al (1988) at Oxford a comparison was made with an Edinburgh community study of depressed women; similar case-finding criteria having been used by the two research teams. However, the Present State Examination which was used in both studies is a semi-structured interview which determines whether or not defined psychiatric symptoms have been present in the previous *month* and is perhaps less sensitive to the lower levels of psychiatric morbidity which are characteristic of postnatal depression. The Oxford and the Edinburgh comparison samples were group-matched for age and number of children, but not for marital status. The results of Cooper's study, however, showed a bunching of new onset depression in the first three months of the first postpartum year, although the point prevalence of psychiatric disorder at six months (8.8%) was no greater than in the comparison group. Their data has also indicated that, despite the similar proportions of *overall* psychiatric cases in the two studies, more women had depressive symptoms and loss of interest and concentration in the postpartum group than in the Edinburgh comparison sample.

These studies have therefore initiated a long overdue debate about the clinical features and frequency of postnatal depression and have pointed out the limitations of knowledge at the present time which is largely based on earlier prospective studies. The question as to whether or not there is an increased risk of new onset depression postpartum should at present therefore be regarded as unanswered.

However, for readers of this chapter who are not concerned with the minutiae of psychiatric research methodology, it is important to re-emphasize that whether or not there is more depression postpartum than in a control non puerperal group, almost all studies have shown that *at least* one in ten women suffer from a clinically important depression three months after childbirth, which is a higher proportion than expected by many obstetricians and general practitioners, and indeed by some psychiatrists.

There are at least eight studies, including those of O'Hara (1989) and Cooper et al (1988), which have found that 9–13% of women suffer from a prolonged postnatal depression, a disorder distinct from the blues which are confined to the emotionalism of the first two weeks postpartum, and substantially more common than the psychoses which follow only one in 500 live births. There can be little doubt therefore that postnatal depression 'exists' and that for at least one in ten families the puerperium is not characterized by being a time of calm, joyful contentment.

What are the causes of postnatal depression?

Many health professionals have their own explanation for the causes of postnatal depression. Popularist theories link the cause of postnatal depression to the feminist movement, the unavailability of parents for support or to other aspects of Western family life.

Psychological considerations

Breen (1975) has described childbirth either as a 'hurdle' to be overcome or a more 'continuous process' which could lead to irreversible physical and psychological change. She prefers the 'process' theory because it links the understanding of pregnancy to the process of puberty, as both are 'biosocial' events which necessitate a reassessment of personal relationships as well as an acceptance of a new biological role. Thus the young primigravida has to re-negotiate her relationship with her husband and mother and also establish an entirely new bond with her baby.

An awareness of these cross-generational links are useful in clinical work as they help in understanding the reasons for an excessive preoccupation with the baby or an overwhelming need for the woman to include her own mother in aspects of child care. If there is a hostile relationship with her mother she may find that the process of 'identification' has made it unexpectedly difficult to be a 'good enough' mother herself. This conflict is then projected onto her baby, who is regarded as being unwanted or maybe rejected altogether. Wolkind and colleagues (1976) have found some research evidence to support these theories and found that women who were themselves deprived of attention in childhood had greater difficulty in accepting their maternal role.

The Swedish research carried out by Nilsson and Almgren (1970) also found that postpartum psychiatric disorder was more likely in women with a poor relationship with their mother or in those who were uncertain of their own female identity.

Other psychological theories include the 'learned helplessness' theory of Seligman (1975), in which depression is thought to be a result of the inability to avoid unpleasant experiences; the mother believes that she will always fail to look after her baby and that adverse consequences will result from this failure; she is then in a state of 'learned helplessness' or depression.

Another influential theory has been put forward by Beck et al (1961) which states that depressed mood is not itself the primary process in depres sion, but is a result of the negative way in which the individual views herself or the environment. A woman who always regards herself as being 'incompetent' has this attitude reinforced. Beck has devised a scheme of 'cognitive therapy'; in this form of psychotherapy the patient is instructed to notice and write down such repetitive negative 'automatic thoughts' about herself, others and the world, and is then exhorted to correct them through a process of rational discussion with a therapist. (A more detailed account of psychological treatments is given in Chapter 11.)

Interestingly these theories assume that the personality attributes are acquired in childhood and that a subsequent life stressor such as childbirth provokes a depression in the susceptible woman. Tetlow (1955) has summarized how such personality factors may relate to the onset of postnatal depression:

1. The 'Achilles heel' theory. There are some women who have a *specific* difficulty with mothering or with their own sexuality which then predisposes them to a psychiatric disorder associated with childbirth.
2. For women who are 'always worriers' childbirth is *another* life event which can cause mental illness; there is no particular vulnerability to the birth event itself and such women are similarly at risk of depression following any other major stress.

Social considerations

It is generally recognized that women are more carefully scrutinized during child-bearing than any other time; the under-utilizers of obstetric services were studied by McKinley (1970) and were found to belong to lower social classes and to have an increased risk of obstetric and psychological complications. Milio (1975) suggested that one reason for not attending the antenatal clinic is that the obstetric services are middle class institutions organized for middle class women and that working class mothers therefore feel alienated. No definite relationships, however, have been found between social class and *postnatal* depression, although this association is established for depression at other times. Thus in Brown and Harris' study (1978) in Camberwell, working class women were more at risk of depression at any time, and women with three or more children under the age of 14 years and who lacked a confidante were found to be particularly vulnerable to the impact of life events.

Women with depression in pregnancy in my African and Scottish studies were more likely to be single, separated or divorced; an illegitimate pregnancy was particularly stigmatized in Uganda as the baby could not be named or placed in the family or clan (Cox, 1979; Cox et al, 1982).

Although the relationship of postnatal depression to hospital delivery cannot now be investigated in the UK, it is likely that the increasing medicalization of childbirth has interrupted to some extent the postpartum social 'rules' (taboos) which previously were more prominent. In Cox (1988), I drew attention to the way in which these rituals and taboos may protect against depression. Pillsbury (1978), for example, has provided one of the most specific accounts of the postpartum Chinese custom of 'doing the month' and has shown how in the month following childbirth the mother has several defined rules of behaviour which include the avoidance of washing, not to go outside during the entire month, not to eat any raw or cold food, to eat chicken, not to be blown by the wind or to move about, not to go to another person's home, not to have sexual intercourse, and not to read or cry. These proscriptions are still practised in Chinese society and allow the mother to receive extra assistance from her family as well as to encourage rest. In this way she is rewarded for the effort of childbirth and given the sanction 'to be idle in bed for an entire month'. These Chinese mothers may therefore receive more attention than women in the United States; Pillsbury concludes that this may prevent Chinese women from having postpartum depression.

Jamaican women also have a period of ritual seclusion for the first nine nights after delivery and Kitzinger (1982) has described this separation of the mother from her family as being similar to the seclusion which follows bereavement. This primary seclusion is then followed by a less restricted seclusion for a further 31 nights, during which the new mother remains at home and is looked after by her own mother. In India, among lower castes in particular, such postpartum seclusion may last for a similar period of time (40 days), during which the new mother is regarded as impure and so must remain alone in confinement. In a study of the Punjabi community in the UK by Homans (1982), the extent of the 'confinement' was found to be modified according to the availability of others to help as well as by the need to obtain employment.

Kelly (1967) has likewise described how a Nigerian mother and baby are placed in a special hut within the family compound for two to three months where they are looked after by the baby's grandmother, a custom which allows the woman to rest and the baby to receive specific attention. Kelly has concluded that these postpartum customs may protect against postpartum depression.

In the UK, Okley's (1975) study of gipsies found that childbirth was regarded as polluting and delivery in hospital was therefore encouraged to prevent contamination. Any assistance with cooking from other women or from older children would prevent contamination of the food by the puerperal mother.

Stern and Kruckman (1983) have also put forward this challenging hypothesis that it is the absence of postpartum behavioural norms in Western society which is important in the causation of postnatal depression. The period of time when special attention is given to the mother is no longer even two to three days; the mother can be 'discharged' home immediately after delivery and may be expected to resume full domestic responsibilities. This abrupt change of environment is associated with the 'loss' of the midwife who assisted her so intimately in pregnancy and may have delivered her baby. The health visitor, obstetrician and general practitioner may show more concern for her child rather than for herself. Another change in Western society is linked to the reduction of support brought about by the ambiguity in role of the partner—whether, for example, he should be present at delivery (traditionally a woman's place) and the extent of his assistance after childbirth. In Sweden this ambiguity is illustrated by the legislation for 'paternity leave', which can be shared with his partner, taken wholly by her or taken entirely by himself. Yet studies show that there has not been a major change in the tasks that husbands actually carry out, the mother tending still to undertake tasks most intimately linked to the practical aspects of baby care. In Western society there are only vestigial remains of a 40-day 'lying in' period; even the postnatal clinic, which also took place at six weeks, is now less commonly held, and baptism and a 'churching' ceremony which occurred at 40 days is less frequently held now than formerly. Thus, although family and obstetric rituals do still occur (Jones and Dougherty, 1982), they are now generally more fragmented and less likely to be enforced; quite often they are ignored altogether.

In what way could this lack of postpartum structure in our Western society relate to the increased awareness of depression postpartum? Seel (1968) has addressed this fascinating question and regards childbirth rituals as part of a *'rite de passage'* which in the West is incomplete. The change in status from a childless women to mother is a major role change which needs to be marked by a public change in social status and by carrying out an appropriate *'rite de passage'*. There are three components of this *'rite de passage'*; the rite of 'separation' (including cleansing and purifying), the 'liminal' period when there is no status and there may be private humiliation, and the 'rite of incorporation' when the subject moves back to a new status. Seel believes that the first two stages of this rite are highly elaborated in Western obstetrics, but that there is little or no 'rite of incorporation': 'We leave the rite of passage unfinished; the new mother and father are left in limbo, having to fend for themselves as best they can. The consequences of this incompleteness may be quite serious for some parents.'

Conflicting advice is given to the mother because there are now no norms for the amount of domestic activities that should be undertaken and no consensus as to when sexual relationships, for example, should be resumed. Her status is therefore ambiguous and her role as 'mother' is less valued by society than formerly. Her husband's role is also uncertain, which makes it more difficult to determine the type of support to give his wife.

This theory suggests that it is the absence of these routine behaviours and rituals which relate to the onset of depression by *lowering* a mother's self-esteem, causing uncertainty about the availability of social support, increasing physical fatigue, as well as stressing the relationship to her husband. Furthermore, as this lack of 'structure' postpartum represents ambivalence about mothering, this uncertainty will exacerbate further her role conflict and increases the threat to her self-esteem, and so predispose to clinical depression. Her baby can also then become a 'long-term difficulty', which may also lead to clinical depression.

Biological factors

The possibility that postnatal depression is caused by neuroendocrine changes has received some direct and indirect support from the literature and is more fully reviewed in Chapter 10. For example, Pitt (1968) found an association between premenstrual tension and postnatal depression and both of these conditions could be caused by hormonal changes. Reich and Winokur (1970) found a one in three risk of a postnatal mental illness occurring if there is a previous and family history of psychiatric disorder, which would suggest a strong genetic predisposition to puerperal mental illness. It is likely that the genes will exert their main effect through their control of neurotransmitter release at central brain synapses, and it is recognized that dopamine receptors are sensitive to the abrupt changes in circulating steroid hormones. However, such biological explanations are likely to be more cogent for early onset puerperal psychoses than the non-psychotic postnatal depression described in this chapter which occurs later in the puerperium.

The interaction between biological, psychological and social factors is complex, and there is also a need to consider the causal impact of life events *other* than childbirth such as house moving, an altered relationship to the partner or the loss of a previously valued work role.

Further progress towards understanding the causes of postnatal depression will occur when neurobiological research is carried out in close collaboration with social scientists. The way in which the birth event is rated as a 'life event' also needs to be carefully reconsidered and the social and personal meaning of childbirth, and the success or otherwise with which the rite de passage is negotiated, taken into account.

How important is it to detect and treat depression?

Most women who have experienced a puerperal depression of moderate to severe degree will readily recall this depression at a subsequent antenatal clinic and then request information about the likelihood of a recurrence. They are often very anxious about the possibility of a second postpartum mental illness and such anticipatory anxiety may increase the risk of obstetric complications, as 'maternal distress' is a well-established risk factor for obstetric complications. The alleviation of antenatal anxiety, which is so often linked with depression, may therefore not only increase the likelihood of good obstetric outcome but could also diminish the risk of a depressive illness postpartum.

Leverton and Elliott (1989) have shown that vulnerable women can be identified in pregnancy and if given instruction and support the risk of postnatal depression in first-time mothers can be reduced. The women known to be at high risk are those who experience excessive antenatal anxiety, have a family history of psychiatric disorder, and have had a previous postpartum depression or psychosis themselves. Poor social supports and adverse social circumstances are also important. In such women the risk of a mental illness occurring after childbirth can be as high as one in five. Since obstetricians and midwives are in regular contact with women during pregnancy there is therefore a responsibility to detect this high-risk group and to arrange appropriate prophylaxis. Such high-risk factors can indeed be as clearly recognized as those for eclampsia or for an assisted delivery and so should be routinely recorded during antenatal attendance. These vulnerable women can then be counselled by obstetric staff and/or referred to a psychologist, psychiatrist or psychiatric nurse so that the optimum strategy for prevention can be determined. Such intervention may include:

1. Giving additional psychological and practical support before and after delivery.
2. Advising against undertaking other life events such as a house move or job change if at all possible.
3. Ensuring that the family supports are mobilized and that the husband is fully briefed about the risk factors and of the need for his practical and psychological assistance.
4. For women at particularly high risk of manic or depressive psychosis, lithium carbonate can be an effective prophylaxis if a mother is not breast-feeding. I have found that thioridazine 50 mg three times daily given after childbirth has been effective and may have prevented a psychosis occurring.

Several studies have shown that about 10–15% of women with postnatal depression also had been depressed *prior* to delivery and that this depression may merge into a postnatal depression without interruption; the recognition of antenatal depression is therefore an important first step in prevention. If such antenatal depression is recognized, then there should be counselling available from a health professional who understands the mother's fears about the threat of recurrence, and careful consideration should also be given to the use of prophylactic medication such as antidepressants though not in the first trimester. A 'wait and see' attitude is rarely appropriate in this circumstance unless delivery is imminent; it should not be assumed that antenatal depression will be cured by the delivery itself. An assumption that a mother will become more cheerful after the birth of her baby may result in postnatal depression not being recognized; when the baby is born to a mother who is already depressed then the risk of a prolonged depression increases substantially.

A mother with severe postnatal blues is also more at risk of developing a prolonged postnatal depression after returning home; a quarter of women with at least three days of tears and distress within ten days of delivery became depressed in our Edinburgh study (Cox et al, 1982). These women therefore benefit from the blues being acknowledged as distressing, and also from receiving advice and reassurance. They also require support from community midwives, health visitors and general practitioners when discharged. There is a sub-group of women with *early onset* (within four weeks) postnatal depression and it is likely that it is in this sub-group that women with a manic/depressive diathesis are found. Obstetricians should therefore be specifically mindful of this possibility, especially when a mother is reported as having 'severe blues' or when there are symptoms suggestive of the early development of depressive illness such as extreme guilt, self-blame, unexpected rejection of the baby, and severe sleep disturbance.

Although most studies find no consistent association between antenatal or postnatal obstetric complications and psychiatric disorder, there is evidence that women who have had a caesarean section are slightly more vulnerable to puerperal psychoses than those who have had a vaginal delivery. Kendell et al (1987) found that twin deliveries were not more likely to be associated with postpartum mental illness but found that perinatal death clearly was. These authors concluded that as the high-risk factors included unmarried women experiencing a first pregnancy with inadequate social support, psychological factors were at least as important, and probably more important, than physical factors in the causation of severe postpartum depression. There is also a sub-group with early-onset psychoses for whom the illness occurs 'out of the blue' with no psychological vulnerability; it is in these women that biological factors, such as an increased sensitivity of the dopamine system to steroids, are likely to be most important in aetiology.

Is it life threatening?

A postpartum psychiatric disorder may place the mother at greater risk of death than from a postpartum haemorrhage and can also be a direct and indirect threat to the well-being and life of the baby. A severe depressive illness may lead to suicide (six cases were reported to the Association for Postnatal Mental Illness in the last year) and may be a contributory factor to some instances of non-accidental injury. In the study by Smith et al (1973), 48% of women who had carried out physical abuse were suffering from a 'neurosis', and it is probable that a proportion of these women were depressed.

These serious consequences are more likely to occur when an early-onset severe depressive illness has not been identified and when an illness which started as an apparently minor depression has developed into a psychotic illness with delusions of self-blame and guilt and a belief that the baby would be disadvantaged to remain alive.

When these events occur they can have a devastating effect on the family and are stressful to the health professionals who provided assistance. We are fortunate that in Britain the infanticide legislation recognizes the specific psychosocial circumstances relevant to the death of a baby within 12 months of childbirth. The Infanticide Law modifies the charge of murder to that of manslaughter and it is usual for a non-custodial sentence to be given. There are, however, several States in North America where no such legislation exists and where a mother may have a long-term prison sentence because of this offence. It is in these circumstances that the lack of a diagnostic category of puerperal psychosis may be extremely harmful to these women and their families.

Does postnatal depression always occur after obstetricians have handed over the management of their patients to primary care workers?

In general this is indeed the situation although, as already described, the identification of high-risk women and those with the onset of psychiatric disorder within two weeks of delivery remains a major routine responsibility for obstetric services.

Screening for postnatal depression at the postnatal clinic should also be carried out; if there is doubt about the value of this clinic from the point of view of customary obstetric practice, then an adequate justification is that this may be the only occasion when psychiatric disorder can be screened for and depression diagnosed.

The development of the Edinburgh Postnatal Depression Scale has allowed this screening to be a practical proposition; the development of this scale has been documented elsewhere (Cox et al, 1987). It has satisfactory psychometric properties (86% sensitivity and 79% specificity) and is superior to the Beck Depression inventory (Beck et al, 1961). It was as successful in detecting depression as established structured personal interview schedules (Harris et al, 1989). The scale can also be used to confirm the diagnosis in a mother who is regarded as a 'problem' patient by the primary care worker or specialist obstetrician or psychiatrist.

Can postnatal depression be prevented?

Some of the components of primary prevention have already been discussed. Parentcraft classes are an optimum time to instruct women about psychiatric disorder and there is no evidence that such instruction upsets or harms the mother. If such beliefs *are* held then they are likely to reflect the anxieties of health professionals rather than of the woman herself.

If primary prevention is to be carried out effectively then there is a need for a substantial increase in the education available for midwives and health visitors, and for refresher courses for general practitioners and possibly also for obstetricians and gynaecologists. Each health district should consider appointing a community psychiatric nurse and/or a psychiatrist who has acquired this extra experience and can then be a local educator able to liaise with the local obstetricians.

Secondary prevention

Early intervention in the treatment of postnatal depression is now feasible and the development of the Edinburgh Postnatal Depression Scale has accelerated this possibility. Occasionally a health visitor is anxious about Item 10 of the scale, which relates to self-harm, but these anxieties are not usually experienced by the mother herself.

Can postnatal depression be treated?

To an extent the treatment of postnatal depression is similar to that for a depressive illness occurring at other times, although because of the presence of a baby, specific treatment facilities may be necessary. There is now substantial evidence (Holden et al, 1989) that supportive counselling by a health professional is effective in at least a third of women with postnatal depression and that health visitors, and possibly community midwives, generally welcome the awareness that these professional skills can in themselves be effective. However, there is at least another third of women who require *other* treatments in addition to counselling/listening therapy, and it is for this group that availability of a mental health professional, such as a psychiatrist, is of particular importance (see Chapter 12).

Medication

Antidepressants, when prescribed in appropriate dosage, are the first line of management; there is no evidence that antidepressants prescribed in normal dosage can adversely affect the baby, even if the mother breast-feeds. However, compliance with antidepressants can be extremely poor and increasingly women are worried that such treatments are addictive and have fears that the baby or themselves will be harmed. Nevertheless, the doctor should ensure that such treatment is complied with if at all possible. Failure of depression to respond to both counselling and antidepressant medication, can have serious consequences, the most common being that the depressive disorder lasts on and becomes 'accepted' by the family and care workers. Persisting depressive symptoms are thus assumed to be the normal way of functioning and yet continue to have adverse consequences on the family and on the well-being of the children. The marriage becomes stressed, temporary separations occur and there is an increased likelihood that the development of the child may be adversely affected. Of yet more serious consequence is that such untreated depression may develop into a depressive psychosis with its associated risk of suicide and infanticide. Every attempt should therefore be made to prevent this situation occurring. Early intervention with electro-convulsive therapy treatment can be extremely effective for the severely depressed; this treatment can be arranged as a day-patient, but if this is not possible then inpatient admission is advisable.

The development of a day unit is a desirable compliment to the domiciliary care carried out by the general practitioner, health visitor or community midwife, and allows some women to be treated in a less stigmatizing environment than would otherwise occur if they had been admitted to an acute psychiatric ward or to an inpatient mother and baby unit.

Public policy considerations

Our present knowledge about postnatal mental illness is now sufficient to recommend certain changes in public policy and in curriculum design:

1. There should be identified within each health district at least two community psychiatric nurses who have a particular concern for the prevention and treatment of postpartum mood disorder and can provide essential back-up to other health professionals such as health visitors and midwives. Every attempt should be made to train general practitioners and hospital consultants such as paediatricians, psychiatrists and obstetricians in the treatments available for postnatal depression. General practitioners are usually well aware of the problem and, when given advice about methods of detection and the effectiveness of

treatment, will collaborate to a much greater extent than is commonly recognized.

2. Day units, either specifically designated for this client group or as a component of an established psychiatric day hospital, should be established. The central aspect of this development is the availability of a nursery so that the mother can attend with her baby and have space away from the child whilst she participates in therapy. The Parent and Baby Day Unit in Stoke-on-Trent has been described by Cox et al (unpublished data) and receives about six new referrals a week, several referrals coming from obstetricians at the North Staffordshire Maternity Hospital.

3. To function optimally these community day units also require the back-up from an inpatient mother and baby unit. In a district of 400 000, two such beds are required, with a flexible nurse management system—when there are no patients in the unit the nurses can be deployed elsewhere but then return to the unit at short notice. The larger mother and baby inpatient units, as well as the specifically designated parent and baby day units, fully justify their extra resource by the publicity they provide for this client group, as well as by the research and education that becomes possible. Oates (1988) has shown that in a health district of 500 000 a consultant psychiatrist who sees all referred women with children under one year can be fully and purposefully occupied for five days a week.

Conclusions

This chapter has highlighted some aspects of the academic literature on postnatal depression, but has also been based on my clinical experience and discussions with obstetric colleagues. This latter liaison task is vital and is perhaps best carried out by a general psychiatrist who has a specific interest in psychosomatic obstetrics and psychiatry. However, assistance from a child and adolescent psychiatrist who is specifically sensitive to the impact of maternal depression on the baby and siblings can also be valuable.

It is clear, however, that it is the obstetrician who is in the most important 'pivotal' position to seek improvement in the treatment facilities for mothers with antenatal or postnatal psychiatric disorder. Even if these managements are carried out by other health professionals, acknowledgement by obstetricians that these disorders commonly occur and that knowledge about their diagnosis and management is a component of professional training is important. It is the influence and leadership of obstetricians and not psychiatrists which may largely determine whether or not there will be a widespread overall improvement in treatment facilities for women with postnatal mental illness. Furthermore, their recognition that one in ten women attending a postnatal clinic or in the weeks that follow will have a depressive illness encourages other health professionals to take a greater interest in this disorder.

Obstetricians may not have the diagnostic and treatment expertise to manage the most severe cases of postpartum mood disorder; nevertheless, this chapter has underlined the need when training specialists for a greater knowledge of mental illnesses, especially non-psychotic disorders.

Frequent face-to-face conferences between obstetricians, psychiatrists and psychologists can be extremely useful for mutual education, for deciding on the details of management for women known to be at high risk of mental illness, and in identifying those who are presently suffering from psychiatric disorder.

It is to be hoped that the Royal College of Obstetricians and Gynaecologists and the Royal College of Psychiatrists will goad each other into action and provide a necessary and reciprocal education about postnatal depression, a serious and neglected postpartum complication.

REFERENCES

Beck AT, Ward CH, Mendelson M et al (1961) An inventory for measuring depression. *Archives of General Psychiatry* **4**: 53–63.

Breen D (1975) *The Birth of a First Child*. London: Tavistock.

Brown G (1989) Discussant. In Cox JL, Paykel E & Page ML (eds) *Childbirth as a Life Event*, p 53. Southampton: Duphar Medical Publications.

Brown GW & Harris T (1978) *Social Origins of Depression*. London: Tavistock.

Cooper PJ, Campbell EA, Day A et al (1988) Non-psychotic psychiatric disorder after childbirth: a prospective study of prevalence, incidence, course and nature. *British Journal of Psychiatry* **152**: 799–806.

Cox JL (1979) Psychiatric morbidity and pregnancy: a controlled study of 263 semi-rural Ugandan women. *British Journal of Psychiatry* **134**: 401–405.

Cox JL (1988) The life event of childbirth: sociocultural aspects of postnatal depression. In Kumar R & Brockington IF (eds) *Motherhood and Mental Illness, Vol II*. London: Wright.

Cox JL, Connor YM, Kendell RE (1982) Prospective study of psychiatric disorders of childbirth. *British Journal of Psychiatry* **140**: 111–117.

Cox JL, Rooney A, Thomas PF & Wrate RW (1984) How accurately do mothers recall postnatal depression? Further data from a 3-year follow-up study. *Journal of Psychosomatic Obstetrics and Gynaecology* **3**: 185–189.

Cox JL, Holden JM & Sagovsky R (1987) Detection of postnatal depression: development of the 10-item Edinburgh postnatal depression scale (EPDS). *British Journal of Psychiatry* **150**: 782–786.

Esquirol E (1845) *Mental Maladies: a Treatise on Insanities Trans*. Philadelphia: EK Hunt and Blanchard.

Harris B, Huckle P, Thomas R, Johns S & Fung H (1989) The use of rating scales to identify post-natal depression. *British Journal of Psychiatry* **154**: 813–817.

Holden JM, Sagovsky R & Cox JL (1989) A controlled study in the treatment of postnatal depression in primary care. *British Medical Journal* **298**: 223–226.

Homans H (1982) Pregnancy and birth as rites of passage. In MacCormack CP (ed.) *Ethnography of Fertility and Birth*, pp 231–268. London: Academic Press.

Jones AD & Dougherty C (1982) Childbirth in a scientific and industrial society. In McCormack CP (ed.) *Ethnography of Fertility in Birth*, pp 269–290. London: Academic Press.

Kelly JV (1967) The influences of native customs on obstetrics in Nigeria. *Obstetric and Gynecology* **30**: 608–612.

Kendell RE, Rennie D, Clarke JA & Dean C (1981) The social and obstetric correlates of psychiatric admission in the puerperium. *Psychological Medicine* **11**: 341–350.

Kendell RE, Chalmers L, Platz C (1987) The epidemiology of puerperal psychoses. *British Journal of Psychiatry* **150**: 662–673.

Kitzinger S (1982) The social context of birth: some comparison between childbirth in Jamaica and Britain. In MacCormack CP (ed.) *Ethnography of Fertility and Birth*, pp 181–203. London: Academic Press.

Kumar R & Brockington IF (eds) (1988) *Motherhood and Mental Illness, Vol. 2*. London: Wright.

Leverton TJ & Elliott SA (1989) Transition to parenthood groups: a preventive intervention for postnatal depression? In van Hall EV & Everaerd W (eds) *The Free Woman. Women's Health in the 1990s*, pp 479–486. Amsterdam: Parthenon Publishing.

McKinlay JB (1970) The new latecomers for antenatal care. *British Journal of Preventive and Social Medicine* **24:** 52–57.

Marcé LV (1858) *Traite de la Folie des Femmes Enceintes des Nouvelles Accouches et des Nourrices*. Paris: Baillière.

Menzies WF (1893) Puerperal insanity. An analysis of 140 consecutive cases. *American Journal of Insanity* **50:** 148–185.

Milio N (1975) Values, social class and community health services. In Cox C & Mead A (eds) *A Sociology of Medical Practice*, pp 49–61. London: Collier-MacMillan.

Nilsson A & Almgren PE (1970) Paranatal emotional and adjustment—a prospective investigation of 165 women. *Acta Psychiatrica Scandinavica Supplement* **220.**

Oates M (1988) The development of an integrated community-orientated service for severe postnatal mental illness. In Kumar R & Brockington IF (eds) *Motherhood and Mental Illness, Vol. 2*. London: Wright.

O'Hara MW, Zekoski EM, Philipps LH & Wright EJ (1989) A controlled study of postpartum mood disorders: comparison of childbearing and nonchildbearing women. *Journal of Abnormal Psychology* (in press).

Okley J (1975) Gipsy women: models in conflict. In Ardener S (ed.) *Perceiving Women*, pp 55–86. Dent: London.

Pillsbury BLK (1978) 'Doing the Month': confinement and convalescence of Chinese women after childbirth. *Social Science and Medicine* **12:** 11–22.

Pitt B (1968) 'Atypical' depression following childbirth. *British Journal of Psychiatry* **114:** 1325–1335.

Reich T & Winokur G (1970) Postpartum psychosis in patients with manic depressive disease. *Journal of Nervous Diseases* **151:** 60–68.

Seel RM (1968) Birth rite. *Health Visitor* **59:** 182–184.

Seligman MP (1975) *Depression, Development and Death*. San Francisco: Freeman.

Smith SM, Hanson R & Noble S (1973) Parents and battered babies: a controlled study. *British Medical Journal* **4:** 388–391.

Snaith RP, Constantopoulous AA, Jardine MY & McGuffin P (1978) A clinical scale for the self-assessment of irritability. *British Journal of Psychiatry* **132:** 164–171.

Stern G & Kruckman L (1983) Multi-disciplinary perspectives on postpartum depression: an anthropological critique. *Social Science and Medicine* **17:** 1027–1041.

Tetlow C (1955) Psychosis of childbearing. *Journal of Mental Science* **101:** 624.

Wolkind SN, Kevk S & Chaves LP (1976) Childhood experiences and psychosocial status in primiparous women: preliminary findings. *British Journal of Psychiatry* **128:** 391–396.

10

Endocrine aspects of postnatal mental disorders

ANGELIKA WIECK

Postnatal mental disorders hold a special position in psychiatry since they follow an event which not only has profound psychosocial implications but is also associated with massive biological changes. A significant role for physiological and in particular hormonal factors in the pathogenesis of these disorders has long been suspected. However, our understanding of the mechanisms by which the endocrine system and the central nervous system may interact has only recently made substantial progress owing to advances in biochemical techniques and behavioural animal models. With the advent of radio-immunoassays it has become possible to measure plasma concentrations of hormones with great specificity, sensitivity and precision. Thus it was discovered that the release of hormones from the pituitary is regulated by central monoamine neurotransmitters which are thought to have a critical role in the pathogenesis of affective disorders and schizophrenia. This neuroendocrine connection has become a major focus of research in psychoneuroendocrinology and is being utilized as a 'window into the brain' to explore neurotransmitter function in psychiatric patients. The elaboration of accurate assay systems also brought new insights into possible hormonal effects on brain function. Thus, hypothalamic peptides, which were initially believed to be solely involved in the control of the pituitary, have been discovered in extra-hypothalamic regions of the central nervous system. Pituitary and peripheral hormones have also been encountered in defined areas of the brain and have been shown to influence neuronal activity in electrophysiological, biochemical and behavioural experiments. Perhaps equally important is the recent recognition that psychological symptoms are common in, and may be the earliest manifestations of, endocrine disorders.

During pregnancy the production of many hormones rises gradually and substantially. After parturition, however, changes are more dramatic and complex; ovarian steroid and cortisol levels, for example, fall precipitously within the first few days and prolactin and oxytocin are secreted in large bursts, whereas the hypothalamic–pituitary–gonadal axis remains inactive for several weeks. The enquiry into the endocrine aetiology of postnatal psychiatric disorders can be approached on the basis of two general hypotheses. Firstly, the primary abnormality may be hormonal, which then impairs neurochemical function and finally leads to psychiatric symptoms. Secondly, the primary cause may be a pre-existing neurochemical abnormality, which is amplified by normal postnatal changes and thus reaches the threshold for symptom formation. Most studies to date have been based on the former assumption and tested for differences in single hormone measurements between postpartum women with psychiatric symptoms and those without.

The purpose of this chapter is to review these clinical studies for both major and minor postnatal mental illness and to highlight recent research evidence for an influence of hormones relevant to child-bearing upon brain function. The chapter begins with an account of the major current neurotransmitter hypotheses of affective disorders and schizophrenia. The following sections address endocrine factors which may have a role in the causation of postnatal mental illness and are divided into the discussion of steroids, peptide and thyroid hormones. Finally, possible reasons why biological studies in postnatal mental disorders have as yet contributed little to the understanding of their pathogenesis are considered and an attempt is made to identify promising areas for future research.

MONOAMINE HYPOTHESES OF MAJOR PSYCHIATRIC DISORDERS

Monoamine neurotransmitters

Over the past three decades much of the biological literature on affective disorders has been concerned with monoamine neurotransmitters, and in particular with the function of central noradrenergic and serotonergic systems in depression. Noradrenaline (norepinephrine; NA) derives from the amino acid tyrosine, and serotonin (5HT) is synthesized from the amino acid tryptophan. These monoamine neurotransmitters are stored in vesicles close to the synaptic membrane and are released into the synaptic cleft when an action potential arrives. The translation of the electrical signal into cellular events is mediated via binding of the transmitter to its postsynaptic receptor. Each monoamine can elicit different cellular responses depending on the receptor subtype present at the particular synapse. In the human brain four noradrenergic (β_1 and β_2, α_1 and α_2) receptor subtypes and at least three major classes of 5HT receptors (5HT-1A, 5HT-1B and 5HT2) have been demonstrated. β-Receptors are located on postsynaptic membranes and when activated stimulate the formation of the second messenger cyclic AMP (cAMP), whereas α_2- and probably also 5HT1-receptors are pre- and post-synaptic and inhibit the formation of cAMP; α_1- and 5HT2-receptors are postsynaptic and their stimulation generates two second messengers, inositol triphosphate and diacylglycerol. Following receptor activation the transmitter is either degraded by the enzyme monoamine oxidase or cleared from the synapse by re-uptake into the nerve terminal, where it is recycled into the storage vesicles. On a biochemical level neurotransmission is regulated via the direct feedback effects of the transmitter on its synthesis and via its presynaptic receptor. Activation of this receptor inhibits further transmitter release.

Affective disorders

The hypothesis that NA and 5HT are involved in the pathogenesis of depression originated from the discovery that a number of antidepressant drugs increase the intrasynaptic concentration of these monoamines by blocking their re-uptake into the nerve terminal or inhibiting the activity of monoamine oxidase. Thus it was thought that depression is caused by a lack of NA and/or 5HT at strategically important central synapses. However, the pharmacological effect occurs within hours of drug administration and cannot explain why the therapeutic response in depressed patients is delayed until after at least two weeks of continuous therapy. Subsequently the chronic administration of antidepressant treatments to experimental animals was found to induce changes at monoamine receptors at about that time. The pattern of changes varies with the type of drug and includes a decrease in the number and sensitivity of β-receptors and presynaptic α_2-receptors and an enhanced responsiveness of α_1- and probably also 5HT-receptors (for review see Baldessarini, 1989). On the basis of these results several new hypotheses were formulated.

Sulser et al (1978), for example, proposed that a hypersensitivity of β-receptors may contribute to the pathogenesis of depression and that the therapeutic effect of antidepressant drugs depends on their desensitization. However, a number of pharmacological and clinical observations have been reported which are inconsistent with this concept. Others suggested that the net effect of prolonged antidepressant therapy is to facilitate noradrenergic neurotransmission by desensitizing hyperresponsive presynaptic α_2-receptors (Leonard, 1980) or by enhancing the sensitivity of α_1-receptors (Menkes et al, 1983). These hypotheses have stimulated a large number of receptor studies in depressed patients. Until recently the assessment of monoamine receptor function in man has been dependent on the use of indirect research strategies. Blood platelets possess α_2-receptors which are pharmacologically similar to those found on neurones and a number of investigators have measured the binding of α_2-agonists and antagonists to platelets obtained from depressed patients and normal controls. The results of such studies have been conflicting. In contrast, neuroendocrine investigations with the α_2-agonist clonidine have in most studies shown a blunted growth hormone (GH) response in drug-free patients with endogenous depression, indicating a reduced sensitivity of postsynaptic α_2-receptors in the hypothalamus, whereas indices of the function of presynaptic α_2-receptors have been reported to be unchanged in the same patients (Checkley et al, 1986). This postsynaptic α_2-receptor subsensitivity seems to persist when patients have fully recovered and thus may represent a trait marker (Matussek, 1988; Mitchell et al, 1988). Its role in the pathogenesis of depressive illness, however, is as yet uncertain. Test systems for the evaluation of α_1-receptor function have not yet been developed.

Investigations of the 5HT system in depression have produced relatively consistent results and have indeed pointed towards a reduced activity in depression as originally suggested. Findings include a decrease in 5HT turnover and 5HT uptake into platelets as well as a lower number of imipramine binding sites on platelets and in post-mortem brain of patients with major depressive disorders (Deakin and Crow, 1986; Wood, 1986; Langer and Shoemaker, 1988). Imipramine binding sites are closely associated with the 5HT re-uptake system and are thought to modulate 5HT transport.

Dopamine (DA) neurotransmission is not acutely affected by the majority of antidepressant drugs and as a result this monoamine was omitted for several years from consideration as a mediator for affective disorders. However, there is now some evidence that chronic antidepressant treatment enhances the responsiveness of mesolimbic DA receptors (Willner, 1985). In addition, clinical evidence points to a role of DA in manic illness. Neuroleptic drugs which reduce dopaminergic neurotransmission are effective antimanic agents and drugs which enhance dopaminergic neurotransmission have been shown to precipitate manic episodes in predisposed patients.

Schizophrenia

For many years the hypothesis of excessive dopamine neurotransmission has been at the centre of attempts to understand the pathophysiology of schizophrenia. It is based on the observation that dopamine-releasing drugs such as amphetamine induce schizophrenia-like states and on the well-established antipsychotic effect of drugs which block dopamine neurotransmission. Investigations of dopamine metabolism in schizophrenia, however, have not provided consistent support for this concept. Post-mortem brain studies indicate that patients with schizophrenia may have an increased number of central dopamine receptors of the D_2 type (Lee et al, 1978; Owen et al, 1978). It is not clear at present whether these changes are indeed part of the disease process or result from chronic drug treatment. New neuroimaging techniques are now available which permit the measurement of dopamine receptors in vivo in patients who have never received neuroleptic drugs. However, the two published studies using positron emission tomography techniques (Wong et al, 1986; Farde et al, 1987) have not yet resolved this issue.

In summary, pharmacological evidence suggests that the DA system mediates the therapeutic effect of antipsychotic drugs and that one or more monoamine systems are involved in the therapeutic response to antidepressant drugs. The hypothesis that abnormal function in these systems contributes to the pathophysiology of major psychiatric illness has not consistently been supported by biological studies in drug-free patients. Progress is to be expected from several areas. For example, ligands with higher receptor specificity are being developed which may provide 'cleaner' test systems for in vivo neuroendocrine and receptor binding studies. The rapid progress in biochemical techniques has also made it possible to look at events downstream from the receptor level. The mood-stabilizing drug lithium has for example, been found to inhibit the recycling of inositol triphosphate. By disrupting this process the drug may diminish the effects of neurotransmission through the many receptor types linked with this second messenger system. Genetic linkage studies may also provide guidance for promising areas of neurochemical research.

STEROID HORMONES

Ovarian steroids

Total oestradiol and progesterone concentrations in maternal plasma increase gradually during gestation and at term are 100–200 times higher than average levels during the luteal phase of the menstrual cycle (Willcox ct al, 1985a; Bourque et al, 1986). About 1 to 3% of circulating ovarian hormones is unbound to plasma proteins and therefore free to enter the brain. Within the individual woman this proportion remains unchanged throughout pregnancy (Willcox et al, 1985a). After delivery there is a precipitous fall in total oestradiol and progesterone levels. Very low values are reached within one week postpartum (Bonnar et al, 1975; Willcox et al, 1985b) and levels remain low until a maturing ovarian follicle resumes steroid production several weeks or months later. Whether there are significant changes in the percentage of free steroids in the postpartum period is not known.

Hormonal studies in women with postnatal psychiatric disorders have almost exclusively relied on measuring total circulating steroid levels. No significant relationships have emerged between postpartum oestradiol levels and the maternity blues (Nott et al, 1976; Kuevi et al, 1983), postnatal depression (Butler and Leonard, 1986; Harris et al, 1989) or puerperal manic-depressive psychosis (Hatotani et al, 1979). However, a different result was obtained by Feksi et al (1984), who measured steroid concentrations in saliva, which are thought to reflect the free fractions in plasma and allow non-invasive repeated sampling. Four saliva samples were collected over 24 hours during the first five days postpartum. Mean concentrations of oestradiol and progesterone were significantly higher in blues-sufferers on the day when symptoms occurred than in matched symptom-free controls. Studies of plasma levels of total progesterone have yielded conflicting results for the maternity blues (Nott et al, 1976; Ballinger et al, 1982; Kuevi et al, 1983; Metz et al, 1983). A deficit of progesterone as an aetiological factor in postnatal depression has been advocated by Dalton (1980) who, in an open study, reported successful prophylaxis with daily administration of progesterone from delivery until two months postpartum or until the return of menstruation. The effectiveness of such treatment remains to be demonstrated in double-blind controlled studies. Butler and Leonard (1986) and Harris et al (1989) found no association between plasma progesterone levels and depressed mood at six to eight weeks postpartum. However, Harris et al (1989) also measured progesterone concentrations in saliva collected three times over one day at six to eight weeks postpartum. In bottle-feeding women salivary progesterone at each time-point correlated positively with several indices of depression and, within this group, was higher in subjects who were taking oral contraceptives than in non-pill users. Conversely, in breast-feeders salivary progesterone correlated negatively with ratings of depression and pill-takers were less likely to score as depressed than non-pill takers. This indicates that both too little and too much progesterone may enhance the vulnerability to postnatal depression. If it were to be replicated by other research groups this finding would have important implications for the use of steroid treatment in postnatal mothers.

Due to their lipophilic structure ovarian hormones have unrestricted access to the brain. Little is known about the interactions of progesterone with the central nervous system and the focus of the following sections will therefore be on oestrogenic effects. Although oestrogens have been demonstrated to act directly upon nerve cell membranes, their main effect involves entering the cell and binding to receptor proteins. The oestrogen-receptor complex moves to the nucleus, where the hormone interacts with the genome and alters the expression of specific genes. Thus oestrogens can modulate the synthesis of enzymes, peptides, neurotransmitters and receptors. Oestrogen receptors are distributed throughout the central nervous system. Apart from the pituitary and the hypothalamus, high densities have been found in limbic forebrain structures and monoaminergic neurones of the brainstem. This suggests that oestrogens are not only involved in the modulation of hormone release and reproductive behaviour but also may influence the function of the monoaminergic systems which are thought to have a role in the pathogenesis of major psychiatric illness.

Oestrogen and dopamine

Various oestrogen-induced alterations of central dopaminergic function have been described. The effects upon the tuberoinfundibular dopamine (TIDA) system have been studied in particular detail. Hypothalamic DA is a potent inhibitor of prolactin secretion from the pituitary, whereas oestrogens stimulate its release. In ovariectomized rats, chronic treatment with high doses of oestrogens has in most studies been shown to suppress TIDA neuronal activity, reduce the number of DA receptors on the lacto-troph cell and attenuate the DA-induced inhibition of adenylate cyclase. The function of DA systems originating from the midbrain may also be influenced by ovarian steroids as suggested by clinical evidence. In women with Parkinson's disease, symptom severity has been reported to vary with the menstrual cycle phase (Quinn and Marsden, 1986) and in women with a previous history of chorea or rheumatic fever, symptoms are known to recur during pregnancy or during treatment with oral contraceptives (Lewis and Parsons, 1966; Nausieda et al, 1979). These observations have stimulated extensive research work into the effects of oestrogen treatment upon the function of nigrostriatal and mesolimbic DA systems in animals. Results are conflicting and depend on the particular part of the systems under investigation, the dose being used and the interval between oestrogen administration and experiment. The topic has been comprehensively reviewed by Van Hartesveldt and Joyce (1986). In a study of ovariectomized rats treated with high doses of oestrogen, Gordon and Perry (1983) found that the behavioural response to the DA agonist apomorphine was significantly enhanced at 72 hours after administration of the last dose, suggesting an increased sensitivity of DA receptors. On the basis of these results our research team is currently investigating the hypothesis that puerperal psychosis may be triggered by the effects of oestrogen withdrawal upon central DA systems. The function of hypothalamic D_2-receptors is being assessed on the fourth day postpartum in women at high risk of developing a puerperal psychosis, using the GH response to the DA agonist apomorphine as the test system. Results obtained so far from 12 drug-free patients and 14 controls indicate a significantly enhanced GH response in the 'high risk' group (Wieck et al, 1989). This suggests that D_2-receptor hypersensitivity in the early puerperal period may contribute to the development of severe postnatal mental disorder. Whether this is indeed induced by oestrogen withdrawal needs further investigation.

Oestrogen and noradrenaline

In the noradrenergic system long-term oestrogen exposure has been shown to reduce the number of noradrenergic β-receptors in the rat cerebral cortex (Biegon et al, 1983). The functional significance of such a change is uncertain. Although desensitization of β-receptors is a mechanism common to most antidepressant treatments, it is probably not central to their therapeutic effect, since β-receptor blocking drugs have no antidepressant properties. Human platelet $α_2$-receptors have been reported to fluctuate across the menstrual cycle and during treatment with oral contraceptives. In a prospective study Best et al (1988) measured platelet [^{3}H]-yohimbine binding as an index of $α_2$-receptor numbers in over 100 women before and after childbirth. All women showed a postpartum drop in the number of $α_2$-receptors but blues-sufferers had significantly more binding sites on days 10 and 20 postpartum than women without the blues. Thus in predisposed women the postpartum period may induce changes of $α_2$-receptors which contribute to the development of postpartum mood disturbance. However, whether these changes are caused by withdrawal from steroids needs to be further examined.

Oestrogen and serotonin

There is also evidence for a role of both oestrogen and progesterone in the modulation of 5HT function in areas of the brain which are not primarily involved with the control of hormone secretion and sexual behaviour. In rat cerebral cortex ovarian steroids have been shown to facilitate the down-regulation of 5HT2 receptors induced by the antidepresant drug imipramine (Kendall et al, 1982). Likewise, in another study (Biegon et al, 1983) chronic treatment with either oestradiol or progesterone induced an increase in 5HT2-receptor numbers in rat cerebral cortex, but also decreased the density of 5HT1-receptors. Thus the net effect of oestrogens on serotonergic transmission is unknown. Stockert and de Robertis (1985) reported that ovariectomy in rats leads to a marked increase in imipramine binding sites in several areas of the central nervous system except for the cerebral cortex and the brainstem. However, chronic treatment of ovariectomized rats with oestrogen also increased the number of imipramine binding sites (Rehavi et al, 1987). In this study only frontal cortex and hypothalamus were examined. Thus it is possible that oestrogenic effects vary in different parts of the brain.

In a study of the function of platelet imipramine binding sites of pregnant and postnatal women, Katona et al (1985) found a significant decrease in receptor affinity at three to seven days postpartum but no changes in binding capacity. The design of this study was cross-sectional and a preparation of lysed platelets was used. This may explain the difference to the results obtained by Best et al (1988). In this longitudinal study the binding capacity of intact platelets significantly decreased on day 10 postpartum and returned to antenatal values on day 20. The affinity of the binding sites did not change over time. Unfortunately, it is not yet known how alterations in binding characteristics are related to the function of serotonergic systems in vivo.

The hypothalamic–pituitary–adrenal axis

The production and secretion of cortisol from the adrenal cortex is stimulated by the pituitary peptide adrenocorticotrophic hormone (ACTH), which is secreted into the systemic circulation principally in response to the stimulatory action of the hypothalamic peptide corticotrophin-releasing hormone (CRH). Cortisol plasma levels are highest in the morning, decline throughout the day and rise again during late sleep. This circadian pattern is produced by periodic changes in CRH release which are determined by an endogenous rhythm in the central nervous system. CRH and ACTH release are further regulated by neurotransmitters, feedback effects of cortisol and stress.

The function of the hypothalamic–pituitary–adrenal (HPA) system is of particular interest in psychiatry. Addison's disease and Cushing's syndrome or treatment with high doses of corticosteroids are frequently associated with psychiatric disturbances ranging from mild depression and apathy to severe psychotic illness. Their pathogenesis may be mediated by changes in central glucocorticoid receptors which have a high density in certain areas of the limbic system. It is well known that in many endogenously depressed patients the 24-hour production of cortisol is enhanced and cortisol levels are more often resistant to dexamethasone feedback inhibition than in other psychiatric patients or normal controls. A number of other functional abnormalities in the HPA system have now been identified in depression, and the pattern of changes best fits the model of a chronic increase in hypothalamic CRH release and secondary compensatory changes in other parts of the system. It is not clear, however, whether the enhanced CRH drive should be regarded as a marker of a primary pathology or rather as an adaptive response to recurrent stress.

Only about 10% of the total amount of circulating cortisol is not bound to plasma proteins and therefore free to enter the brain. During pregnancy total and free cortisol levels and corticosteroid-binding globulin gradually increase until term and then fall precipitously within the first few days postpartum (Cousins et al, 1983; Willcox et al, 1985b; Potter et al, 1987). A similar time course has been reported for CRH and ACTH, which are thought to be of both central and placental origin (Rees et al, 1975; Csontos et al, 1979; Shibasaki et al, 1982).

Several research groups have examined the relationship between cortisol levels and postpartum mood changes and results are conflicting. In the study of Handley et al (1977), elation correlated positively with plasma cortisol levels over the first postpartum week. Similarly, Ballinger et al (1982) reported that women who experienced positive postpartum mood changes had significantly higher total cortisol levels on the first day after delivery than women whose mood remained stable. Significantly elevated cortisol levels have also been found in blues-sufferers at 38 weeks of pregnancy and five days after delivery (Handley et al, 1980) and at three to four days postpartum (Okano, 1989). However, in two other studies no significant associations emerged between plasma cortisol levels and blues symptoms (Kuevi et al, 1983; Brinsmead et al, 1985). An important reason for this lack of agreement may be that single cortisol measurements yield unreliable results because of the episodic nature of its release, with particularly high peaks in the morning. Measurements of the free cortisol fraction may be more informative, but available methods are time-consuming and costly. These problems may be circumvented by measuring the 24-hour urinary secretion of free cortisol which provides a fairly reliable estimate of adreno-cortical activity over time. Another possibility is the estimation of cortisol content in saliva. Using this method Feksi et al (1984) did not find any significant differences in diurnal cortisol profiles between women with a high blues score and women who exhibited no postpartum mood changes. In the study of Harris et al (1989) no consistent differences were found in saliva levels between depressed and non-depressed women at six to eight weeks postpartum.

Pregnancy is associated with a decreased response to the dexamethasone suppression test (DST), which in the majority of women persists up to the second or third postpartum week and is not associated with postnatal psychiatric morbidity (Greenwood and Parker, 1984; Owens et al, 1987). The dissociation between the rapid fall of cortisol and ACTH after parturition and the late recovery of feedback mechanisms is intriguing. One may speculate that this indicates a pregnancy-induced down-regulation of central glucocorticoid receptors which, in the presence of low postpartum cortisol levels, may enhance the vulnerability to psychiatric disorder.

PEPTIDES

Gonadotrophin-releasing hormone and pituitary gonadotrophins

Gonadotrophin-releasing hormone (GnRH) is probably the most important mediator of central nervous system influences upon reproduction. It is synthesized in neurones of the mediobasal hypothalamus, secreted into the portal circulation and transported to the anterior pituitary. Here it binds to specific receptors and thus activates the synthesis and release of follicle-stimulating hormone (FSH) and luteinizing hormone (LH). FSH is responsible for the maturation of an ovarian follicle and ovarian steroid secretion, whereas LH induces ovulation and the formation of the corpus luteum. Gonadotrophins are released in pulses in direct response to episodic secretory discharges of GnRH. A number of neurotransmitters have been reported to control the activity of GnRH neurones. These inputs are subject to the feedback effects of ovarian steroids which modulate pulse frequency and amplitude. At the pituitary level the responsiveness of gonadotroph cells is regulated both by ovarian steroids and a positive feedback of GnRH onto its own receptors. In the follicular phase of the menstrual cycle these influences result in low-amplitude LH pulses which increase in frequency towards ovulation. In contrast, the luteal phase is characterized by a pattern of infrequent high-amplitude pulses, often with long intervals when gonadotrophin levels remain low and non-pulsatile. Pharmacological studies suggest that endogenous opioid peptides (EOP) are an important mediator for the slowing of the pulse generator in the luteal phase. Thus administration of the opioid receptor antagonist naloxone increases the frequency and amplitude of pulsatile LH release (Veldhuis et al, 1983). The observation that naloxone includes high LH responses in the luteal phase but only low responses in the early follicular phase suggests that ovarian steroids modify the activity of EOP (Quigley and Yen, 1980). This may be an important mechanism for the suppression of gonadotrophin secretion during pregnancy. After delivery the majority of lactating women have abnormally low-frequency and low-amplitude LH release during the period of full postpartum ovarian suppression (Glasier et al, 1984). Ishizuka et al (1984) reported that in the early puerperium naloxone induces significant LH and FSH increments. These findings suggest that increased opioid activity is enhanced in the postpartum period despite low ovarian hormone levels and that it contributes to postpartum amenorrhoea. A possible role for EOPs in postnatal mental disorders is discussed below.

Axons of GnRH neurones are not confined to the median eminence. There are widespread projections to limbic and other extra-hypothalamic areas of the brain including the ventral tegmental area of the pons (Silverman and Krey, 1978). This region also contains the cell bodies of the mesolimbic DA system, which is thought to be involved in the pathogenesis of psychoses and to be a target site of antipsychotic drugs. In rats, GnRH has been shown to stimulate male and female mating behaviour by direct action upon the central nervous system. GnRH has also been reported to increase libido and potency in impotent or hypogonadotrophic men. McAdoo et al (1978) administered GnRH intravenously to normal men and found an enhancement of alertness and speed of performance and a decrease in anxiety and fatigue. However, it has not been established whether in man GnRH-induced effects occur independently from elevation of plasma testosterone levels. Thus it is possible that the GnRH system modulates aspects of human behaviour and that a dysregulation in the postpartum period results in psychological symptoms. Direct information on hypothalamic GnRH secretory activity, however, can only be obtained by measuring the peptide in the portal circulation, which is obviously impossible in humans. Nott et al (1976) and Kuevi et al (1983) measured plasma concentrations of pituitary gonadotrophins after delivery and found no significant correlations with the occurrence of maternity blues. FSH and LH themselves are not known to have behavioural functions.

Endogenous opioid peptides

A large number of endogenous peptides have over recent years been shown to act as ligands for opiate receptors. Opioid peptides can conveniently be divided into three families according to their precursor molecules. Encephalins and dynorphins derive from proencephalin A and B, respectively. They are present in perikarya and fibres in many areas of the brain. β-Endorphin is produced by enzymatic cleavage from pro-opiomelanocortin, which also contains ACTH and a number of other peptides. β-Endorphin-containing neurones are mainly located in and around the arcuate nucleus of the hypothalamus and their fibres project both to other hypothalamic nuclei and to more distant target sites. The widespread distribution in the CNS suggests that EOPs have multiple physiological functions. Their analgesic properties and their role in neuroendocrine regulation are well established, but little is known about possible effects on mood, behaviour or cognitive function in man. In drug addicts opiates have been reported to reduce anxiety and depression, which may be related to the relief from distressing withdrawal symptoms rather than to a primary pharmacological effect. In unaddicted pain-free subjects, opiate drugs frequently induce unpleasant experiences including dysphoria and anxiety.

β-Endorphin is also produced by the pituitary and during pregnancy possibly by the placenta. Levels in maternal plasma rise steeply during labour and quickly fall again after delivery (Csontos et al, 1979; Newnham et al, 1984). Whether substantial changes in plasma levels occur before term is controversial. Fletcher et al (1980) and Goland et al (1981) found no difference between women at various stages of pregnancy and non-pregnant control subjects. In contrast, Newnham and colleagues (1983, 1984) reported a gradual and significant increase from the first trimester onwards and put forward the hypothesis that postpartum opioid withdrawal may be a cause of the postnatal blues syndrome. However, they found a negative correlation between β-endorphin levels at 36 weeks of pregnancy and the postnatal blues score and no significant correlations between β-endorphin levels during labour or the rate of postpartum decline and blues symptoms. A similar study by Brinsmead et al (1985) also failed to demonstrate significant correlations between changes in β-endorphin concentrations and several measures of blues symptoms. In contrast, George and Wilson (1983) reported a significant correlation between plasma β-endorphin levels and symptoms of depression, anxiety and tension over the first week postpartum. One problem with these studies is that radio-immunoassay methods cannot distinguish between the active and inactive forms of β-endorphin, which both exist in plasma. In addition, the functional role of circulating opioid peptides is uncertain. β-Endorphin is released from the pituitary in response to stress and may be involved in peripheral adaptive processes. However, central effects are unlikely to be mediated by peripheral opioids since they only poorly pass the blood–brain barrier.

As pointed out earlier, there is good evidence that inhibition of GnRH release during the luteal phase of the menstrual cycle is mediated by increased hypothalamic opioid activity. Facchinetti et al (1988) examined LH release in response to the opiate antagonist naloxone in women with premenstrual syndrome (PMS), women with premenstrual migraine (PMM) and normal controls. During the mid-luteal phase naloxone induced a large rise in LH release in all groups. Close to the onset of menses, controls maintained this response, whereas women with PMS and PMM exhibited a marked drop in their responsiveness. Interestingly, in the premenstrual phase the LH response correlated negatively with negative affect in the PMS group and with pain in the PMM group. Thus the authors suggest that a transient failure of central opioid tone may increase the vulnerability to premenstrual depression and migraine. The opioid system involved in GnRH inhibition is β-endorphinergic (Wehrenberg et al, 1982) and one of its extra-hypothalamic projections terminates at noradrenergic neurones in the pons (Bloom et al, 1978). This connection is intriguing since the noradrenergic system has been implicated in the pathogenesis of affective disorders and in the production of opiate withdrawal symptoms. Since the postpartum period is also character-ized by increased opioid inhibition of GnRH release, Deakin (1988) proposed that a dysfunction in this system could be an aetiological factor in postnatal mental disorders. Studies of LH pulsatility or naloxone responsiveness have not yet been carried out within this context.

A series of remarkable findings has been reported by a Swedish research group. Lindstroem et al (1978, 1984) identified an opioid peptide in the cerebrospinal fluid and plasma of lactating women with puerperal psychosis which was not present in lactating healthy mothers. The physicochemical properties of this peptide were closely similar to those of β-casomorphins. These are opioid peptides which derive from enzymatic degradation of the milk protein β-casein. In a subsequent study the content of this protein was found to be reduced in the breast-milk of psychotic mothers, whereas the levels of opioid peptides were increased compared with normal controls, suggesting an enhanced proteolytic degradation (Nyberg et al, 1988). The authors proposed that abnormally high levels of opioid peptides derived from milk proteins may contribute to organic symptoms of puerperal psychosis. These preliminary findings are intriguing since the maternity blues and the onset of many cases of puerperal psychosis coincide with the initiation of lactation.

Prolactin

During pregnancy there is a gradual and progressive increase in prolactin (PRL) serum concentrations until term, when levels are about ten times higher than during the menstrual cycle (Tyson et al, 1972). They remain remarkably high in the early puerperium, but in non-breast-feeding mothers return to the prepregnant range by about the third week postpartum (Tolis et al, 1974). In regularly nursing mothers, basal PRL levels slowly decrease as lactation progresses (Johnston and Amico, 1986), the rate of decline depending on the frequency of breast-feeds (Howie et al, 1981).

PRL has often been suspected to be aetiologically relevant to the various somatic and psychological changes which some women experience during the premenstrual period. In general, clinical studies have revealed that the incidence of hyperprolactinaemia in women with premenstrual syndrome is very low and not greater than in normal populations. Evidence for a link between this hormone and psychiatric symptomatology comes from investigations of patients recruited from endocrinology clinics (Kellner et al, 1984; Buckman and Kellner, 1985). In these studies hyperprolactinaemic patients scored significantly higher on depression, anxiety and hostility scales than carefully selected control groups. Symptom ratings fell markedly when PRL secretion was suppressed by the dopamine agonist bromocriptine. George et al (1980) measured basal serum PRL levels in 38 women during the first postpartum week and reported a significant positive correlation with symptoms of depression, anxiety and tension as elicited by a standardized psychiatric interview. However, two other research groups (Nott et al, 1976; Kuevi et al, 1983) failed to find significant differences in PRL levels between blues and non-blues sufferers. Whereas Nott et al (1976) did not measure baseline values, methodological differences between the two other studies are not directly apparent. In a carefully designed study Alder et al (1986) examined the relationship between PRL and postnatal depression. Baseline serum levels were measured at fortnightly intervals from week 4 to 24 postpartum. Every week each woman rated on visual analogue scales how she had felt during the previous week. In the 14 women who were breast-feeding for more than six weeks and did not use oral contraceptives, hormone levels were not correlated with weekly mood ratings. In contrast, Harris et al (1989) found significantly lower PRL levels in six breast-feeding mothers with depression than in 12 breast-feeders who remained well. In this study sampling time was not controlled with regard to the last breast-feed. This is important since suckling-induced PRL secretion remains at a high level for at least 120 minutes after feeding has begun (Noel et al, 1974). Systematic studies of PRL have not been carried out in women with puerperal psychosis. A relationship is unlikely to emerge since prolactin-secreting tumours are not known to be associated with major psychiatric illness.

Clearly more investigations are required which should be designed according to the hypothesis to be tested. For an estimate of total daily prolactin secretion it may be useful to measure hormone levels during and at an appropriate interval after a breast-feeding episode and to carefully record nursing frequency. As mentioned above, pituitary PRL secretion is under the inhibitory control of the TIDA system and is often used to assess the function of hypothalamic DA receptors. Thus the suppression of PRL secretion is measured after administration of a DA agonist. Studies in postpartum women at high risk of developing a major psychiatric illness are currently in progress.

Oxytocin

Circulating oxytocin levels are usually low during pregnancy but rise in association with labour and breast-feeding episodes. The primary function of oxytocin is to augment uterine contractions during labour and to stimulate lactation by its action on the myoepithelial cells of the mammary gland. The peptide is synthesized as part of a large precursor molecule in the cell bodies of the supraoptic and paraventricular nuclei of the hypothalamus. During transport along the axon toward the nerve terminal in the posterior pituitary the molecule is cleaved into oxytocin and a number of other peptides, including oestrogen-sensitive neurophysin (ESN). Oxytocin and ESN are released simultaneously into the systemic circulation.

Several lines of evidence suggest that, apart from its peripheral actions, the peptide may also have a role in modulating central nervous system function. Thus oxytocin-containing nerve terminals are located throughout the mammalian nervous system. Among the brain areas with the highest density are those which contain DA-producing neurones such as the substantia nigra and ventral tegmental area, but significant amounts have also been found in the noradrenergic and serotonergic nuclei of the brain stem (Sofroniew, 1983). There is some evidence that oxytocin influences monoamine neurotransmission by altering DA and NA turnover (Kovacs and Telegdy, 1983). The behavioural effects of oxytocin which have so far been observed in animals are of potential interest for the study of postnatal mental disorders. The peptide facilitates maternal behaviour in virgin rats (Pedersen and Prange, 1979). De Wied and Bohus (1979) have also suggested that oxytocin has amnesic properties, although others have argued that these are due to non-specific mechanisms.

Whalley et al (1982) measured oxytocin-like immunoreactivity in plasma in three women at high risk of puerperal psychosis at the end of pregnancy and at several time-points in the postnatal period. Nine blood samples were taken on each test day and results compared with two normal control subjects. The one patient who relapsed postpartum showed considerably higher values for oxytocin-like immunoreactivity in all blood samples taken before delivery than the other four subjects. However, further investigation revealed that the very high levels were probably caused by cross-reacting placental oxytocinase. This is a relatively unspecific enzyme which degrades a number of peptides. The authors suggest that the loss of high plasma oxytocinase activity after delivery may participate in the development of psychotic symptoms due to abnormal patterns of centrally active peptides.

In recent studies the measurement of ESN in peripheral blood has been preferred to that of oxytocin because of its longer half-life. Electroconvulsive therapy (ECT) induces ESN release and Scott et al (1989) reported that the percentage increase in ESN levels after the first treatment was significantly higher in depressed patients who made a good recovery than in those who responded poorly to treatment. The significance of this result is as yet unclear. The authors have suggested that it may represent a dysregulation of the neurotransmitter control of oxytocin release in ECT responders or that the peptide itself may have a therapeutic effect. However, whether and to what extent peripheral oxytocin can reach a central site of action has not been established. Administration of oestrogen leads to a dose-dependent increase in ESN secretion and this response is currently being used as a model to assess oestrogen receptor function in women at high risk for severe postnatal psychiatric disorder (Bearn et al, 1986).

THYROID SYSTEM

Transient thyroid dysfunction is surprisingly common in the postpartum period. Epidemiological surveys have reported an incidence of 5.5–11.3% (Amino et al, 1982; Nikolai et al, 1987). Most of these cases can be attributed to 'painless thyroiditis'. This syndrome is characterized by an initial thyrotoxic and often asymptomatic phase occurring between the second and fourth month postpartum followed by a more prolonged hypothyroid phase and a return to euthyroid function by six to twelve months after delivery (Walfish and Chan, 1985). During the hypothyroid phase painless swelling of the gland may be prominent but other physical signs of hypothyroidism are often missing. Complaints of fatigue, weight gain and loss of libido are frequent but difficult to distinguish from normal postpartum experiences (Jansson et al, 1988). Thyroid microsomal antibodies are usually present and the condition is thought to be due to the postpartum enhancement of immunoreactivity in women predisposed to autoimmune thyroiditis.

It is now well established that psychological changes are almost universal in patients presenting with thyroid disorder. Hyperthyroidism is associated with hyperactivity, anxiety and mood lability, but severely depressive affect is uncommon. Psychotic illnesses are probably not caused by thyroid over-activity. Psychological disturbances associated with hypothyroidism include mood changes and mental and motor slowing of varying degrees. In long-standing or severe cases a typical picture of endogenous depression, organic psychosis or dementia may develop. The biochemical mechanisms by which thyroid hormone imbalances may cause such diverse psychiatric symptoms are ill understood. Mood changes have been related to the effect of thyroid hormones on the sensitivity of noradrenergic receptors (Whybrow and Prange, 1981).

These observations suggest that thyroid dysfunction may be aetiologically relevant in some cases of postnatal mental disorder and in particular those which begin in the late puerperium. Recently Steward et al (1988) investigated 30 women who developed a puerperal psychosis within one year of childbirth and 30 normal controls matched for age and time after delivery. Values for total triiodothyronine (T_3) and thyroxine (T_4), T_3 resin uptake, free thyroxine index and thyroid-stimulating hormone (TSH) were all within the normal range in the nine patients with an early onset of psychosis (within four weeks postpartum) and the 21 patients with a late onset. Testing for thyroid microsomal antibodies in the latter group revealed a seropositive result for only one woman. Jansson (1984) also found no indication of abnormal thyroid function in seven cases of puerperal psychosis. George and Wilson (1983) reported that correlations between TSH levels and mood ratings over the first postpartum week were not significant. In a study by Okano (1989), TSH, total T_3 and T_4 levels did not differ significantly between blues sufferers and non-blues sufferers, but at one month postpartum the four women who developed a major depression according to DSM III criteria had significantly lower total T_3 levels than the 39 control subjects. However, free thyroid hormones were not determined. In a prospective study Harris et al (1988) recruited 65 women who were seropositive for thyroid microsomal or thyroglobulin antibodies at delivery and assessed their mood state at six to eight weeks postpartum. At this timepoint eight women had evidence of thyroid dysfunction as judged by free and total hormone and TSH measurements and three of these scored as depressed on all three rating scales employed.

Considering the high incidence of postpartum painless thyroiditis with the typical appearance of abnormal hormone levels from the second month onwards and the usually mild degree of dysfunction, women with postnatal depression are the most likely to show evidence of thyroid disease. Clearly further studies with larger numbers of subjects and measurements of TSH and both total and free thyroid hormones are required.

SUMMARY

Biological research in postnatal mental illness has only a short history and few encouraging data have yet emerged. The most promising positive findings are perhaps preliminary evidence for an increase of postnatal depression in women with postpartum thyroid dysfunction, some evidence for an enhanced sensitivity to changes in progesterone levels in postnatal depression, and the presence of an opioid peptide with unknown function in the cerebrospinal fluid of women with puerperal psychosis. Although steroid hormones are generally thought to be aetiologically relevant since they freely enter the brain and are known to interact with central monoamine neurotransmitter systems, attempts to demonstrate abnormal levels in postnatal disorders have been disappointing. An important reason for this outcome may be the usually employed approach of isolated hormone measurements. Ovarian steroid levels show marked interindividual variations. Thus significant between-group differences may only be obtained when large numbers of subjects are tested. Since only the unbound fraction can enter the brain, its measurement should be included in such studies. In the case of cortisol, single values are insufficient because of the pulsatile nature and the circadian pattern of its release. Thus serial sampling over 24 hours is more appropriate to detect secretory abnormalities. Measurements of circulating peptides are difficult to interpret since the amount reaching the brain is at best small. What is needed here are estimations of peptides in the cerebrospinal fluid which, however, pose ethical problems. Another explanation for the dearth of consistent positive data may be that women with postnatal mental disorders react to normal postnatal changes differently to women who remain well after childbirth.

There is already evidence that patients at high risk of puerperal manic-depressive illness develop a hypersensitivity of central D_2 receptors which may be related to the effects of oestrogen withdrawal on the function of DA systems. Further investigations of central neurotransmitter function are needed.

In many ways postnatal mental disorders provide a unique opportunity for psychosomatic research since their onset can almost be predicted and follows an event which is associated with changes in many physiological systems. Results of recent neuropharmacological and behavioural investigations into the central effects of steroid and peptide hormones provide the basis for a multitude of pathogenetic hypotheses to be tested in postnatal mental disorders and research in this area may see exciting times ahead.

Acknowledgements

The material described in this chapter is drawn from a review for submission to *Psychological Medicine* which has been prepared during work on a MRC funded project on puerperal psychosis.

REFERENCES

Alder EM, Cook A, Davidson D, West C & Bancroft J (1986) Hormones, mood and sexuality in lactating women. *British Journal of Psychiatry* **148:** 74–79.

Amino N, Mori H, Iwatani Y et al (1982) High prevalence of transient post-partum thyrotoxicosis and hypothyroidism. *New England Journal of Medicine* **306:** 849–852.

Baldessarini RJ (1989) Current status of antidepressants: clinical pharmacology and therapy. *Journal of Clinical Psychiatry* **50:** 117–126.

Ballinger CB, Kay DSG, Naylor GJ & Smith AHW (1982) Some biochemical findings during pregnancy and after delivery in relation to mood change. *Psychological Medicine* **12:** 549–556.

Bearn J, Fairhall S & Checkley S (1986) A new marker for oestrogen sensitivity with potential application to post-partum depression. *Proceedings of the Third International Conference of the Marcè Society* (abstract).

Best NR, Wiley M, Stump K, Elliott JM & Cowen PJ (1988) Binding of tritiated yohimbine to platelets in women with maternity blues. *Psychological Medicine* **18:** 837–842.

Biegon A, Reches A, Snyder L & McEwen B (1983) Serotonergic and noradrenergic receptors in the exposure to ovarian hormones. *Life Sciences* **32:** 2015–2021.

Bloom F, Battenberg E, Rossier J, Ling N & Guillemin R (1978) Neurons containing enkephalin: immunocytochemical studies. *Proceedings of the National Academy of Sciences of the USA* **75:** 1591–1595.

Bonnar J, Franklin M, Nott PN & McNeilly AS (1975) Effect of breast-feeding on pituitary–ovarian function after childbirth. *British Medical Journal* **iv:** 82–84.

Bourque J, Sulon J, Demey-Ponsart E, Sodoyez JC & Gaspard U (1986) A simple, direct radioimmunoassay for saliva progesterone determination during the menstrual cycle. *Clinical Chemistry* **32:** 948–951.

Brinsmead M, Smith R, Singh B, Lewin T & Owens P (1985) Peripartum concentrations of beta-endorphin and cortisol and maternal mood states. *Australian and New Zealand Journal of Obstetrics and Gynaecology* **25:** 194–197.

Buckman MT & Kellner R (1985) Reduction of distress in hyperprolactinemia with bromocriptine. *American Journal of Psychiatry* **142:** 242–244.

Butler J & Leonard BE (1986) Post-partum depression and the effect of nomifensine treatment. *International Clinical Psychopharmacology* **1:** 244–252.

Checkley SA, Corn TH, Glass IB, Burton SW & Burke CA (1986) The responsiveness of central alpha$_2$ adrenoceptors in depression. In Deakin JFW (ed.) *The Biology of Depression*, pp 100–120. London: Gaskell.

Cousins L, Rigg L, Hollingsworth D et al (1983) Qualitative and quantitative assessment of the circadian rhythm of cortisol in pregnancy. *American Journal of Obstetrics and Gynecology* **145:** 411–416.

Csontos K, Rust M, Hoellt V et al (1979) Elevated plasma β-endorphin levels in pregnant women and their neonates. *Life Sciences* **25:** 835–844.

Dalton K (1980) *Depression after Childbirth*. Oxford: Oxford University Press.

Deakin JFW (1988) Relevance of hormone–CNS interactions to psychological changes in the puerperium. In Kumar R & Brockington IF (eds) *Motherhood and Mental Illness 2: Causes and Consequences*, pp 113–132. London: Wright.

Deakin JFW & Crow TJ (1986) Monoamines, reward and punishments: the anatomy and physiology of the affective disorders. In Deakin JFW (ed.) *The Biology of Depression*, pp 1–25. London: Gaskell.

De Wied D & Bohus B (1979) Modulation of memory processes by neuropeptides of hypothalamic-neurohypophyseal origin. In Brazier MAB (ed.) *Brain Mechanism in Memory and Learning: From the Single Neuron to Man*, pp 139–149. New York: Raven Press.

Facchinetti F, Martignoni E, Sola D et al (1988) Transient failure of central opioid tonus and premenstrual symptoms. *Journal of Reproductive Medicine* **33:** 633–638.

Farde L, Wiesel FA, Hall H et al (1987) No D$_2$ receptor increase in PET study of schizophrenia. *Archives of General Psychiatry* **44:** 671–672.

Feksi A, Harris B, Walker RF, Riad-Fahmy D & Newcombe RG (1984) 'Maternity blues' and hormone levels in saliva. *Journal of Affective Disorders* **6:** 351–355.

Fletcher JE, Thomas TA & Hill RG (1980) β-Endorphin and parturition. *Lancet* **ii:** 310.

George AJ & Wilson KCM (1983) β-Endorphin and puerpheral psychiatric symptoms. *British Journal of Pharmacology* **80:** 493P.

George AJ, Copeland JRM & Wilson KCM (1980) Prolactin secretion and the postpartum blues syndrome. *British Journal of Pharmacology* **70:** 102–103.

Glasier A, McNeilly AS & Howie PW (1984) Pulsatile secretion of LH in relation to the resumption of ovarian activity postpartum. *Clinical Endocrinology* **20:** 415–426.

Goland RS, Wardlaw SL, Stark RI & Frantz AG (1981) Human plasma β-endorphin during pregnancy, labor, and delivery. *Journal of Clinical Endocrinology and Metabolism* **52:** 74–78.

Gordon JH & Perry KO (1983) Pre- and postsynaptic neurochemical alterations following estrogen-induced striatal dopamine hypo- and hypersensitivity. *Brain Research Bulletin* **10:** 425–428.

Greenwood J & Parker G (1984) The dexamethasone suppression test in the puerperium. *Australian and New Zealand Journal of Psychiatry* **18:** 282–284.

Handley SL, Dunn TL, Baker JM, Cockshott C & Gould S (1977) Mood changes in puerperium, and plasma tryptophan and cortisol concentrations. *British Medical Journal* **ii:** 18–22.

Handley SL, Dunn TL, Waldron G & Baker JM (1980) Tryptophan, cortisol and puerperal mood. *British Journal of Psychiatry* **136:** 498–508.

Harris B, Fung H, McGregor A & Hall R (1988) Postpartum thyroiditis and depressive illness. *Proceedings of the Fourth International Conference of the Marcè Society*.

Harris B, Johns S, Fung H et al (1989) The hormonal environment of postnatal depression. *British Journal of Psychiatry* **154:** 660–667.

Hatotani N, Nishikubo M & Kitayama I (1979) Periodic psychoses in the female and the reproductive process. In Zichella L & Panchevi P (eds) *Psychoneuroendocrinology in Reproduction*, pp 55–68. Amsterdam: North Holland/Elsevier.

Howie PW, McNeilly AS, Houston MJ, Cook A & Boyle H (1981) Effect of supplementary food on suckling patterns and ovarian activity during lactation. *British Medical Journal* **283:** 757–759.

Ishizuka B, Quigley ME & Yen SSC (1984) Postpartum hypogonadotrophinism: evidence for an increased opioid inhibition. *Clinical Endocrinology* **20:** 573–578.

Jansson R (1984) Autoimmune thyroiditis (Doctoral thesis). *Acta Universitatis Upsaliensis* **492.**

Jansson R, Dahlberg PA & Karlsson FA (1988) Postpartum thyroiditis. *Baillière's Clinical Endocrinology and Metabolism* **2(3):** 619–635.

Johnston JM & Amico JA (1986) A prospective longitudinal study of the release of oxytocin and prolactin in response to infant suckling in long-term lactation. *Journal of Clinical Endocrinology and Metabolism* **62:** 653–657.

Katona CLE, Theodorou AE, Missouris CG et al (1985) Platelet $_3$H-imipramine binding in pregnancy and the puerperium. *Psychiatry Research* **14:** 33–38.

Kellner R, Buckman MT, Fava GA & Pathak D (1984) Hyperprolactinemia, distress and hostility. *American Journal of Psychiatry* **141:** 759–763.

Kendall DA, Stancel GM & Enna SJ (1982) Imipramine: effect of ovarian steroids on modifications in serotonin receptor binding. *Science* **211:** 1183–1185.

Kovacs GL & Telegdy G (1983) Effects of oxytocin, des-glycinamide-oxytocin and anti-oxytocin serum on the α-MPT-induced disappearance of catecholamines in the rat brain. *Brain Research* **268:** 307–314.

Kuevi V, Causon R, Dixson AF et al (1983) Plasma amine and hormone changes in 'post-partum blues'. *Clinical Endocrinology* **19:** 39–46.

Langer SZ & Shoemaker H (1988) Platelet imipramine binding in depression. In Sen AK & Lee T (eds) *Receptors and Ligands in Psychiatry*, pp 327–346. Cambridge: Cambridge University Press.

Lee T, Seeman P, Tourtelotte WW, Farley IJ & Hornykeiwicz O (1978) Binding of $_3$H-neuroleptics and $_3$H-apomorphine in schizophrenic brains. *Nature* **274:** 897–900.

Leonard BE (1980) Pharmacological properties of some 'second generation' antidepressant drugs. *Neuropharmacology* **19:** 1175–1183.

Lewis BV & Parsons M (1966) Chorea gravidarum. *Lancet* i: 284–296.

Lindstroem LH, Widerloev L-M, Wahlstroem A & Terenius L (1978) Endorphins in human cerebrospinal fluid: clinical correlations to some psychotic states. *Acta Psychiatrica Scandinavica* **57:** 153–164.

Lindstroem LH, Nyberg F, Terenius L et al (1984) CSF and plasma β-casomorphin-like opioid peptides in postpartum psychosis. *American Journal of Psychiatry* **141:** 1059–1066.

Matussek N (1988) Catecholamines and mood: neuroendocrine aspects. In Ganten D — Pfaff D (eds) *Current Topics in Neuroendocrinology*, vol. 8, pp 141–182. Berlin: Springer.

McAdoo BC, Doering CH, Kraemer HC et al (1978) A study of the effects of gonadotropin-releasing hormone on human mood and behaviour. *Psychosomatic Medicine* **40:** 199–209.

Menkes DB, Aghajanian GK & Gallagher DW (1983) Chronic anti-depressant treatment enhances agonist affinity of brain alpha$_1$ adrenoceptors. *European Journal of Pharmacology* **87:** 35–41.

Metz A, Cowen PJ, Gelder MG et al (1983) Changes in platelet α$_2$-adrenoceptor binding post partum: possible relation to maternity blues. *Lancet* ii: 495–498.

Mitchell PB, Bearn JA, Corn TH & Checkley SA (1988) Growth hormone response to clonidine after recovery in patients with endogenous depression. *British Journal of Psychiatry* **152:** 34–38.

Moore KE, Lookingland KJ & Gunnet JW (1988) Effects of gonadal steroids and pituitary hormones on the activity of tuberoinfundibular dopaminergic neurons. In Genazzini AR (ed.) *The Brain and Female Reproductive Function*, pp 117–125. Carnforth: Parthenon.

Nausieda PA, Koller WC, Weiner WJ & Klawans HL (1979) Chorea induced by oral contraceptives. *Neurology* **29:** 1605–1609.

Newnham JP, Tomlin S, Ratter SJ, Bourne GL & Rees LH (1983) Endogenous opioid peptides in pregnancy. *British Journal of Obstetrics and Gynaecology* **90:** 535–538.

Newnham JP, Dennett PM, Ferron SA et al (1984) A study of the relationship between circulating β-endorphinlike immunoreactivity and the postpartum 'blues'. *Clinical Endocrinology* **20:** 169–177.

Nikolai TF, Turney SL & Roberts RC (1987) Postpartum lymphocytic thyroiditis. *Archives of Internal Medicine* **147:** 221–224.

Noel GL, Suh HK & Frantz AG (1974) Prolactin release and breast stimulation in postpartum and non-postpartum subjects. *Journal of Clinical Endocrinology and Metabolism* **38:** 413–423.

Nott PN, Franklin M, Armitage C & Gelder MG (1976) Hormonal changes in the puerperium. *British Journal of Psychiatry* **128:** 379–383.

Nyberg F, Lindstroem LH & Terenius L (1988) Reduced beta-casein levels in milk samples from patients with puerperal psychosis. *Biological Psychiatry* **23:** 115–122.

Okano T (1989) Clinico-endocrine study of maternity blues. *Mie Medical Journal* **39:** 189–200.

Owen F, Cross AJ, Crow TJ et al (1978) Increased dopamine receptor sensitivity in schizophrenia. *Lancet* **ii**: 223–226.

Owens PC, Smith R, Brinsmead MW et al (1987) Postnatal disappearance of the pregnancy-associated reduced sensitivity of plasma cortisol to feedback inhibition. *Life Sciences* **41**: 1745–1750.

Pedersen CA & Prange AJ (1979) Induction of maternal behaviour in virgin rats after intracerebroventricular administration of oxytocin. *Proceedings of the National Academy of Sciences of the USA* **76**: 661–665.

Potter JM, Mueller UW, Hickman PE & Michael CA (1987) Corticosteroid binding globulin in normotensive and hypertensive human pregnancy. *Clinical Science* **72**: 725–735.

Quigley ME & Yen SSC (1980) The role of endogenous opiates on LH secretion during the menstrual cycle. *Journal of Clinical Endocrinology and Metabolism* **51**: 179–182.

Quinn NP & Marsden CD (1986) Menstrual-related fluctuations in Parkinson's disease. *Movement Disorders* **1**: 85–87.

Rees LH, Burke CW, Chard T, Evans SW & Letchworth AT (1975) Possible placental origin of ACTH in normal human pregnancy. *Nature* **254**: 620–622.

Rehavi M, Sepcuti H & Weizman A (1987) Upregulation of imipramine binding and serotonin uptake by oestradiol in female rat brain. *Brain Research* **410**: 135–139.

Scott AIF, Whalley LJ & Legros J-J (1989) Treatment outcome, seizure duration, and the neurophysin response to ECT. *Biological Psychiatry* **25**: 585–597.

Shibasaki T, Odagiri E, Shizume K & Ling N (1982) Corticotrophin-releasing factor-like activity in human placental extracts. *Journal of Clinical Endocrinology and Metabolism* **55**: 384–386.

Silverman AJ & Krey LC (1978) The luteinizing hormone-releasing hormone (LH-RH) neuronal networks of the guinea pig brain. 1. Intra- and extra-hypothalamic projections. *Brain Research* **157**: 233–246.

Sofroniew MV (1983) Vasopressin and oxytocin in the mammalian brain and spinal cord. *Trends in the Neurosciences* **6**: 467–472.

Steward DE, Addison AM, Robinson GE et al (1988) Thyroid function in psychosis following childbirth. *American Journal of Psychiatry* **145**: 1579–1581.

Stockert M & de Robertis E (1985) Effect of ovariectomy and estrogen on ^{3}H-imipramine binding to different regions of rat brain. *European Journal of Pharmacology* **119**: 225–257.

Sulser F, Vetulani J & Mobley PL (1978) Mode of action of anti-depressant drugs. *Biochemical Pharmacology* **27**: 257–261.

Tolis G, Guyda H, Pillorger R & Friesen HG (1974) Breast-feeding: effects on the hypothalamic pituitary gonadal axis. *Endocrine Research Communication* **1**: 293–303.

Tyson JE, Hwang P, Guyda H & Friesen HG (1972) Studies of prolactin secretion in human pregnancy. *American Journal of Obstetrics and Gynecology* **113**: 14–20.

Van Hartesveldt C & Joyce JN (1986) Effects of estrogen on the basal ganglia. *Neuroscience and Biobehavioral Reviews* **10**: 1–14.

Veldhuis JD, Rogol AD, Johnson ML & Dufau ML (1983) Endogenous oppiates modulate the pulsatile secretion of biologically active luteinizing hormone secretion in man. *Journal of Clinical Investigation* **72**: 2031–2040.

Walfish PG & Chan JY (1985) Postpartum hyperthryoidism. *Clinics in Endocrinology and Metabolism* **14(2)**: 417–447.

Wehrenberg WB, Wardlaw SL, Frantz AG & Ferin M (1982) β–Endorphin in hypophyseal portal blood: variations throughout the menstrual cycle. *Endocrinology* **111**: 879–881.

Whalley LJ, Robinson ICAF & Fink G (1982) Oxytocin and neurophysin in post-partum mania. *Lancet* **ii**: 387–388.

Whybrow PC & Prange AJ (1981) A hypothesis of thyroid–catecholamine–receptor interaction. Its relevance to affective illness. *Archives of General Psychiatry* **38**: 106–113.

Wieck A, Hirst AD, Marks MN et al (1989) The growth hormone response to the dopamine agonist apomorphine is enhanced in women at high risk of puerperal psychosis. *Proceedings of the Joint Annual Meeting of the British Association for Psychopharmacology and the Canadian College of Neuropsychopharmacology* (abstract).

Willcox DL, Yovich JL, McColm SC & Schmitt LH (1985a) Changes in total and free concentrations of steroid hormones in the plasma of women throughout pregnancy: effects of medroxyprogesterone acetate in the first trimester. *Journal of Endocrinology* **107**: 293–300.

Willcox DL, Yovich JL, McColm SC & Phillips JM (1985b) Progesterone, cortisol and oestradiol-17β in the initiation of human parturition: partitioning between free and bound hormone in plasma. *British Journal of Obstetrics and Gynaecology* **92:** 65–71.
Willner P (1985) *Depression: A Psychobiological Synthesis*. New York: John Wiley & Sons.
Wong DF, Wagner HN, Tune LE et al (1986) Positron emission tomography reveals elevated D_2-dopamine receptors in drug-naive schizophrenics. *Science* **234:** 1558–1563.
Wood K (1986) 5HT transport and the mediation of action of anti-depressants. Do anti-depressants facilitate 5HT transport? In Deakin JFW (ed.) *The Biology of Depression*, pp 1–25. London: Gaskell.

11

Psychological strategies in the prevention and treatment of postnatal depression

SANDRA A. ELLIOTT

The psychological well-being of most recently delivered mothers is significantly determined by their psychosocial 'world', in particular by how others relate to them before, during and after childbirth. This is an oversimplified statement but one of appealing 'face validity' which, until recently, lacked the theoretical underpinning and experimental data to warrant much page space in obstetric textbooks. However, recent advances have served to stimulate the development and evaluation of new approaches to the psychological disorders encountered by the maternity services.

The most researched psychological complication of pregnancy is postnatal depression. Whilst the symptomatology of depressive disorder in the puerperium is essentially the same as in depressive disorders at other times, postnatal depression does have special features in aetiology, phenomenology and, of course its consequences. For many women the birth, the baby and the new role act as stressors contributing to the onset or exacerbation of depression. The baby also features in the manifestation of the depression. In psychotic disorders the mother may hold delusions such as thinking the baby can fly or is a reincarnation of the devil, whilst the cognitive distortions of neurotically depressed mothers include excessively negative views of their mothering and potential as 'good enough mothers'. In addition, they typically hold an understandable fear that because they do not love the baby at present, then they will never love this child for whom their responsibility will continue for at least 20 years. Professional help is usually required to attain the insight that such loss of affect is a symptom of depression, but few women obtain such help (see Chapter 9). Finally, depression affects the sufferer's behaviour, particularly social behaviour, yet the puerperium is of special, unrepeatable significance in the mother's developing relationship with her child. It is not surprising, therefore, that depression in the puerperium has special consequences not shared by depression at other times. Depression after childbirth may:

1. Fundamentally and enduringly undermine a woman's self-esteem, particularly her confidence in her ability to be a 'good enough' mother.
2. Be a permanent and well-remembered source of regret, since women describe having 'missed the first year' of their child's life.

3. Delay the development of mother–infant attachment and mutually satisfying interactive behaviours.
4. Lead to long-term effects on the child's behaviour or cognitive ability, as well as the mother/child relationship, if the mother's 'withdrawal' is not adequately compensated for by the father or other suitable persons.
5. Lead to marital stress and, if this remains unresolved, eventually divorce.

Depression is one of the most distressing conditions to experience and can involve complications ranging from the relatively trivial, such as personal neglect, to serious consequences such as suicide and infanticide. It also carries the risk of long-term effects on other family members and on family relationships. The special experiential and consequential features of depression in the puerperium demand particular attention to its prevention and treatment. It is extremely fortunate, therefore, that puerperal women have a special relationship with the health services, not only during the relevant risk period but for nearly nine months before it begins.

It is, perhaps, not surprising that most published initiatives to date have arisen within groups that see the consequences of undetected and untreated depression, i.e. psychiatrists, psychologists and mothers. However, now that these groups have developed communicable, if not complete, models of postnatal depression, suggestions can be offered to those health professionals who would rarely see the postnatal disorders but who are nevertheless best placed to prevent them—obstetricians and midwives.

The review of existing treatment and prevention programmes in this chapter, all of which are mother or mental health profession led, is therefore followed by a discussion of the implications for 'postnatal depression sensitive' maternity services.

PREDICTING AND PREVENTING POSTNATAL DEPRESSION

Studies relating to the prevention of low mood postnatally date back nearly 30 years and have not all been directly targeted on the group now defined within psychiatry as 'depressed' postnatally. However, there have been so few controlled trials that they are all worthy of mention.

Antenatal classes

The authors of one such study were concerned with emotional distress in the first ten postnatal days, the period when the so-called 'blues' is common. Halonen and Passman (1985) used the simple strategy of offering primiparae who had attended antenatal classes an extension to the labour-specific relaxation training which forms part of such classes. Two sessions of relaxation training and practice were given alongside instruction on the use of the relaxation procedure as a coping strategy to be employed whenever they felt upset during the postpartum period. A refresher session was given two days postnatally, and then the Beck Depression Inventory was given daily until the tenth day. Scores were significantly lower from the seventh to tenth postnatal day in the groups receiving the additional relaxation training.

As early as 1960, Gordon and Gordon expressed their concern about the effect of unpreparedness for parenting on the postnatal experience of couples having their first child. They devised a very simple educational approach which was added on as two 40-minute sessions to the antenatal education for the two randomly selected experimental classes. The two control groups were also apparently 'selected randomly in advance' from existing classes, although they were 'matched by background history questionnaires and were essentially the same in make-up as those in the experimental groups'.

The more important points included in these extra talks were:

1. The responsibilities of being a mother (and not a martyr) are learned, hence get help and advice.
2. Make friends of other couples who are experienced with young children.
3. Don't overload yourself with extra, less important tasks.
4. Don't move soon after the baby arrives.
5. Don't be too concerned with appearances when other things are more important.
6. Get plenty of rest and sleep.
7. Don't be a nurse to elderly relatives at this period.
8. Confer and consult with husband, family and experienced friends, and discuss your plans and worries.
9. Don't give up your outside interests, but cut down the responsibilities and rearrange your schedules.
10. Arrange for babysitters in advance.*
11. Learn to drive a car.*
12. Get a family doctor now.

(* Some of these suggestions presuppose a level of income out of reach of a substantial minority of British mothers.)

The 50 participating obstetricians, who were blind to the treatment condition of their patients, rated them on a four point scale of emotional distress six to eight weeks after delivery. Women receiving the extra instruction ($n = 85$) were significantly less likely to be described as emotionally distressed (15%) than the controls (37%, $n = 76$).

Preparation for parenthood has seen a revival of interest in the 1980s, with a variety of more elaborate approaches being reported in the literature (Duncan and Markman, 1988). None of these have included postnatal depression in their outcome measures. However, one well-designed controlled study (Cowan and Cowan, 1987) included a preparation programme focused on the changes in the couple's relationship which had long-term benefits for marital adjustment (e.g. no separations or divorces compared with 12.5% of controls), self-esteem and life satisfaction—all factors which might be expected to be protective against depression.

Psychotherapy

Shereshefsky and Yarrow's study went for the more intensive (and expensive) approach of prenatal counselling by a psychiatric caseworker (Liebenberg, 1973; Shereshefsky and Lockman, 1973). Half of the 62 married primiparae were randomly assigned to the counselling group, who received bi-weekly 'ego-supportive' therapy sessions, though the precise nature of the counselling varied between counsellors. A comparison of the total counselled group with the controls failed to find differences on 'maternal adaptation' or 'infant adaptation', although the marital relationships of the control group had deteriorated at six months postnatally while the marital relationships of the counselled group remained at the level of the first antenatal assessment. However, an interesting finding emerged when the counselled group was divided according to the type of therapy received. Therapy apparently fell into three types: clarification of feelings and interpersonal relationships, insight-oriented psychodynamic therapy, and anticipatory guidance as preparation for potentially stressful parenting situations. Comparisons within the counselled group showed the highest level of 'maternal adaptation' in the group receiving anticipatory guidance. It is possible that this was due to differences between counsellors rather than between techniques. On the other hand, it seems reasonable to suggest that it provides some support for Gordon and Gordon's (1960) educational approach to prevention. One cautionary note relates to the lack of data on the importance of how the preparation is conducted. Halonen and Passman (1985) found that simply describing potential post-partum stressors to pregnant women does not reduce depressed mood in the 'blues' period and may even reduce the elation common on the second and third postnatal days. This would suggest that exposure to the realities of parenthood is insufficient, or even potentially harmful, and needs to be accompanied by some discussion of how stressful situations can be avoided or managed. Studies comparing different styles of anticipatory guidance or preparation for parenthood are required.

Prevention of postnatal depression in vulnerable women

The studies reported above used unselected groups so that the great majority of women receiving the intervention would not be expected to experience postnatal depression with or without the preventive intervention. A smaller sample could be used if the research was targeted on more vulnerable women. Unfortunately developing and prospectively testing a measure of risk is a time-consuming and expensive procedure. One option seemed to be to take a chance with an unproven vulnerability measure and incorporate a check on the validity of such a procedure within the study of a preventive intervention. Leverton (Leverton and Elliott, 1988) chose items scaled on five psychological and social variables: psychiatric history (broadly defined), marital relationship, confiding relationship, anxiety score on the Crown Crisp Experimental Index, and previous postnatal depression. These had been positively associated with postnatal depression in at least two previous prospective studies (Todd,

1964; Pitt, 1968; Blair et al, 1970; Dalton, 1971; Meares et al, 1976; Martin, 1977; Braverman and Roux, 1978; Zajicek and Wolkind, 1978; Hayworth et al, 1980; Oakley, 1980; Paykel et al, 1980; Kendell et al, 1981; Playfair and Gowers, 1981; Cox et al, 1982; Elliott, 1982; Kumar and Robson, 1984; Watson et al, 1984). These items were then expressed as 'user friendly' questions and embedded within a fuller questionnaire of obvious relevance to women attending for their first hospital antenatal clinic visit. The questionnaire was piloted until a version was achieved which could be easily filled in within ten minutes of waiting time in the clinic, and which women found acceptable. First- and second-time mothers participating in the research project subsequently received a detailed interview at three months postpartum. Part of this interview consisted of a standardized psychiatric assessment, the Present State Examination, to which fixed criteria for diagnosis of depressive disorders could be applied. Forty per cent of the women with identified vulnerability factors ($n = 50$) were judged to have experienced definite or borderline depression at some time in the first three postnatal months. This was significantly more than the 16% ($n = 90$) in the group without identified vulnerability factors (Leverton and Elliott, 1988). The results of this prospective study confirm that groups can be successfully differentiated antenatally according to their level of vulnerability to post-natal neurotic depression. The immediate need of research was served since the higher the predicted base rate for depression, the smaller the sample size needed to test the efficacy of an intervention aimed at reducing the prevalence of postnatal depression. Obviously, we also anticipated benefits for clinical practice; postnatal depression has the unusual advantage of being preceded by an event which can be predicted up to nine months in advance and the event is one which is generally known to a variety of health professionals with whom the individual has regular contact.

A note of caution must be added before any vulnerability questionnaire is indiscriminately used in obstetric practice. Whilst it is unreasonable to expect every clinician who wants to follow up this approach to reinvent measures from first base, there are certain questions which must be addressed afresh for each clinical setting.

First and foremost is '*why?*' In other words, what will be done with the information once it is obtained? What extra service will be provided and for what purpose? Some initiatives will be service-driven whilst others will be condition-oriented. The recent trend to liaison posts means that a new service may be made available, such as from a liaison psychiatrist or psychologist. A system will then be required to ensure that the full range of appropriate referrals reaches them whilst simultaneously preventing inappropriate referrals from flooding the waiting list. In other instances, funds are allocated for the prevention of a particular condition, such as postnatal depression, which will demand more specialized assessment procedures. These examples will require different antenatal assessments.

Simpler to answer is '*when?*' Generally this will be as early as possible. At the very least it must be early enough to achieve delivery of the minimum service believed to be effective.

At least three questions relate to personnel: '*who assesses?*', '*who *accesses?*' and '*who acts?*'. Whilst assessing at the point of maximum convenience to staff and client is essential to successful adoption as a routine policy, it is also important that the 'shopfront' for this approach should be managed with sensitivity and the appropriate interpersonal skills. For example, undue pressure to complete a vulnerability questionnaire 'because everyone has to' will not achieve the ultimate message of this approach, which is that 'we are interested in your emotional wellbeing', particularly if the client's initial reluctance is a function of anxiety or depression!

Sensitive information will be obtained during these assessments. Respect for privacy may therefore dictate that access to this information is limited to a specified group of people. Furthermore, assurances of such confidentiality may encourage women to reveal information that they would otherwise be reluctant to mention. Finally, the 'vulnerable' label may itself be stigmatizing and should be communicated with caution.

It must be made clear who is responsible for acting on the information obtained. Will one named person, such as the antenatal liaison health visitor, be requested to identify all vulnerable women and then to select from amongst various available agencies in order to make an appropriate referral? Alternatively, will it be open to all professionals in contact with the pregnant woman to make referrals to one named treatment agency such as the obstetrics and gynaecology liaison team in the district mental illness service?

It is the nature of such new or existing referral systems which should largely determine *how* the assessment is made. Where referrals are all channelled through a liaison health visitor who meets all women in the antenatal clinic, a few well chosen questions may be included into the interview. In a system channelling referrals to a liaison team from any one of the maternity services personnel, questionnaires could be handed out by the clinic receptionist and returned in sealed envelopes to the 'antenatal support service' (avoiding the term 'psychiatric'). Alternatively, tear-out sections could be included in the midwive's first interview, but this may require revalidating since sensitive information may not be revealed as readily as in an anonymous questionnaire and responses may vary according to the interviewing style of the midwife.

Equally (or perhaps more) important is the matter of *how it is presented* to the participating women. Informed consent demands that women are aware that they are participating in an assessment for a described service. Misinformation can cause unnecessary anxieties or lead to dismissal of a potentially useful service. It is therefore vital that all personnel are clear what is, and what is not, involved. To take the example of a questionnaire for vulnerability to postnatal depression, staff must understand that:

1. Prediction in the individual case is impossible.
2. Even on a group basis, the more vulnerable group identified by existing instruments are not a 'high-risk' group. More than half of the more vulnerable group will not be depressed.
3. Postnatal depression is not 'puerperal psychoses' nor is it the 'blues'. Whilst there are individuals whose experiences blur the distinction between psychoses and postnatal (i.e. neurotic) depression and

between the short-term blues and depression, the manifestation and prognosis as well as incidence of these conditions varies greatly. It is important that women are not led into the mistaken belief that they have been identified as 'at risk' of 'going mad', when in fact they have simply been allocated to the group more vulnerable to postnatal depression. Staff must be able to correct misunderstandings about postnatal depression such as those which periodically arise in the media (e.g. Kilroy, BBC TV, March 1989).

4. The term 'at risk' should not be used because of connotations relating to child abuse registers.

Accurate but non-threatening information is also a crucial part of a research programme if couples are going to be encouraged to participate. In our research project, care was taken not only to inform the staff involved in antenatal and postnatal care for the participants about the prevention approach, but also to provide carefully worded letters and handouts describing the support groups for the participants themselves. Since it is known that women are reluctant to take up services under the title 'psychiatry' or 'psychotherapy' (Robinson and Young, 1982), the educational aspects were emphasized in the invitation to groups. The titles 'Preparation for Parenthood' and 'Surviving Parenthood' were used for first- and second-time mothers' groups respectively. These terms were chosen to be reminiscent of the customary antenatal classes, although the handout emphasized that these groups would be additional to the traditional classes, would cover the postnatal rather than the antenatal and perinatal period, and would aim for informal discussion between participants. It was also made clear that there would be six monthly meetings after the birth as well as the five meetings scheduled during the pregnancy.

Participation is also influenced by the timing of meetings and the convenience and comfort of the setting. This is particularly true for multiparae who will be encouraged to attend by the provision of attractive play facilities in a crèche for their toddlers and will be discouraged by long journeys, particularly in the last trimester of pregnancy and first postnatal trimester. Yet this is a crucial time with respect to postnatal depression and its prevention, and it is also a time at which an extra service is often required to compensate for the lack of continuity in relationships with the health care staff. Midwives and obstetricians that the woman may have come to know during her pregnancy terminate their contacts with her a few days or weeks after the birth, often before the health visitor has made her first contact. Consequently, health visitors were asked to make an antenatal visit in mid-pregnancy in order to establish contact as early as possible.

To summarize, our intervention combined the social support approach to promotion of positive mental health currently gaining popularity (particularly in the USA) (Elliott et al, 1988; Gottlieb, 1988) with the preparation for parenthood advocated by Gordon and Gordon (1960). One of the innovations was the addition of an antenatal session devoted to psychological problems. Other differences from traditional hospital antenatal classes include:

1. *Emphasis on continuity of care over the child-bearing period*, with monthly meetings beginning as soon as possible (fourth or fifth months of pregnancy) and continuing to six months postpartum.

2. *Easy access to extra individual help* from or through the group leader. This was based on the assumption that women would seek help earlier from someone they already knew and if they did not have to have a diagnosable mental illness to be entitled to it. Less intervention would then be required at this early stage, when the full descent of the viscious spiral could be prevented, than later when lengthy treatment would be required to 'dislodge' someone from the viscious circle of physical symptoms, mood and negative thoughts which exists at the bottom of that 'pit of depression' (Elliott, 1989).

3. *Emphasis on the development of social support over education.* Not only was the room informally organized, but also discussion between the women was facilitated and maintained even at the expense of leaving out the educational material for the session. This demands group work skills rather than teaching skills from the leader.

4. *Restricted membership of groups.* The groups were 'closed', i.e. invitations were restricted to a predefined list and new members were not permitted to join at a later stage. The groups were confined to women with partners (single mothers had social-worker-run support) and to first-and second-time mothers, who met in separate groups. This was to facilitate the sense of going through a life stage with others in similar circumstances. Restricting the groups to women with expected dates of confinement within a six-week period was also essential for fostering this group identity. Even with this limit, the failure (!) of babies to strictly follow the 40-week gestation rule resulted in some sessions with a mix of postnatal and pregnant women. Such women clearly have very different issues so the number of such mixed sessions is best restricted to one, which can be focused on new babies being introduced to the group. (For the research design, seasonal effects were minimized by the choice of six week blocks roughly one third and two thirds through the range of expected delivery dates of the women scheduled for research interviews.) However, the restriction to more vulnerable women was not made to facilitate this 'similar other' comparison process. It was simply a strategy to reduce the cost of research psychiatrists by limiting the number of interviews on low vulnerability women. (The latter were, by definition, less likely to contribute to the prevalence of depression which was the key outcome variable for the intervention and control comparison.) The group leader was kept 'blind' to the Leverton questionnaire responses, including those on the vulnerability factors. These factors were not raised by the leader in the groups (although of course, issues relating to them may have arisen during discussions). There is, therefore, no reason why low vulnerability women should not be invited to, and benefit from, positive health promotion groups such as these. Indeed they may prove to be a valuable source of support for the more vulnerable women.

5. *Focus of the groups beyond the birth.* The informal discussion format

inevitably left open the option for some discussion of pregnancy and labour (particularly previous labour experiences in second-time mothers). However, the expressed purpose of the groups enabled the discussion to centre on postnatal parental issues.

It is clear, therefore, that these group meetings must be in addition to, not instead of, traditional antenatal classes which have their own important 'agenda'. Nevertheless, these elements were easy to combine so the result was a single programme not demanding excessive amounts of expensive professional time. It was therefore satisfying to find that the prevalence of depression, defined by the use of the Bedford College Criteria applied to a standardized psychiatric interview (the Present State Examination), in the more vulnerable women offered this service ($n = 48$) was significantly lower (19%) than in the more vulnerable women not offered this service (40%; $n = 50$.) This would appear to confirm the belief that psychosocial interventions can prevent postnatal depression. Purist researchers will now wish to replicate this small scale study using more complex designs to determine the effective components. In the meantime, however, I hope that clinicians will not wait for sophisticated research before considering how the philosophy of such preventive interventions can be enacted within their own routine services.

PSYCHOLOGICAL TREATMENTS FOR POSTNATAL DEPRESSION

There have been many initiatives around the world for dealing with postnatal depression in the community, once it has been recognized, ranging from self-help to specific psychotherapeutic interventions. Research has not kept pace with these initiatives and I am aware of only one published controlled trial which undertook to confirm the widespread view that such psychological strategies can be effective in treating postnatal depression (Holden et al, 1989).

There have, of course, been a number of well-designed studies of specific psychotherapies for depression, such as cognitive therapy which directly tackles the 'faulty thinking' which is exerting a negative influence over mood and behaviour (Blackburn et al, 1981; Murphy et al, 1984; Teasdale et al, 1984), and books on finding an appropriate therapist are widely available (e.g. Edwards, 1987). Since postnatal depression shares many of the clinical features found in other depressions (Cooper et al, 1988; O'Hara and Zekoski, 1988), there is every reason to assume that these therapies would be as effective in puerperal women as in non-child-bearing-women and men. It is tempting, therefore, to review such empirical studies here because of their convincing methodology. However, these studies have been adequately reviewed elsewhere (e.g., Williams, 1984; Mathews, 1987), whilst few comprehensive reviews of treatment for postnatal depression have been produced. There have been many exciting, original initiatives specifically developed in response to the clinical needs of new mothers.

References to these are scattered throughout the psychological, psychiatric and other literature, with little cross-referencing and few methodologically sound clinical trials. In summarizing this literature, it is hard to avoid the conclusion that many people all over the world have been 'reinventing the wheel'. The purpose of the following review is therefore to document the nature of existing services and some of the problems experienced in developing these. The aim is both to stimulate controlled evaluations and to aid those setting up new services.

Self-help and support for all parents

Postnatal depression is often managed in the community without referral to specialist treatment agencies. Services are not limited to women diagnosed as depressed but are offered for any problems new parents may have. Support and advice can be offered from one supporter allocated to the new mother (e.g. National Childbirth Trust postnatal supporters in Britain), in groups (e.g. Meet-a-Mum Association in Britain, Postpartum Education for Parents in California) and from 24-hour telephone helplines to deal with specific parenting problems (Parents Anonymous and Crysis in Britain). Further details on organizations such as these are given in lay books (e.g. Dix, 1986; Comport, 1987).

Self-help for those with postnatal depression

The first organization set up specifically for postnatally depressed mothers would seem to be the Pacific Postpartum Support Society (Robertson, 1980; Handford, 1985). In 1973 women experiencing postpartum depression met informally to give each other support. This evolved into a professional-led self-help programme offered by the British Columbia Ministry of Human Resources, but funding ceased in 1983 'as a result of the government's fiscal restraint measures'. It has continued as a charity utilizing volunteers. This group decided that 'in general, psychiatrists are not knowledgeable about what it means to be at home and to take care of small children' (Handford, 1985). They have concluded that the treatment model which is most useful to the postpartum depressed women is one which encourages talking, in confidence, to other women who have experienced the same difficulties. These exchanges take place by telephone initially until the woman is ready to attend support group meetings. It is not clear how, or indeed whether, referral is made to specialist agencies of individuals for whom this approach is insufficient or inappropriate.

In Britain an organization was formed independently but seems to share a similar philosophy regarding the value of discussion with women who have experienced postnatal disorder themselves (Association for Postnatal Illness). However, from the outset this organization had close liaison with psychiatrists who were experts in the field of motherhood and mental illness, consequently this organization caters for women who are experiencing, or have experienced puerperal psychoses (for which formal psychiatric help would also be required) as well as those with neurotic postnatal depression (who are often not in contact with mental illness services).

For women keen on self-help but unable to reach one of these organizations, a paperback written by Welburn in 1980 is still the most readable and least threatening description of the experience of postnatal depression.

Mental health services

In theory, departments of the health service are always able to cross refer. In practice, communications are enhanced and the speed and quality of referral are improved when formal links are established. In North America psychiatrists began establishing such Special Consultation Liaison Services to Obstetrics and Gynaecology Units over 20 years ago (Stewart, 1986). Recently Britain has been following suit (Riley, 1986; Appleby et al, 1989). In Norway, specialist mental health services have been taken one step further with the establishment in 1985 of the Institute of Tocology and Family Psychology which takes referrals for crisis intervention during the perinatal period (ITF, 1986).

Most published reports of these specialist services have focused on the nature of the client groups and the referral systems rather than the treatment used. Recently two psychologists have described their therapeutic approach in detail (Morris, 1987; Brierley, 1988).

Morris (1987) conducted group psychotherapy for seven postnatally depressed women with three cotherapists (a GP, an occupational therapist and a community nurse). Meetings of one and a half hours each were held weekly for 11 months and a crèche was run at the same time in the surgery. After the group therapy terminated the group continued as a self-help group for over a year. Initially the group was depressed and uncommunicative but the use of psychodrama techniques enabled discussion to get underway. The discussions centred on issues raised by the clients themselves including the role of the GP, marital and sexual problems, and hostility towards parents, including a sense of being unloved by their own mothers. It emerged that these women carried a considerable burden of guilt. They considered themselves to be inadequate mothers just as their own mothers had been and hated themselves for it. Psychoanalysts concerned with the transition to parenthood frequently encounter reports of such difficulties with the client's own parents, not only when the presenting problem is psychological disturbance in the mother, but also when young children are referred to the child psychotherapists for problems such as sleep disturbance (e.g. Daws, 1989). The difficulty lies in determining whether such reports reflect the cause or the effect of the psychological disturbance.

Outcome in this small uncontrolled study was assessed using the Beck Depression Inventory (BDI) for depressive symptomatology and a Repertory Grid as a measure of the woman's conceptualization of her personal world. Scores on the BDI dropped significantly between the beginning and end of therapy. This was accompanied by shifts in constructs relating to self, ideal self, mother, children and self as mother (i.e. favourable changes on the adjectives used to describe her personal images of herself as she is and as she would like to be and her images of other relevant people). This was a very labour intensive therapy using weekly meetings of up to four therapists with seven women with no 'waiting list' or 'minimal intervention' controls. However, it is important to note that a significant reduction in depression was achieved with a group of women with chronic postnatal depression. All of the women offered the group psychotherapy had already been depressed for more than a year, whilst most episodes of postnatal depression resolve in less than six months (Watson et al, 1984; Cooper et al, 1988).

Clinical psychologists in primary care settings will routinely receive referrals of postnatal women experiencing anxiety and depression. Brierley (1988) describes in detail the cognitive–behavioural approach she has found to be successful with 18 women, seven of whom experienced problems in relating to their baby as well as depression. Mothers were typically seen individually for therapy, although all the mothers were strongly encouraged to attend support groups once they had sufficiently overcome their feeling of worthlessness to make this possible.

The focus of therapy was on understanding the psychological mechanisms maintaining the depression rather than the psychological or hormonal factors which may have contributed to the initial dysphoric moods. Mothers were shown a diagram (see Figure 1) of the kinds of psychological mechanisms which can operate in postnatal depression. The discussion emphasized that not all conditions applied to every mother and enabled them to find a train of events with which they could personally identify. This demystified the unexpected and bewildering experience of depression, coming just when one has had a healthy baby and expected to be happy. Recognizing that they are not alone in the experience of postnatal depression lessens the sense of guilt and isolation. The diagram was used because the author believed that it would enable women to see that there may be contributing factors which could be identified and changed. This recognition would, in turn, decrease their immobilizing sense of hopelessness. The therapy, geared to individual needs identified from the discussion of the diagram, could then include:

1. The opportunity to express feelings of resentment and hostility such as towards her own mother for her style of mothering or towards the baby for all the losses having a baby has brought (job, personal freedom, etc.).
2. Discussion of their view that their feelings should be hidden from everyone because they have no 'right' to feel this sad. This may require assurance that other mothers also feel fatigue, anxiety, depression, etc., so that they have no need to feel guilty because motherhood and their mothering isn't as wonderful as they expected.
3. Helping mothers to recognize their own negative thoughts which keep a negative feedback loop going. (Negative thoughts lead to low mood, low moods increase the frequency of negative thoughts.) Weekly activity schedules were used to record such thoughts for later discussion in therapy.
4. Scheduling into their diary half-an-hour per day of activity for their own pleasure.

5. Making it safe to express innermost resentments or fears about their baby (e.g. if they resembled someone the woman disliked).
6. Reducing the feelings of failure and indifference towards their baby by understanding it as a 'phobic' type response to a subjectively traumatic situation (i.e. encouraging women to see the anxiety aspect of their postnatal depression as analogous to so-called 'post-traumatic shock', and then blaming this shocked state, rather than enduring personal qualities, for their perceived 'failings').
7. Challenging the irrational beliefs underlying negative thoughts about the relationship with the baby. This generally took the form of a belief in the 'perfect' mother who always got things right.
8. Anxiety management techniques and relaxation training to provide women with strategies to deal with panicky feelings.
9. Therapist play with the baby to encourage a playful response from a baby who has become withdrawn and avoids eye contact or other responses to adults because her depressed mother often failed to respond in the past (see Chapter 12). The mother is then brought into a three-way interaction to build up positive feelings of success, enjoyment and pleasure with the baby.
10. An early appointment with the partner to explain about his wife's depression and the commonest accompanying feelings such as anxiety, irritability and lack of sexual interest, and to encourage social time for the couple away from the baby.

The therapy which the mothers received 'was perceived as some help in alleviating this distress' (Brierley, 1988). Brierley provides a description of an existing clinical service and no information was offered on the recovery rate in comparable women not receiving the therapy. That her therapy is effective is assumed from the fact that it was based on cognitive–behavioural therapies which have been submitted to controlled trials in non-puerperal samples. It will be several years before the results of the first controlled trial of cognitive-behavioural therapy (and other therapies) for postnatally depressed women becomes available (L. Murray and P.J. Cooper, personal communication).

Services to disadvantaged mothers

These services typically cater for families with under fives and not just postnatal mothers. The aims of such services are often stated in terms of preventing child abuse and/or breaking the cycle of child abuse and neglect across generations. These services are relevant here, however, because most users of such services are, in fact, depressed and have a child under one year of age (Mills and Pound, 1986).

In Britain many such services were set up around the country in the early 1980s, including Home Start, Cope and Newpin. Newpin, the New Parent–Infant Network, will be described in some detail because it is a model service subjected to extensive descriptive study (Pound and Mills, 1985; Mills and Pound, 1986) and worthy of experimental evaluation (although the latter is

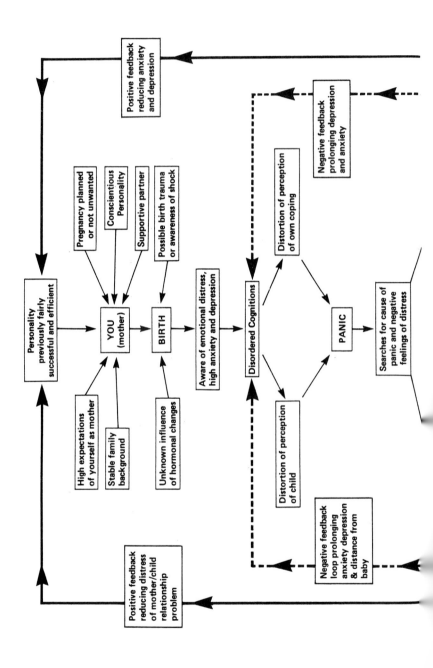

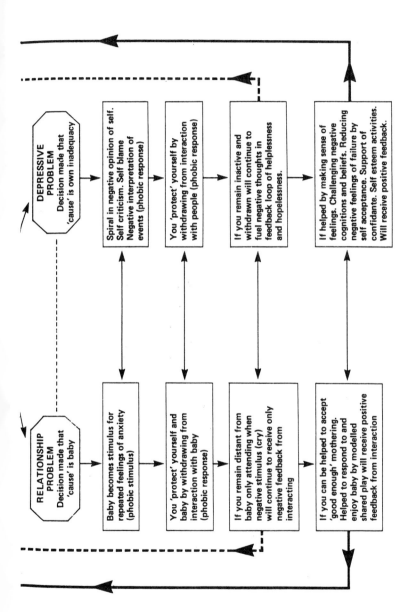

Figure 1. Postnatal distress in the absence of obvious predisposing factors (possible psychological mechanisms and ways forward). Courtesy of Eileen Brierley

unlikely because of the ethical and practical problems of achieving a comparable untreated control group).

This service was set up in a deprived inner city area in South East London with one of the countries highest rates of reported child abuse. It was targeted on families with extremely limited resources in an area with high rates of unemployment and many single-parent families. Such parents left school early themselves and 'lack the internal resources and experience to keep a young child happy and occupied and meet their needs. The results are whingeing, trying children and dysphoric parents. All this in the context of a media that constantly sells the joys of motherhood' (Mills and Pound, 1986). Newpin was set up in 1982, with voluntary money. It is run by a professional co-ordinator but the service is provided by volunteers from the same background as the women they befriend. Interestingly, the befrienders may themselves have been referred to Newpin for help but the co-ordinator may decide that the best help for them would be to take part in the training and to assist others. This consists of one-day-a-week training over four months, and includes a therapy group to provide support and advice while they are befriending as well as 'an opportunity to explore themselves'. The co-ordinator then matches them to a newly referred person for whom she becomes an 'official friend'. The 'contracts' between such pairs vary but are likely to include support in stressful situations such as going to the Social Security office, bringing mothers to the Newpin Centre to meet and chat with other mothers and watch how they handle the children, and use of the nursery to allow time for themselves. Disapproval and criticism is always avoided and the aim is to change a woman's self-esteem and understanding of her own feelings and those of others. Women who reach Newpin tend to be those with no family support or very unhelpful families. Newpin acts as a substitute family with rules and expectations of respecting, tolerating and trusting others and giving them personal space, which is very different from the family of origin, where basic human obligations were not met and children were harshly criticised, mistreated or abandoned (Mills and Pound, 1986).

All volunteers and referrals were interviewed on entry to the Newpin project for a small pilot study. Pound and Mills (1985) found that the mothers referred to Newpin were indeed an exceedingly disadvantaged and vulnerable group of women in their teens and early twenties. In addition to widespread financial, housing, family and social problems, 'most had long-standing emotional problems, commonly depression and anxiety'. Twelve volunteers and eleven matched referrals were reinterviewed six to twelve months after entry to the project. Whilst no control group was available, the authors had seen from their own previous research that it is uncommon for women in difficult circumstances to recover from their depression. On this basis they judged that involvement in Newpin not only improved the way the mothers felt about themselves, but enabled them to function at a level and enjoy a quality of life that they had not seen in their previous research study of depressed mothers in the same area of London, where no such intervention was available. More relevant in this context was that one third of those who were found to be clinically depressed at initial interview had completely recovered and the remainder had improved by the follow-up interview six to twelve months after entry into the project.

Treating 'new mother' anxiety

Whilst middle-class mothers may not suffer the deprivation-related distress of the disadvantaged mothers catered for by services such as Newpin, many middle-class first-time mothers will experience anxiety about the life change. Indeed, they may experience more anxiety because of the greater contrast of maternal role to the nature of their previous professional job and the tendency of that earlier occupation to keep them out of the company of mothers and babies. Many postnatal depressions are accompanied by anxiety (Cooper et al, 1988) or indeed may be preceded by antenatal anxiety (Elliott et al, 1983; Watson et al, 1984).

Barnett and Parker (1985) recently reported on a carefully controlled study of the treatment of anxiety identified as soon as possible after the birth. Married primiparae were given the Spielberger trait and state anxiety scales on the third or fourth postnatal day to enable a high anxiety group to be identified for random allocation to three subgroups for a controlled treatment trial. The women were then interviewed at home within three weeks before being allocated to one of five groups; low-anxiety, moderate-anxiety, high-anxiety non-professional intervention, high-anxiety professional intervention, and high-anxiety controls. All women were posted questionnaires at three, six, nine and twelve months and reinterviewed at twelve months postpartum.

Non-professional intervention involved allocation to an experienced mother who met the 'authors requirements for a support figure who would offer common sense advice, support and practical help, but avoid proselytizing any particular narrow model of mothering'. Professional intervention comprised assistance from a social worker experienced in working with mothers and children. Guidelines were given to the social workers on the provision of support, specific anti-anxiety measures, the promotion of self-esteem and confidence, a reduction in intensity of the mother–infant interaction (if appropriate), and promotion of mother–father and father–child interactions. Contacts were made by telephone as well as through visits to or from the client. It is not clear how many contacts therapy typically involved, although non-professionals apparently made more contacts than professionals. It is also not clear how long therapy lasted. The 12-month interview is referred to as a 'follow-up' interview but no time for termination of therapy was specified. In the non-professional intervention group, anxiety scores dropped rapidly in the first three months but the scores over the twelve months did not differ significantly from the high anxiety controls. The anxiety scores in the professional intervention group reduced more slowly but by 12 months postpartum were significantly lower than the high-anxiety controls and similar to the moderate-anxiety controls. This is a finding worthy of further investigation, even though this report itself gives insufficient information about the time and cost of the therapy or the clinical significance of the change (i.e. whether anxiety reduced from levels disruptive to daily life to comfortable levels).

Health visitor counselling for postnatal depression

The one controlled trial of treatment for postnatal depression was not of the small minority of postnatally depressed women who find their way into the psychiatric services. It built on the unusual ability of the maternity services to reach a total population in the community. Since all health authorities in Britain have a statutory duty to provide a home visitation service for all newly delivered mothers, all women in Britain are assigned a health visitor. (Health visitors have trained as nurses and midwives but now work in the community with a health promotion role which includes immunizations, developmental checks, regular weighing of babies under three months and advice on feeding as well as support to the mother.) The time and place of contacts varies between authorities, but invariably the most frequent client contacts are within the first few postnatal months. Holden and her colleagues (Holden et al, 1989) capitalized on this by asking health visitors in Edinburgh and Livingstone (Scotland) to give the screening questionnaire for postnatal depression described by Cox (Chapter 9) to all women at around six weeks postpartum.

The women who obtained a high score on their Edinburgh Postnatal Depression Scale were interviewed by a psychiatrist and those diagnosed as depressed according to Research Diagnostic Criteria (RDC) applied to the Goldberg Standardized Psychiatric Interview were assigned to the research programme. In the meantime, health visitors received a manual and three sessions of instruction on postnatal depression and on non-directive counselling. Routine health visiting involves 'counselling' in the broadest sense of that term, but the aim is usually to identify specific needs and to offer appropriate specific advice (such as feeding practices). Training in non-directive counselling for health visitors therefore places emphasis on 'the importance of listening to clients and encouraging them to make decisions based on their own judgement rather than giving advice' (Holden et al, 1989). Once a diagnosis of depression was made, the depressed women were randomly assigned to two groups. The health visitors were notified of the diagnosis of depression only if the women were in the treatment group. They were asked to visit these women at a pre-arranged time for eight successive weeks. Support and supervision were provided to health visitors throughout the programme on request. When all the women were re-assessed by the psychiatrist three months later, 18 (69%) of the 26 depressed women in the treatment group showed no evidence of having a depressive illness, whereas only 9 (38%) of the 24 women in the control group had recovered.

As with the prevention studies, it would appear that relatively small changes in professional contacts with child-bearing women may result in a reduction in suffering from postnatal depression. Once again, purist researchers will seek to determine the most effective element of this health visitor intervention as well as to undertake controlled trials of the more sophisticated therapies available to the mental health professionals receiving referrals of more severe cases.

Meanwhile, maternity services personnel have to choose between waiting for the results of such thorough research or attempting to integrate what can already be gleaned from studies of postnatal depression into their existing practice. Since existing practice has been little researched in relation to postnatal psychological outcomes, postnatal depression researchers will opt for the latter option. Clinicians, however, do not have the luxury of ignoring the fact that existing practices are directed to serve other purposes and will continue to use what are seen to be 'tried and tested' systems for achieving the main goals of that service. The ultimate test of the value of postnatal depression intervention research may therefore be its compatibility with existing essential services.

INTEGRATING SERVICES FOR POSTNATAL DEPRESSION

Health visitors

Prevention and treatment are not mutually exclusive strategies for the management of postnatal depression. The treatment programme developed by Holden and her colleagues (1989) has been combined with primary prevention into one training programme designed to enable health visitors to maximize their potential to promote the positive mental health of mothers. If this training is successful in the trial areas of London, Edinburgh and Stoke, then a programme will be developed to train trainers in all British health districts.

Obstetricians and midwives

Whilst the timing of postnatal depression puts its management largely in the hands of health visitors and other members of the primary care team, the greatest opportunity for prediction and prevention is typically with the obstetrician and midwives. It will often not be feasible, or even desirable, to set up elaborate services targeted on postnatal depression. Rather the aim would be for all maternity staff to acquire an understanding of the complex aetiology of depression following childbirth, thus facilitating the incorporation of an empowering and enabling philosophy into routine service delivery.

At its most simplistic, the current 'model' suggests that the onset of depression depends on what has happened to people and how they perceive it. Prevention can focus on helping to prevent the events themselves, on changing the perception of them, or on support to facilitate coping with such events. Prevention begins antenatally and falls firmly under the influence of obstetricians and midwives providing antenatal care and classes as well as those involved in perinatal and postnatal care. Prevention of postnatal depression need not demand expensive additional services. A slight shift in emphasis within existing services could achieve a great deal. As a start, education about postnatal disorders need not take up more than an hour of antenatal classes, but it would enable parents to recognize disorders sooner and to seek appropriate help (see Chapter 11) as well as to take steps to prevent it. Some midwives and obstetricians have been reluctant to introduce such topics because of fears of unnecessarily raising anxieties or of creating a self-fulfilling prophesy by mentioning the possibility of postnatal psychological problems. It is important therefore to utilize material which makes clear the reasons for antenatal education on the topic and to include partners (or other relatives in single mothers' groups) who will be the best placed to recognize and refer any disorders which may arise postnatally. Enquiry should be made as to anxieties raised, towards the end of the session. These must then be dealt with in the group session or, if the anxieties relate to an individual's recognition of the risk of relapse of a previous psychiatric disorder, in a separate meeting with the group leader or a mental health professional. In our experience, such raised anxieties are rare and the majority of participants welcome the information and the opportunity to constructively consider these outcomes. Besides, Esther Rantzen and others have made strenuous efforts to keep postnatal depression in the media so 'blissful ignorance' is no longer a real option, whilst the risk of 'misinformation' or misunderstood information is increasing.

Preparation for parenthood based on the Gordon and Gordon (1960) model demands only two sessions of an antenatal class. Open discussion in these sessions should begin the process of identifying and challenging expectations of the baby, of parenthood and of one's emotions. It will also provide expectant couples with the opportunity to revise their plans in order to minimize the number of stressful demands they place on themselves during the postnatal period.

The opportunity to develop social support networks can be provided by running antenatal clinics and classes in such a way as to facilitate the development of relationships (e.g. waiting area chairs facing not in rows, the same people coming to the whole course of classes, etc.).

Support from professionals can be improved by attention to the question of continuity of care, permitting the development of a trusting relationship prior to the psychological 'shake up' that comes with gaining a new little family member. Such caring relationships can offer not only practical and emotional support but also vital 'self-esteem support' (Wandersman et al 1980) by facilitating the client's own decision making (Newton, 1989). To this end, it is vital to avoid conflicting advice, which is a source of considerable dissatisfaction and which may reduce self-esteem in vulnerable women (Ball, 1981, 1987). Ball (1988) has attempted to translate 'sensitive emotional support' into specific midwifery practices* including:

1. 'All mothers should be encouraged to set their own pace in taking responsibility for the various aspects of care required by a newborn baby; they should not be subjected to routine patterns of care which assume that all mothers can cope equally well.' (p. 29)

---

* Reproduced by kind permission of Jean Ball and the *Nursing Times*, where these quotes first appeared on 27 April 1988.

2. 'Women with low self-esteem are enriched by having their opinions sought and acknowledged as important, and by being encouraged to make their own decisions. Seeking opinions should not take the form of questions which imply the required answer, or which assume that the mother is willing and able to fall in with a pre-planned pattern of care.' (p. 29)
3. 'When a woman is feeding her baby, whether by breast or bottle, she is not simply providing him with nutrients, but is conveying to him love and protection. It is crucial, therefore, not to show disapproval of the feeding method chosen by the mother or to express doubts about her ability to 'do it properly'. (p. 30)
4. 'As soon as it is suitable after the birth, a discussion should take place between the mother and the midwife in order to plan an agreed programme of care.' (p. 30)
5. 'The midwife may invite the mother to discuss her labour and the delivery of her baby, which will give the mother an opportunity to explore her feelings about the birth. There is evidence that providing women with an opportunity to integrate and make sense of their birth experience, by answering questions and explaining actions and events which may not have been understood at the time, is beneficial in stengthening psychological processes (Affonso, 1984).' (p. 30)
6. 'Conflicting advice can be overcome when the details of individual care plans are used as a basis for discussion and when midwives and others take the trouble to check what advice has been given by their colleagues, to build on, rather than to contradict it.' (p. 30)
7. 'The development of primary nursing care models and the team care of mothers throughout pregnancy, labour and the puerperium also serve to reduce the incidence of conflicting advice and provide emotionally integrated support (Hooton, 1984; Flint, 1985, 1987).' (p. 30)
8. 'Each mother should be provided with a 'Do not disturb' card, to be used whenever she wishes to rest or to be left alone.' (p. 30)
9. 'The atmosphere of postnatal wards can be changed from that in which mothers are expected to conform to pre-set patterns of activity to one which is dictated by the needs and desires of the mothers occupying the ward.' (p. 31)

Obstetricians and midwives have a unique opportunity not usually available to psychiatrists and psychologists in the management of pregnancy, labour and delivery. The attending staff have a direct input into the nature of events and, just as important, into how they are perceived. There is a rapidly expanding literature in sociology and cognitive psychology on the relation between events, how they are perceived and ensuing depression (e.g. Abramson et al, 1978; Brown and Harris 1978; Teasdale, 1985) and this applies equally well to the event of childbirth and depression in the puerperium (Oakley, 1980; Elliott, 1989). In so far as procedures increase uncontrollable pain, discomfort, sleeplessness, fear, helplessness or low self-esteem, it is reasonable to assume that they increase the risk of subsequent depression. Clearly life-saving procedures can't be avoided simply because they are unpleasant. As Vandenbergh (1980) emphasized in his overview of postnatal depression, 'stressful environmental conditions should be kept in perspective as primarily the triggering factors that interact with the patient's own internal conflicts'. The important message to take from cognitive psychology is that how events are understood by the individual is crucial to their role in the genesis of depression. This is borne out by recent research on the event of childbirth which confirms that it is not the number of interventions, nor whether interventions are major, which determines their relationship with emotional well-being six weeks after the birth. Rather, it is whether the woman believes that the 'right thing happened' which is related to later emotional well-being (Green et al, 1988). This, in turn, is related to the amount of information given. This can be best understood within Seligman's 'learned helplessness' theory of depression (Abramson et al, 1978). If an unpleasant and unexpected procedure is used on a labouring woman she may feel that events have passed out of her control, and this will lead to feelings of helplessness which in turn may lead to depression if it activates helpless feelings learnt in the past. On the other hand, if information about the procedure, and the medical indications for its use, is supplied to the woman she will feel that she is participating in the decision process and therefore retaining some control. This is true even if her choice is to ask no further questions and place the immediate decision in the hands of her qualified carers. She perceives herself to be in control of to whom she gives control. In emergencies explanation will obviously be clipped, but this does not preclude full explanation as early as possible after the event; indeed the general anaesthetic which will be required for many emergencies will increase the woman's need for information about the sequence of events. For example, a woman will be much reassured to learn that an emergency caesarean was performed because of the unusual presentation of her baby rather than her 'failure' to push hard enough.

Obstetricians and midwives who decide that they should include prevention of the common complication of depression alongside the prevention of physical complications can pick up many useful guidelines from recent descriptive research reports relating specific midwifery and obstetric practices to emotional well-being (e.g. Ball, 1987; Green et al, 1988), as well as from the reports of the controlled trials of psychological strategies for postnatal depression described earlier.

SUMMARY

Prevention or treatment of most postnatal psychological disorders currently demands the manipulation of psychosocial not biological variables. How we treat women matters in terms of the emotional outcome of pregnancy and ultimately the family outcome. This is confirmed by two types of studies. Firstly, there are the controlled trials of psychological strategies aimed at the prevention or treatment of postnatal mood disturbance. Secondly, there are the studies of the relationship between the type of obstetric and midwifery care and emotional well-being following the birth. There have been far too few of either type of study. Since the rapid advances in medicine which relate to physical outcome have peaked, with mortality rates at an all-time low, the 1990s should see more clinical and research effort devoted to psychological outcomes. Perhaps some progress can now be made in reducing postnatal psychiatric and psychological morbidity.

Acknowledgements

I am grateful to Melissa Fenton, Tessa Leverton, Adam Rodin and Helen Turner for their comments on earlier drafts of this paper and to Yvonne Hedderman for typing the same numerous drafts.

This paper was written whilst the author was in receipt of a grant from the Gatsby Charitable Foundation.

REFERENCES

*Indicates key references.

Abramson LY, Seligman MEP & Teasdale JD (1978) Learned helplessness in humans: critique and reformulation. *Journal of Abnormal Psychology* 87: 49–74.

Affonso DD (1984) Post partum depression. In Field PA (ed) *Perinatal Nursing*. Edinburgh: Churchill Livingstone.

Affonso DD & Arizmendi TG (1986) Disturbances in postpartum adaptation and depressive symptomatology. *Journal of Psychosomatic Obstetrics and Gynaecology* 5: 15–32.

Appleby L, Fox H, Shaw M & Kumar R (1989) The psychiatrist in the obstetric unit: establishing a liaison service. *British Journal of Psychiatry* 154: 510–515.

Ball J (1981) Effects of present patterns of maternity care on emotional needs of mothers. Parts 1 and 2. *Midwives Chronicle* 95: 198–202.

*Ball J (1987) *Reactions to Motherhood: The Role of Postnatal Care*. Cambridge: Cambridge University Press.

Ball J (1988) Mothers need nurturing too. *Nursing Times* 84: 29–30.

Barnett B, Parker G (1985) Professional and non-professional interruption for highly anxious primiparous mothers. *British Journal of Psychiatry* 146: 289–293.

Blackburn I, Bishop S, Glen A, Whalley J & Christie J (1981) The efficiency of cognitive therapy in depression. A treatment trial using cognitive therapy and pharmacotherapy, each alone and in combination. *British Journal of Psychiatry* 138: 181–189.

Blair RA, Gilmore JS, Playfair HR, Tisdall MW & O'Shea C (1970) Puerperal depression. A study of predictive factors. *Journal of Royal College of GP's,* 19: 22–25.

Braverman J & Roux JF (1978) Screening for the patient at risk for postpartum depression. *Obstetrics and Gynaecology* 52: 731–736.

*Brierley E (1988) A cognitive-behavioural approach to the treatment of post-natal distress. *Marce Bulletin* 1: 27–41.

Brown GW & Harris T (1978) *Social Origins of Depression*. London: Tavistock.

Comport M (1987) *Towards Happy Motherhood: Understanding Postnatal Depression*. Corgi: London.

Cooper PJ, Campbell EA, Day A, Kennerley H & Bond A (1988) Non-psychotic psychiatric disorder after childbirth: a prospective study of prevalence, incidence, course and nature. *British Journal of Psychiatry* 152: 799–806.

Cowan CP & Cowan PA (1987) A preventive intervention for couples becoming parents. In Boukydis CFZ (ed.) *Research on Support for Parents and Infants in the Postnatal Period*. Norwood, New Jersey: Ablex.

Cox JL, Connor YM & Kendell RE (1982) Prospective study of the psychiatric disorders of childbirth. *British Journal of Psychiatry* 140: 111–117.

Dalton K (1971) Prospective study into puerperal depression. *British Journal of Psychiatry* 118: 689–692.

Daws D (1989) *Through the Night. Helping Parents and Sleepless Infants.* London: Free Association Books.

Dix C (1986) *The New Mother Syndrome: Coping with Stress and Depression,* London: Allen & Unwin.

Duncan SW & Markman HJ (1988) Intervention programs for the transition to parenthood: current status from a prevention perspective. In Michaels GY & Goldberg WA (eds) *The Transition to parenthood: Current Theory and Research,* Cambridge: Cambridge University Press.

*Edwards H (1987) *Psychological Problems: Who can Help?* British Psychological Society and Methuen.

Elliott SA (1982) *Mood change in pregnancy and early motherhood.* PhD thesis, University of London.

Elliott SA (1989) Postnatal depression: consequences and intervention. In Demers LM, McGuire JL, Phillips A & Rubinow DR (eds) *Premenstrual, Postpartum and Menopausal Mood Disorders.* Maryland: Urban & Schwarzenberg.

Elliott SA, Rugg AJ, Watson JP & Brough DI (1983) Mood change during pregnancy and after the birth of a child. *British Journal of Clinical Psychology* 22: 295–308.

*Elliott SA, Sanjack M & Leverton TJ (1988) Parents' groups in pregnancy: a preventive intervention for postnatal depression? In Gottlieb BJ (ed.) *Marshalling Social Support: Formats, Processes, and Effects.* California: Sage.

Flint C (1985) Labour of love. *Nursing Times* 81(5): 16–18.

Flint C (1987) *Sensitive Midwifery.* London: Heinemann Medical Books.

Gordon RE & Gordon KK (1960) Social factors in prevention of postpartum emotional problems. *Obstetrics and Gynecology* 15: 433–438.

*Green JM, Coupland VA & Kitzinger JV (1988) *Great Expectations: A Prospective Study of Women's Expectations and Experiences of Childbirth,* Vol. 1. Monograph of Childcare and Development Group, University of Cambridge.

Gottlieb BJ (1988) (ed) *Marshalling Social Support: Format, Processes and Effects.* California: Sage.

Halonen JS & Passman RH (1985) Relaxation training and expectation in the treatment of postpartum distress. *Journal of Consulting and Clinical Psychology* 53: 839–845.

Handford P (1985) Postpartum depression: what is it, what helps? *The Canadian Nurse* **January:** 30–33.

Hayworth J, Little BC, Bonham Carter S et al (1980) A predictive study of post-partum depression: some predisposing characteristics. *British Journal of Medical Psychology* 53: 161–167.

*Holden JM, Sagovsky R & Cox JL (1989) Counselling in a general practice setting: controlled study of health visitors' intervention in treatment of postnatal depression. *British Medical Journal* 298: 223–226.

Hooton P (1984) The team approach to midwifery care. RCM Professional Day papers. *Midwives Chronicle* 97: 161, 5–8(supplement).

ITF (1986) Institute of Tocology and Family Psychology. *Marce Bulletin* 2: 11.

Kendell RE, Rennie D, Clarke JA & Dean C (1981) The social and obstetric correlates of psychiatric admission in the puerperium. *Psychological Medicine* 11: 341–350.

Kumar R & Robson KM (1984) A prospective study of emotional disorders in childbearing women. *British Journal of Psychiatry* 144: 35–47.

Leverton TJ & Elliott SA (1988) *Antenatal intervention for postnatal depression.* Paper presented at Autumn Quarterly Meeting of the Royal College of Psychiatrists, London.

Leverton TJ & Elliott SA (1989) Transition to parenthood groups: a preventive intervention for postnatal depression? In Van Hall EV & Everaerd W (eds) *The Free Woman: Women's Health in the 1990s.* Carnforth: The Parthenon Publishing Group.

Liebenberg B (1973) Techniques in prenatal counselling. In Shereshefsky PM & Yarrow LJ (eds) *Psychological Aspects of a First Pregnancy,* pp 123–151. New York: Raven Press.

Martin ME (1977) Maternity hospital study of psychiatric illness associated with childbirth *Irish Journal of Medical Science* 146: 239–244.

*Mathews A (1987) Cognitive therapy of depression. *Practical Reviews in Psychiatry* 2: 9–15.

Meares R, Grimwade J & Wood C (1976) A possible relationship between anxiety in pregnancy and puerperal depression. *Journal of Psychosomatic Research* 20: 605–610.

Mills M & Pound A (1986) Mechanisms of change. The Newpin Project. *Marce Bulletin* 2: 3–7

Morris JB (1987) Group psychotherapy for prolonged postnatal depression. *British Journal of Medical Psychology* **60:** 279–281.

Murphy G, Simons A, Wetzel R & Lustman P (1984) Cognitive therapy and pharmacotherapy singly and together in the treatment of depression. *Archives of General Psychiatry* **41:** 33–41.

Newton J (1989) Empowerment for isolated parents. *Open Mind* **38:** 12–13.

Oakley A (1980) *Women Confined–Towards a Sociology of Childbirth.* Oxford: Martin Robertson.

*O'Hara MW & Zekoski EM (1988) Postpartum depression: a comprehensive review. In Kumar R & Brockington IF (eds) *Motherhood and Mental Illness 2: Causes and Consequences,* 17–57. London: Wright.

Paykel ES, Emms EM, Fletcher S & Rassaby ES (1980) Life events and social support in puerperal depression. *British Journal of Psychiatry* **136:** 339–346.

Pitt B (1968) 'Atypical' depression following childbirth. *British Journal of Psychiatry* **114:** 1325–1335.

Playfair HR & Gowers JI (1981) Depression following childbirth–a search for predictive signs. *Journal of the Royal College of General Practitioners* **31:** 201–208.

Pound A & Mills M (1985) A pilot evaluation of NEWPIN: home visiting and befriending scheme in South London. *Association of Child Psychiatry and Psychology Newsletter* **7:** 13–15.

Riley D (1986) An audit of obstetric liaison psychiatry in 1984. *Journal of Reproductive and Infant Psychology* **4:** 99–115.

Robertson J (1980) Treatment model for postpartum depression. *Canada Mental Health* **28(2):** 16–17.

Robinson S & Young J (1982) Screening for depression and anxiety in the postnatal period: acceptance/rejection of a subsequent treatment offer. *Australian and New Zealand Journal of Psychiatry* **16:** 47–51.

Shereshefsky PM & Lockman RF (1973) Comparison of counselled and non-counselled groups. In Shereshefsky PM & Yarrow LJ (eds) *Psychological Aspects of a First Pregnancy,* pp 151–163. New York: Raven Press.

Stewart D (1989) Puerperal mental illness in North America. *Marce Bulletin* 40–51.

Teasdale JD (1985) Psychological treatments for depression: how do they work? *Behavioural Research and Therapy* **23:** 157–165.

Teasdale JD, Fennel M, Hibbert G & Amies P (1984) Cognitive therapy for major depressive disorders in primary care. *British Journal of Psychiatry* **144:** 400–406.

Todd EDM (1964) Puerperal depression: a prospective epidemiological study. *Lancet* **ii:** 1264–1266.

Vandenbergh RL (1980) Differential diagnosis: postpartum blues. *Clinical Obstetrics and Gynecology* **23(4):** 1105–1111.

Wandersman LW, Wandersman A & Kahn G (1980) Social support in the transition to parenthood. *Journal of Community Psychology* **8:** 332–342.

Watson JP, Elliott SA, Rugg AH & Brough DI (1984) Psychiatric disorder in pregnancy and the first postnatal year. *British Journal of Psychiatry* **144:** 453–462.

*Welburn V (1980) *Postnatal Depression.* London: Fontana.

Williams JMG (1984) *The Psychological Treatment of Depression: a Guide to the Therapy and Practice of Cognitive Behaviour Therapy.* London: Croom Helm.

Zajicek E & Wolkind S (1978) Emotional difficulties in married women during and after the first pregnancy. *British Journal of Medical Psychology* **51:** 379–385.

12

Management of major mental illness in pregnancy and the puerperium

MARGARET OATES

Many recent prospective antenatal and community studies have shown that between 10 and 15% of women become mentally ill following childbirth (Cox et al, 1983; Kumar and Robson, 1984). The majority of these women will be suffering from non-psychotic, minor or neurotic mental disorder and there is some controversy as to whether these conditions are in fact more common after childbirth than at other times (O'Hara, 1986; Cooper et al, 1988). However, there appears to be little doubt that the risk of serious mental disorder is increased following childbirth. Approximately 2% of all women will be referred to a psychiatrist following childbirth, over half of whom are seriously mentally ill (Oates, 1988), and two per 1000 deliveries will require admission to a psychiatric unit, most of whom will be suffering from a puerperal psychosis (Kendell et al, 1987). In addition, a significant minority of women become mentally ill during pregnancy. The majority of these conditions are non-psychotic and will resolve as the pregnancy progresses. However, some will not, with implications for the mental health and functioning of these women after delivery. Women may also present at the booking clinic with past histories of psychiatric disorder, currently well but concerned about the effect that parturition might have upon their mental health. Such women may still be taking medication and may have additional concerns about the effects of this upon the developing fetus. Thus a substantial minority of patients seen by obstetricians and the maternity services (between 15 and 20% of all patients) will have mental health issues which have to be taken into account in their management.

Accurate diagnosis and formulation of all the factors contributing to mental health problems is always important, but especially so in the setting of obstetrics. Close liaison between obstetricians and psychiatrists is essential for the following reasons:

1. A woman's emotional state might be altered from her 'normal' state. The tendency for all women to be more emotionally vulnerable and more 'neurotic' during pregnancy and the puerperium may lead to misdiagnosis of normal emotional changes, or states of distress, as illness. Inappropriate diagnosis and treatment may detract from the understanding of her situation and the support that she needs. The

patient and her family may wrongly see her as abnormal, with subsequent blows to self-esteem and confidence.

2. Although few psychotropic drugs have been proven teratogenic or hazardous to the developing fetus, no such drug has been proven safe. Drug treatment must involve at least a theoretical and potential hazard to the developing fetus or infant directly (through placental transfer or breast-feeding) or indirectly (through diminished alertness). It is therefore particularly important to prescribe medication only when it is necessary to do so.

3. There is evidence that minor mental illness in the puerperium may be predictable and preventable during pregnancy. If it occurs the patient may benefit as much from psychological treatment strategies as from pharmacological ones, and therefore differential diagnosis is very important.

4. Serious mental illness is more common in the puerperium than at other times in a woman's life, and is dangerous both to the woman and her infant. It requires swift medical attention and treatment. As it most commonly occurs in the days and weeks following delivery at a time of high surveillance by both doctors, health visitors and midwives, it is important that these groups are aware of the risk factors for these conditions and of the signs and symptoms of the disturbance. Morbidity and distress may be reduced to a minimum by speedy diagnosis and treatment.

5. The less serious conditions, untreated, may be protracted and may have a damaging effect on both the child and the woman's marriage and other social relationships. It is therefore equally important that the risk factors for these conditions should be familiar and that swift diagnosis, detection and appropriate treatment should be instigated, again not only to relieve distress but also in the best interests of the child and the family.

Thus it is often necessary for obstetricians to call upon the services of a psychiatrist, who should preferably be one experienced in the field. The rates of psychiatric disorder following childbirth are such that most maternity units generate a sufficient 'workload' to justify at least the sessional commitment from a consultant psychiatrist and his team. For example, a maternity unit with 5000 deliveries a year in a health district with standard sociodemographic features produces sufficient referred psychiatric morbidity (at the current rates of psychiatric referral) to occupy the equivalent of half of a full-time consultant psychiatrist (Oates, 1988). If a maternity unit does not already have such a liaison service it may be beneficial to establish one, as a close liaison between maternity services and psychiatry is essential for the well-being of the mentally ill woman and her family.

DIFFERENT TYPES OF PSYCHIATRIC ILLNESS

The distinction between distress and illness, between major illness and minor illness, is not always easy. It may be particularly difficult when the woman's normal state is altered in the pregnancy and the puerperium, with heightened emotions and anxiety. Help from a psychiatrist with a special interest will assist the obstetrician in the differential diagnosis.

Minor mental illness

In minor mental illnesses the signs and symptoms vary only in quantity from those which are part of the normal human experience. Both the timing of the illness and the symptoms are usually understandable as a result of an interaction of the personality with stress. Despite the fact that the symptoms may be very distressing and disabling, there is not usually any impairment of the patient's perception of reality. Symptoms of anxiety tend to predominate. Anxiety states, phobic anxiety states, neurotic ('reactive') depressive illness and obsessional compulsive illnesses are examples of neurotic mental illness. Such illnesses are very common (probably at least 10% of the population suffer from such an illness at any given time). Some people are more vulnerable to developing these illnesses than others, by virtue of personality problems, ongoing social and family problems or recent major stresses ('life events').

In pregnancy

There is probably a slightly increased risk of minor or neurotic mental illness during the first trimester of pregnancy, with about 15% of women suffering from such conditions having been well prior to conception (Kumar and Robson, 1978). Most commonly the clinical picture is of reactive or neurotic depression, or an anxiety state. Eighty per cent of these new episodes will have resolved by the second or third trimester of pregnancy. Women already suffering from neurotic illness, such as phobic anxiety states or obsessional compulsive neurosis, at the time of conception may deteriorate during pregnancy. Those women most at risk include those with previous psychiatric histories of neurosis, chronic marital or social difficulties, ambivalence or unhappiness about the pregnancy and markedly anxious or obsessional previous personalities.

A smaller proportion of women (up to 5%) (Kumar and Robson, 1978) will develop a new episode of minor mental illness, usually a depressive neurosis, during the last trimester of pregnancy.

In the puerperium

Prospective antenatal and community studies reveal that about 10% of women suffer from a new episode of neurotic mental illness in the puerperium, having previously been well. There is some controversy (Cooper et al, 1988; O'Hara and Zekoski, 1988) about whether this represents a true increase in risk; nonetheless these illnesses can be quite severe and disabling and have major implications for the child and the family. They tend to start insidiously in the weeks following birth, and the clinical syndrome is predominantly that of a depressive neurosis with marked anxiety features; less commonly phobic anxiety states and obsessional compulsive neurosis may occur at this time. A full clinical description of this condition can be found in Chapter 9. The majority of these patients are not known to and do not present to the psychiatric services, indeed not even to their general practitioners (Cox et al, 1983). Those most at risk include women with chronic marital and social difficulties, ambivalence or un-happiness about the pregnancy, obstetric anxieties, previous psychiatric histories, or neurotic disorder or depressive syndromes in the last trimester of pregnancy. Many of these 'at risk' women may be detected early in the pregnancy (see Chapter 11).

Relationship between illness in pregnancy and the puerperium

Whilst many of the risk factors for postnatal depressive neurosis may be identified early in the pregnancy, those women suffering from an illness in the first trimester of pregnancy are most likely to recover and are not, apparently, at increased risk of becoming ill after delivery (Kumar and Robson, 1978). However, those women who develop depressive neurosis in the last trimester of pregnancy do appear to be at increased risk of con-tinuing the same illness after delivery.

Major mental illness or psychoses

These are conditions characterized by symptoms that differ in quality from those of ordinary human experience. They usually involve distortions of perception, of both personal and external reality, and major disturbances to bodily and mental functions. Patients may develop hallucinations and delusions, and the term covers such illnesses as manic-depressive illness, major depressive illness, schizophrenia and schizophrenia-like conditions. Approximately 2% of the population suffer from such conditions and probably the major vulnerability factor is genetic, although recent major stress may play an important part.

In the United States these illnesses are called 'major mental illnesses' and the term 'psychotic' is confined to the description of a mental state characterized by either hallucinations or delusions, or major impairment of reality testing. However, in Great Britain and in much of the world, the term 'psychotic' is still used to describe a group of illnesses (e.g. manic-depressive psychosis), even if the person afflicted does not have a psychotic mental state examination. In this chapter the term 'major mental illness' will be used and the term 'psychotic' is used to describe a mental state.

In pregnancy

The risk of developing a new episode of major mental illness (manic-depressive illness or schizophrenia) is much lower during pregnancy than at other times in a woman's life, and dramatically lower than in the puerperium.

Women with past histories of major psychiatric disorder, or those suffering from chronic major psychiatric disorder, are not at a particular risk of relapse or deterioration during pregnancy.

In the puerperium

The risk of developing a major mental illness is greatly increased in the puerperium (see Chapter 8).

Management of major mental illness in pregnancy

It is uncommon for a new episode of manic-depressive illness or schizophrenia to arise in pregnancy in a woman who has previously been well. However, on rare occasions this does occur. It is also uncommon for a woman with a previous history of a chronic condition to relapse during pregnancy. On occasion women may become pregnant whilst still actively ill with large numbers of symptoms and in such situations the diagnosis and development of the pregnancy may produce a deterioration in the woman's mental state. Such pregnancies may be planned and much wanted or may have resulted from behavioural disorganization produced by the illness. If the pregnancy is to continue then the management of the woman's mental illness is complicated by the need to balance the risk to the developing fetus of psychotropic medication and the risk to the developing fetus of the mother's disturbed mental state.

The management of acute episodes of major mental illness during pregnancy necessitates a close collaboration of obstetrician and psychiatrist.

Management of schizophrenia and schizophrenia-like conditions

These patients may have hallucinations, delusions (into which the pregnancy may be incorporated) and disturbances of behaviour and disorganization of personal functioning which may pose an indirect threat to the fetus through problems of nutrition and compliance with antenatal care. The rapid resolution of the disturbance is therefore a high priority for both mother and fetus, and the patient will nearly always need to be contained in a safe environment, usually a psychiatric unit.

In ordinary psychiatric practice, the management of acute schizophrenic illnesses (in non-pregnant cases) would involve the administration of a phenothiazine drug (chlorpromazine, dosage range 50–800 mg daily; trifluoperazine, dosage range 5–30 mg daily). Often, particularly when there is thought to be a considerable risk of relapse in the two years following the resolution of the illness, longer-acting depot preparations such as flupenthixol are given by fortnightly intramuscular injection. When treating an acute schizophrenic illness during pregnancy it is probably better to use a phenothiazine such as chlorpromazine or trifluoperazine because these have a wide dosage range which can be flexibly adjusted as soon as the acute episode has resolved. Inadequately treated, the mother's psychiatric disorder is hazardous to the fetus. Although concern has been expressed for the potential toxicity of phenothiazines to the developing fetus, most studies have concluded that chlorpromazine is safe for both mother and fetus if used at low dosage, and conclude that phenothiazines are not teratogenic. Chlorpromazine has been widely used in all stages of pregnancy since the 1950s for medical reasons. However, there have been some reports that mothers receiving chlorpromazine at around the time of delivery suffer marked and unpredictable falls in blood pressure that could be dangerous to mother and fetus. A full review of phenothiazines in pregnancy is given in Ruben (1987). In other reports mothers receiving large doses of chlorpromazine in the last week of pregnancy have delivered babies who have suffered from extrapyramidal syndromes. It should therefore seem reasonable, once the acute episode has largely resolved, to reduce the level of phenothiazine to the minimum possible dose; this reduction is particularly important in the last month of pregnancy when the mothers should be receiving the minimum possible maintenance dose. Phenothiazine drugs, particularly perphenazine derivatives such as trifluoperazine, may cause acute extrapyramidal syndromes (dystonias) or more chronic and insidious ones, such as rigidity and parkinsonian-like syndrome. In order to reduce these side-effects, anti-parkinsonian agents such as procyclidine 5–10 mg daily or benzhexol (trihexyphenidyl USP 2–5 mg daily are frequently prescribed concurrently. These anti-parkinsonian agents have atropine-like qualities. Although there is no definite evidence that such drugs are teratogenic or harmful to the fetus, it seems reasonable not to prescribe them in the first trimester of pregnancy and thereafter only if they are positively indicated by the appearance of extrapyramidal symptoms.

Management of mania

It is very uncommon for a new episode of mania or hypomania to begin during pregnancy, even if the patient has a past history of such a condition.

On occasion, a manic patient may become pregnant while still actively psychotic or the circumstances of conception (or even the diagnosis of pregnancy) may occasionally precipitate a manic episode. An extreme motor restlessness, over-activity and speeding of both physical and psychological functioning is characteristic of this condition, together with marked insomnia and reduced biological functioning such as eating and drinking. Mania may be hazardous to both mother and fetus and may make compliance with antenatal care difficult. Therefore the rapid resolution of the mother's mental state is a priority and will almost always involve safe containment within a psychiatric unit.

The medication used to produce as rapid symptom relief as possible would be either chlorpromazine, in the dosage range given above, or the butyrophenone haloperidol, dosage range 1.5–40 mg daily in divided doses. As described above these substances are probably not hazardous to the developing fetus, providing the dosage is reduced to the minimum possible as soon as is clinically indicated, and this is particularly important in the weeks before delivery. It is likely that such medication will have to be continued throughout the pregnancy, and for a period of between three an six months at least following delivery, as the risk of a puerperal relapse is substantial.

Lithium carbonate, a substance frequently used in psychiatry both as a prophylactic against the recurrence of manic-depressive psychosis and as a treatment for manic illnesses, should not be used during the first trimester of pregnancy. Lithium freely crosses the placenta and amniotic fluid concentrations exceed maternal serum levels. There is much evidence linking the use of lithium during the first trimester to an increased incidence of congenital defects of the cardiovascular system. The majority of data has been accumulated by the lithium baby register in Denmark (Schou et al, 1973). There have also been frequent reports of lithium toxicity in babies born to mothers receiving lithium in the last trimester of pregnancy. These include hypothyroidism, dysrhythmias and ECG a rmalities, diabetes insipidus, hepatomegaly and gastrointestinal bleeding. For these reasons the use of lithium should be avoided during pregnancy, particularly during the first and last trimester. As it is also excreted into breast milk, it is also contraindicated in breast-feeding mothers.

A full review of lithium in pregnancy and lactation is given in Ruben (1987).

Management of depressive illness

The majority of depressive illnesses that occur during pregnancy (mostly in the first trimester but a small proportion in the last trimester) are neurotic depressive illnesses and will not require medical forms of treatment. However, major depressive illness does sometimes occur for the first time during pregnancy, and occasionally may recur in pregnancy in a woman with a previous history. The differential diagnosis of the depressive illness is of great importance and will usually necessitate a psychiatric referral. The indications for the medical treatment of a depressive disorder during pregnancy are, as at other times, the so-called biological symptoms of depression: early morning wakening, diurnal variation of mood, impaired concentration, interest and ability and a marked slowing of psychomotor functioning, together with morbid and often guilty ideation. As the presence of a depressive illness in the last trimester of pregnancy is related to severe postnatal depressive illness, the accurate diagnosis and speedy treatment of such conditions is important. Conventional well-tried tricyclic antidepressants, such as amitriptyline, dothiepin and imipramine, can probably be safely used during pregnancy. The therapeutic dosage of these drugs is 150 mg daily. The patient is usually started on 50–75 mg daily and the dosage gradually increased over a period of one week. It can be given as a single dose at night or as a divided dose during the day. The therapeutic effect of tricyclic antidepressants does not usually begin before ten days and significant clinical recovery will not take place before two to four weeks. Therefore if the patient is extremely agitated or distressed it may be necessary initially to use adjunctive treatment, such as small doses of chlorpromazine (25–50 mg three times a day). This can be withdrawn as the patient begins to improve. There have been reports of limb reduction anomalies associated with the use of amitriptyline and imipramine in the first trimester of pregnancy. However, larger studies have not confirmed this association (Australian Drug Evaluation Committee, 1973). There is little available evidence on the possible teratogenicity of the newer antidepressants or of monoamine oxidase inhibitors. These substances should therefore not be used in pregnancy. With monoamine oxidase inhibitors there is the potential hazard of interaction with anaesthetic agents, which is an additional reason for avoiding their use during pregnancy.

Electroconvulsive therapy (ECT) is a very effective treatment for profound depressive illnesses. It is also being used successfully for the resolution of manic illnesses (although less so since the introduction of lithium) and for schizophrenic illnesses, particularly those with large affective components. However, because it involves the use of anaesthetic and the induction of a controlled epileptic fit, its use is not to be recommended during the first trimester of pregnancy and should probably be avoided if at all possible during the whole of pregnancy. The use of anaesthetic agents in the first trimester of pregnancy has been implicated in fetal abnormalities and there is a theoretical risk of miscarriage or premature labour.

Tricyclic antidepressants would normally be continued for at least six months following the resolution of a depressive illness. However, in pregnancy there have been some reports of neonatal withdrawal symptoms in babies born to mothers receiving full therapeutic dosage of tricyclic antidepressants (particularly imipramine and clomipramine) in the weeks before delivery. These include neonatal jitteriness and fits, as well as urinary retention. For these reasons the dosage of antidepressant should be reduced to a minimum possible maintenance dose or even stopped before delivery. As there is a substantial risk of relapse in the puerperium, the tricyclic antidepressant should be increased back to therapeutic levels following delivery. Although amitriptyline and imipramine are excreted into breast milk, no studies have detected the substance in the infant's serum, nor is there any evidence that clinical signs of drug activity have been observed in infants who are breast-fed by mothers receiving tricyclic antidepressants. It therefore seems reasonable that the continuation of tricyclic antidepressants is compatible with breast-feeding. A full review of the use of tricyclic antidepressants in pregnancy and lactation is given in Ruben (1987).

Management of the patient on maintenance prophylactic medication

Obstetricians may see patients with past histories of major mental illness (either schizophrenia or schizophrenia-like conditions or manic-depressive illness) who are still on medication. These women may either be seeking advice before conception or may already be pregnant. Decisions about their management should be made in collaboration with a psychiatrist with special experience in this area. If a woman has had a single episode of such an illness more than two years before conception and the psychiatrist feels that the relapse risk is low, the medication should gradually be withdrawn before conception. The risk to the woman of a relapse during pregnancy is low, but the risk of relapse after delivery is high; therefore, she must be closely followed up for the duration of the pregnancy and for the puerperium (see below). It is particularly important that lithium should be withdrawn well in advance of conception.

Management of the pregnant women on medication. If such a woman has had a single episode of manic-depressive illness in the past and is thought to be at low risk of relapse then her medication should be withdrawn. She may well be receiving lithium carbonate and this should be withdrawn immediately. There is some suggestion (Dickson and Kendell, 1986) that the sudden withdrawal of lithium may precipitate a manic illness and therefore her psychiatric status should be closely supervised following the withdrawal of lithium. She may also be receiving a maintenance dose of a phenothiazine such as chlorpromazine or a butyrophenone such as haloperidol. Concurrent anti-parkinsonian medication should be withdrawn immediately, but it is probably safe to withdraw the phenothiazine or butyrophenone more gradually over a period of weeks. If she is receiving antidepressant medication, this too should be slowly withdrawn at the rate of 25 mg a week. A sudden cessation of tricyclic antidepressants may be associated with withdrawal symptoms such as nausea and the somatic symptoms of anxiety.

Patients who have had an isolated episode of a schizophrenia-like illness some years previously and are thought to be at low risk may well be receiving phenothiazines such as chlorpromazine or trifluoperazine or depot preparations such as flupenthixol; these too can be safely discontinued gradually during the first few weeks of pregnancy.

If the patient has chronic schizophrenia or multiple episodes, with evidence of previous relapse on cessation of medication, the psychiatrist may feel that the risk of relapse to the woman is high and, therefore, it is in her best interests and those of the fetus for some medication to be continued. With the exception of lithium it is probably safe to continue phenothiazine or butyrophenone medication at the lowest possible dosage to maintain good health throughout pregnancy. It is particularly important to reduce these medications to a minimum possible level before delivery.

Management of the 'at risk' mother

Patients with family histories of manic-depressive illness and schizophrenia-like disorder, and those with previous histories of such conditions themselves, are at high risk of developing a puerperal psychosis following delivery. They and their families, as well as their medical practitioners, may well be extremely anxious about this possibility. It is, therefore, strongly advisable for such a patient to see a psychiatrist during pregnancy and when discussing the possibility of further pregnancies. This offers the opportunity of advice and counselling and the possibility of risk reduction and perhaps in the future preventative medication. Those who have had previous illnesses, particularly of a manic nature, or previous non-puerperal manias have a particularly high risk of puerperal psychosis. In such circumstances the psychiatrist may well feel there is an indication for giving prophylactic medication after delivery and before the onset of the illness. There is some preliminary work on the use of lithium in this context, but of course this would necessitate the woman deciding not to breast-feed her infant.

Women with chronic or relapsing schizophrenic illnesses should be continued on prophylactic medication during pregnancy and the puerperium and can thus be helped not to have a puerperal relapse. However, other concerns for their well-being and the possible need for help and support in the care of their child will necessitate on-going psychiatric contact.

The use of natural progesterone in late pregnancy and early puerperium to prevent the recurrence of puerperal psychosis or severe postnatal depression has been recommended by Dalton (1980) and has a number of keen disciples. However, properly controlled studies have yet to be undertaken to prove the efficacy of this treatment.

With a general recurrence rate of one in five, perhaps even higher in individual cases, there are few parallels in medicine for such a high and predictable rate of recurrence as occurs in a woman embarking upon her second pregnancy with a past history of puerperal psychosis. Whether or not active preventative treatment is being contemplated, there is an overwhelming advantage, to both patient and psychiatrist, of meeting such a woman during pregnancy when she is well. For the psychiatrist it provides the rare opportunity to understand his patient, her expectations and wishes before the onset of an illness, and to be able to predict and plan for any ramifications of the illness that are likely in the patient's social and family life. For the patient, who is almost always extremely anxious about the possibility of a recurrence anyhow, it provides an opportunity for realistic reassurance, forward planning and the opportunity to meet members of staff who might be involved in her care afterwards. Discussion with her psychiatrist may help her to identify risk factors herself which can be reduced, and help her to plan for adequate rest and support once the baby is born. Handled sensibly, contact with the appropriate psychiatric services before delivery for the 'at risk' woman should not increase anxiety nor make the illness more likely to happen. On the contrary it almost always decreases anxiety and theoretically at least may reduce the possibility of a further illness.

Management of major mental illness in the puerperium

Although only two per 1000 women are admitted to psychiatric units following delivery (most of whom are psychotic), this figure substantially under-represents the proportion of women who suffer from serious mental illness following delivery. Seventeen per 1000 women will be referred to psychiatric services following delivery, at least half of whom attract the diagnosis of schizophrenia, schizophrenia-like conditions or manic-depressive psychosis. The rates of referral following childbirth are approximately ten times higher than for men or women of reproductive age, and the proportion of those referred with serious mental disorder is at least twice as high as for comparable groups of men and women (Oates, 1988). Prospective antenatal studies and community studies reveal that 10% of all recently delivered women will suffer from a depressive illness of a severity that would normally be seen in psychiatric outpatient clinics (Cox et al, 1987). However, we know that few of these women are actually referred to psychiatrists. Whilst it is difficult to gather from many of these community and prospective studies the exact proportion of women suffering from severe or major depressive illnesses (of the type that require medical forms of treatment), a reasonable estimate would be that at least 3% of all women delivered suffer from a severe depressive illness of the type that in the United States is known as 'major depressive illness' and in Europe as 'manic-depressive illness—depressed type'. Taken together, puerperal psychosis (either admitted or managed in the community), referred psychiatric morbidity and major depressive illness represent a substantial serious psychiatric morbidity in relation to childbirth. All of these serious illnesses, either the puerperal psychoses or the major depressive illnesses, begin in the early days or weeks of the puerperium and the majority have become clinically apparent or will have presented by 90 days postpartum and will almost certainly be detectable by the time of the postnatal check at six weeks postpartum. It is therefore very important for obstetricians and general practitioners to be aware of the clinical syndromes, to ensure speedy detection and treatment of these very distressing and disabling conditions.

A full description of these clinical syndromes, their aetiology and epidemiology is given in Chapter 8.

Puerperal psychosis

Clinical presentation

Puerperal psychosis is usually an acute florid illness (related to the manic-depressive psychoses) and tends to present abruptly within the first two weeks of delivery (75%) and almost always within the first 90 days following delivery. It rarely, if ever, occurs within the first 48 hours after delivery—the so-called latent period. In the beginning the illness is an acute undifferentiated psychotic condition, with marked agitation, perplexity, fear and disturbance of bodily and psychological functioning. Often the patients are confused and disorientated as well. These acutely frightened and distressed women are often only a few days delivered and need not only urgent psychiatric assessment but intensive physical and psychiatric nursing. Nutrition, hydration and hygiene need to be closely supervised by the nurse, who will need to be with the patient more or less continuously ('specialling'). The patient should be managed in a quiet well-lit room and not left unattended. The avoidance of large numbers of changing nursing personnel and the presence of a familiar relative will help to reduce the fear and perplexity. Although the mother may require considerable help with feeding and caring for her baby, it should be, if at all possible, in the same room as she is, as prolonged absences from the baby may lead to fears or even delusions that something has happened to her baby or that it has been taken away from her.

After a few days the illness usually becomes more recognizable as an affective psychosis, with a classical manic or depressive ideation and biological features. However, commonly there are also many symptoms often found in schizophrenia and for this reason many of these conditions are known as schizo-affective. Because these women are so profoundly disturbed, both behaviourally and psychologically, they should usually be admitted to a psychiatric unit, together with their babies. In such circumstances the daily visit of a midwife for 14 days and periodically thereafter for 28 days will assist the psychiatric nurses in their management of the newborn infant and its mother, and also provide the same postnatal care that the woman would receive if she were at home.

Medical management

When the psychosis first presents the immediate priority is to sedate the patient with phenothiazines or butyrophenones to a level that allows the patient to be safely containable within her environment, and allows for adequate hydration and nutrition. Such medication will also reduce the perplexity, fear and distress, and over a period of 48 hours should begin to make some impact on hallucinations and delusions. A suggested initial regimen would be 50 mg of chlorpromazine or thioridazine three times daily, together with 75 or 100 mg at night, as frequently their mental state is at its worst during the night. The dose should be 'titrated' up or down, and up to 150 mg or even occasionally 200 mg of either chlorpromazine or thioridazine can be given three or four times a day. Chlorpromazine up to 100 mg can be given as an intramuscular injection. Both chlorpromazine and thioridazine come in syrup form which may aid compliance in a highly disturbed state. Extrapyramidal side-effects are uncommon with these preparations so anti-parkinsonian agents are rarely required. After a few days the clinical picture settles and becomes more clearly manic-depressive or schizophrenia-like.

If the mental state is that of mania, many psychiatrists prefer to use haloperidol. The dose range is between 1.5 and 10 mg in a single dose. This drug commonly produces extrapyramidal side-effects, both parkinsonism and acute dystonias, and an anti-parkinsonian agent such as benzhexol (5–10 mg twice a day) will usually be required. Haloperidol also comes in intramuscular form and 5–10 mg intramuscularly can be given to a patient in a highly disturbed state. Lithium carbonate can also be used to treat acute episodes of mania, as well as its more familiar use as a prophylactic against recurrence of bipolar affective psychosis. Using lithium to treat a manic episode would be particularly indicated if a patient had had a previous episode known to respond to lithium. Lithium may be used as a solitary treatment or as an adjunctive treatment to a phenothiazine other than haloperidol. Many clinicians would be cautious about prescribing lithium and haloperidol concurrently, as there has been some suggestion that lithium may potentiate some of the more unpleasant side-effects of haloperidol and even the occurrence of the malignant neuroleptic syndrome. When using lithium carbonate as a treatment for an acute manic episode, normal thyroid and renal function should first be established. Lithium carbonate should then be given in 400 mg tablets, increasing from one tablet to two or three (1200 mg a day) until a therapeutic serum lithium level is obtained. When treating mania it is usual for the lithium level to be stabilized at the higher end of the therapeutic range (between 0.8 and 1 mmol/l). In the few days before a therapeutic lithium level is produced it will often be necessary to use an adjunctive phenothiazine with sedative properties, such as chlorpromazine 50 mg three times daily.

Tricyclic antidepressants, because they take between seven and ten days to begin their effect, are rarely appropriate as a first-line treatment for a severely disturbed depressive psychosis and these patients should be initially given a phenothiazine. If the patient is not responding within three to seven days of a regimen of regular phenothiazine medication, then for puerperal mania and puerperal depressive psychosis (ECT) is the treatment of choice (Oates, 1986). Most of the schizophrenia-like conditions in the puerperium also have a strong affective component and respond very well to ECT. It is usually given twice a week for approximately six to eight treatment sessions. In cases of extreme disturbance it may be necessary to give ECT as an emergency, particularly if the patient is not eating or drinking and her physical state is in danger.

Major depressive illness. Two-thirds of major depressive illnesses present rather later in the puerperium (between six and twelve weeks). The absence of psychotic features would indicate treating these patients with tricyclic anti-depressants. However, the presence of psychotic features—hallucinations, delusions, suicidal ideation or extreme agitation—would again indicate the use of phenothiazines as well, usually chlorpromazine or thioridazine because of their sedative properties, at a dosage of 25–50 mg three times a day, and possibly ECT. The phenothiazines can then be withdrawn as the psychotic features disappear, but the tricyclic antidepressants will require to be continued for at least 12 weeks after the patient has become symptom-free. States of hopeless despair and suicidal ideation may require admission, but otherwise many of these patients can be managed at home.

Risk of relapse

Many early onset puerperal psychoses, although responding to treatment initially very well, relapse, particularly in the early weeks after recovery. Therefore continuation of the phenothiazines, albeit at a reduced dosage, is probably important for a number of weeks or at least until the baby is three months old.

A patient who has presented with manic psychosis may relapse with a depressive psychosis or a further episode of mania. If this happens on more than one occasion the clinician may well think of using lithium carbonate in an attempt to stabilize the mood over the period of a few months after delivery. This mode of treatment would also be indicated if the patient has a past history of manic-depressive illness or has previously been stabilized on lithium.

When lithium is used as a prophylactic against future manic or depressive episodes, the patient is given 400 mg daily and this is gradually increased over a week up to maximum of 1200 mg daily to achieve a therapeutic serum level of (conventionally) between 0.8 and 1 mmol/l. Recent evidence suggests that a lower serum level, between 0.6 and 0.8 mmol/l, may be just as effective and reduce short-term side-effects, such as nausea and diarrhoea, and longer-term ones, such as thyroid dysfunction (Vestergaard and Schou, 1988). Before treatment is commenced, normal renal function and thyroid function should be confirmed and the serum level should be monitored within three days of initiating treatment and thereafter weekly until a stable serum level is reached. Once the serum level is stable, the levels can be safely checked once every three months. For a patient who has depressive illness only in association with the puerperium, prophylactic lithium therapy would not normally be continued beyond the first year. However, for a patient who has a previous history, lithium prophylaxis may be continued for longer.

Breast-feeding

Many women who present with severe mental illness early in the puerperium are breast-feeding and its continuation is usually very important to them. Stopping breast-feeding because of a mental illness may add to the burden of guilt they feel once they recover. Continuing may help the recovery of their self-esteem and their relationship with their baby once their mental state improves. Continuing breast-feeding requires a great deal of skill on the part of the psychiatric nurse when women are very disturbed. Totally breast-feeding the infant may not be possible in the first few days of a severe puerperal psychosis. Nonetheless it should be possible to maintain lactation with a combination of expressing the milk and frequent suckling of the infant. When it is clearly important to continue breast-feeding the choice of psychotropic medication becomes very important. Lithium should probably not be given to breast-feeding women. The available evidence (see Ruben, 1987) suggests that tricyclic antidepressants in full dosage are safe for breast-feeding. They are only present in very small amounts in breast milk and significant quantities are not detectable in the infant's serum. Pheno-thiazines such as chlorpromazine and thioridazine (Melleril) (in a single dosage of 100 mg and not more than 400 mg a day), haloperidol (in a single dosage of 10 mg and not more than 20 mg a day), or trifluoperazine (in a single dosage of 5 mg and not more than 30 mg a day) are also probably safe for breast-feeding mothers. The infant should be closely monitored and the breast-feeding suspended if the baby is drowsy, does not wake and cry for its feeds, or does not suckle strongly. If the severity of her mental state requires the use of parenteral medication or a single dosage of more than the equivalent of 100 mg of chlorpromazine, it is probably safer to suspend breast-feeding for a period of 12–24 hours and express the milk. Paediatric advice should be sought if the baby is premature, of low birth-weight or jaundiced.

Other aspects of management

The most severe illnesses, puerperal psychoses, tend to present very early— often within days of delivery. These conditions, particularly if associated with life-threatening features and extreme behavioural disturbance, will usually require admission to a psychiatric unit, preferably one which can manage mother and baby together. Mother and baby units can be found in many health districts in Great Britain. Other patients with puerperal psychosis, who are less behaviourally disturbed, can be managed at home by psychiatric teams with community psychiatric nurses, particularly if there are relatives to assist in their care. Other alternatives to admission are specialist day hospitals, which are available in some areas. In the absence of marked suicidal intent, major depressive illnesses too can ideally be managed in this way. Wherever the treatment takes place, in a mother and baby unit, day hospital or at home, the first priority is energetic treatment, as outlined above, to produce as rapid as possible a resolution of the illness. However, equally important is specialist psychiatric nursing. The philosophy of care is to maintain the mother/infant relationship, despite the disturbance of the mother's mental state. This involves maintaining close proximity between mother and infant with frequent physical contact and assistance with those aspects of care which the mother is too ill to perform. As she improves the nurses help her to acquire skills (particularly if she is a first-time mother) and restore self-esteem and autonomy. Later, she is helped to understand what has happened to her and why. Whatever the initial setting of the treatment, frequent and sensitive follow-up is required with continuation of medication beyond clinical recovery. The aim is, therefore, to produce as rapid and as complete a clinical recovery as possible and to reduce to a minimum secondary disability for the woman and her family.

REFERENCES

Australian Drug Evaluation Committee (1973) Tricyclic antidepressants and limb reduction deformities. *Australian Medical Journal* **1:** 768–769.

Cooper PJ, Campbell EA, Day A et al (1988) Non-psychotic psychiatric disorder after childbirth: a prospective study of prevalence, incidence, course and nature. *British Journal of Psychiatry* **152:** 799–806.

Cox JL, Connor YM, Henderson I et al (1983) Prospective study of the psychiatric disorders of childbirth by self-report questionnaire. *Journal of Affective Disorders* **5:** 1–7.

Cox JL, Holden JM & Sagovsky R (1987) Detection of postnatal depression: development of the 10-item Edinburgh postnatal depression scale (EPDS). *British Journal of Psychiatry* **150:** 782–786.

Dalton K (1980) *Depression after Childbirth.* Oxford: Oxford University Press.

Dickson WE & Kendell RE (1986) Does maintenance lithium therapy prevent recurrences of mania under ordinary clinical conditions? *Psychological Medicine* **16:** 521–530.

Kendell RE, Rennie D, Clarke JA et al (1981) The social and obstetric correlates of psychiatric admission in the puerperium. *Psychological Medicine* **11:** 341–350.

Kendell RE, Chalmers C & Platz C (1987) The epidemiology of puerperal psychoses. *British Journal of Psychiatry* **150:** 662–672.

Kumar R & Robson K (1978) Neurotic disturbance during pregnancy and the puerperium: preliminary report of a prospective survey of 119 primiparae. In Sander M (ed.) *Mental Illness in Pregnancy and the Puerperium,* pp 40–51. London: Oxford University Press.

Kumar R & Robson K (1984) A prospective study of emotional disorders in childbearing women. *British Journal of Psychiatry* **144:** 35–47.

Oates MR (1986) The role of electroconvulsive therapy in the treatment of postnatal mental illness. In Cox JL, Kumar R et al (eds) *Current Approaches: Puerperal Mental Illness*, pp 1–12. Southampton: Duphar Medical Relations.

Oates MR (1988) The development of an integrated community-orientated service for severe postnatal mental illness. In Kumar R & Brockington IF (eds) *Motherhood and Mental Illness*, vol. 2, pp 133–158. Sevenoaks: Wright.

O'Hara MW (1986) Social support, life events, and depression during pregnancy and the puerperium. *Archives of General Psychiatry* **43**: 569–573.

O'Hara MW & Zekoski EM (1988) Postpartum depression: a comprehensive review. In Kumar R & Brockington IF (eds) *Motherhood and Mental Illness*, vol. 2, pp 17–63. Sevenoaks: Wright.

Ruben PC (1987) *Prescribing in Pregnancy*. London: British Medical Association.

Schou M, Goldfield MD, Weinstein MR et al (1973) Lithium and pregnancy. A report from the register of lithium babies. *British Medical Journal* **ii**: 135–136.

Vestergaard P & Schou M (1988) Prospective studies on a lithium cohort. *Acta Psychiatrica Scandinavica* **78**: 421–433.

13

The effects of postnatal depression on the infant

LYNNE MURRAY
ALAN STEIN

Studies of the impact of parental depression on preschool and school-age children have consistently reported a variety of adverse effects. For example, there have been findings of raised levels of psychiatric disturbance, greater insecurity in attachment relationships, impairments in attention and lowered IQ (Weissman et al, 1972, 1984; Cohler et al, 1977; Gamer et al, 1977; Welner et al, 1977; Grunebaum et al, 1978; McKnew et al, 1979; Cox et al, 1987).

Epidemiological research carried out in the last decade has shown that approximately 10% of women suffer from non-psychotic depression in the first few months following childbirth. This prevalence rate contrasts with that for postpartum psychotic episodes which, while more severe, occur rarely, affecting only one or two per 1000 women. Since obstetric staff are far more likely, therefore, to encounter those affected by non-psychotic depressions, the present chapter has as its focus the effects on the infant of these more common, neurotic disorders.

In cases of depression with postnatal onset, all the characteristics of depression occurring at other times are present, with irritability, anxiety, concentration impairments, and depressive mood and thoughts being prominent (Nott, 1987; Cooper et al, 1988; Murray and Carothers, 1989). All these features of depression may exert a profound effect on inter-personal relationships, including that established with the infant. Moreover, it is common for some level of symptoms to persist for at least a year beyond childbirth. Since it is the case that, in most cultures, the mother constitutes the infant's primary social environment in these first months, the issue of the effects on the rapidly developing infant of depression occurring at this time is one of special clinical concern. The following chapter reviews studies that have been carried out in recent years to address this question. The implications of the findings for obstetric staff are then considered.

RESEARCH FINDINGS

Maternal reports

Several studies have made indirect child assessments by interviewing mothers, often some years after an episode of postnatal depression, about their child's current behaviour. Zajicek and de Salis (1979) interviewed women who had experienced symptoms in the postnatal period either of a severity to produce impairments in daily functioning and relationships or that were subjectively distressing but not incapacitating. At 27 months the children of these women were reported to be fearful, to have eating problems and to have difficulties in bladder control. Uddenberg and Englesson (1978), using very similar case definitions to those described above, found that the four-and-a-half-year-old children of women who had suffered from postpartum mental disturbance were described as being troublesome, uncontrollable and prone to temper tantrums.

Williams and Carmichael (1985) conducted a study of the effects of maternal depression on infants in a poor, multi-ethnic community in Melbourne, Australia. Amongst the primiparous mothers in their sample, those who became depressed reported significantly more difficulties than well mothers. Two principal patterns of disturbance were found. Several mothers reported that there had been a failure to establish a relationship or routine pattern of management with the baby whilst on the postnatal ward. On their return home, the infant was said to cry persistently, feed poorly, sleep irregularly and only for brief periods, and to be difficult to soothe. This situation itself appeared to cause depressive symptoms in the mothers who became frustrated and angry with their infants. In other mothers, infant sleeping, feeding and crying difficulties developed only *after* the onset, some weeks following delivery, of the depressive episode. Again, a vicious cycle of impaired communication became established. This picture of marked difficulties in infant care and behaviour where the infant was an only child contrasted with that obtained where there were older children in the family. In these circumstances there was no increase in reports of infant behavioural disturbance. Indeed, in a substantial proportion of cases the depressed mothers were protective of their infants and had a good relationship with them. However, significant levels of behaviour problems were found instead amongst the older preschool siblings.

These studies point to an increased risk of child behavioural disturbance and difficulties in the mother–child relationship where there has been psychiatric disturbance in the months following delivery. However, it should be borne in mind that many of the women taking part in the research described above were depressed at the time of interview. Current maternal depression may influence the outcome of these studies in two ways. Firstly, there may be a direct effect of current symptoms on child functioning, making it difficult to determine the effect of *postnatal* depression. Secondly, the mother's current depression may colour her perceptions of the child's behaviour, and hence lead to over-reporting of problems. Thus some caution is required when considering the findings of this series of studies.

A carefully analysed study was carried out by Ghodsian et al (1984), in which account was taken of current symptoms when evaluating the impact on the child of depression occurring during the three-and-a-half years after the birth. Mothers were psychiatrically assessed at 4, 14, 27 and 42 months, and, on all but the first occasion, they were interviewed about their child's behaviour. No effects were found of depression occurring in the first four months. However, there was evidence that depression occurring at 14 months had an independent effect on later behaviour problems.

Wrate et al (1985) interviewed women who had participated in a prospective study of postnatal depression when their children were three years old. As in the study carried out by Ghodsian et al (1984), the data were analysed to take account of current depression, and again no increase in child behavioural disturbance was reported by mothers who had suffered from a postnatal depressive episode. However, women who had had *mild* depressive symptoms in the postnatal period did report more difficulties. These women had earlier shown far greater anxiety about their maternal role, and had often gone on to have depressive episodes in the subsequent two years that focused on anxieties about the child.

Using a similar design to that adopted by Wrate et al (1985), Caplan et al (1989) followed up women who had taken part in a study of depression occurring after childbirth (Kumar and Robson, 1984). When the children were four years old, mothers who were currently depressed reported more child behavioural difficulties. The association seemed to be mediated by disturbed family interactions, since reports of such difficulties were also related to marital conflict and paternal psychiatric history. However, as in the studies of Ghodsian et al (1984) and Wrate et al (1985), no relationship was found between reported child disturbance and clinical depression occurring in the postnatal period.

Evidence from these indirect studies indicates, therefore, that while there have been several reports of an increase in later behavioural disturbance associated with episodes of postnatal depression, when account is taken of current symptoms and the pattern of family relationships, no effects of postnatal depression *per se* are found on these particular dimensions of child outcome.

Direct studies of older children

Two studies have been completed in recent years that have the advantage of direct assessments having been made of the children of women from unselected community samples who had suffered from depression occurring during the postnatal period. Using the same cohort as Caplan et al (1989) above, Cogill et al (1986) examined the children's cognitive functioning. At four years, children whose mothers had been depressed during the first postnatal year had significantly lower scores on the McCarthy Scales of children's cognitive development than children whose mothers had not been postnatally depressed. These differences could not be accounted for by current maternal depression.

A further study has recently been carried out (A. Stein et al, unpublished data) in which the relationship between maternal postnatal depressive disorder and later mother–child interactions was investigated. Two groups of mothers and infants were observed during home assessments when the infants were 19 months old. The index group consisted of mothers who had had a depressive disorder during the postnatal year. By 19 months, half of these mothers had made a full recovery. The control group consisted of mothers who had been free from depression since the child's birth.

The main significant findings from the observational studies were that, compared with the controls, depressed mothers interacted less with their children and showed less facilitation (positive contribution to their child's activity). Their children, in turn, showed less affective sharing (smiling and showing toys to the mother, or smiling and vocalizing during joint play), and greater distress during a planned brief departure of the mother from the room. Similar but reduced effects were seen in the subgroup of families in which the mothers had been depressed postnatally but who were no longer so at the 19-month follow-up.

The index group of mothers had experienced significantly more marital difficulties and social problems mainly concerning housing and finance. Logistic regression analysis revealed that these difficulties were the most powerful predictors of the quality of mother–child interaction at 19 months. An additional contribution was made by maternal depression, both in the first few months and at the time of assessment.

In contrast to research based on maternal reports of frank child behavioural disturbance, these direct studies indicate that maternal depression in the postpartum period may be associated with later lowered scores on cognitive assessments and with less harmonious and mutual mother–child interactions. However, the way in which these specific adverse outcomes arise in the context of postnatal depression remains to be established. To date, prospective, longitudinal evidence from random community samples about the developing relationship between the depressed mother and her infant, and the course of infant progress is not available. However, a few studies have been carried out in recent years in which assessments have been made of early interactions between depressed mothers and their babies. These are reviewed below, along with evidence from developmental psychology about the normal development of mother–child relations. Together these two lines of research provide some indication of the routes by which deviant outcome may be brought about.

Direct studies of early mother–infant interactions

Normal populations

Over the last 20 years a large body of evidence has accumulated from developmental psychology about the interpersonal functioning of infants. One finding to emerge from this work is that, very early on, there is a propensity to be attracted to human forms. For example, even neonates show preferential responsiveness to the sound of the human voice compared with non-human sounds of the same pitch and intensity, and face-like compared with scrambled visual arrays (Friedlander, 1970; Eisenberg, 1975; Goren et al, 1975). Furthermore, there is a tendency in the infant to develop a preference for the particular qualities of the person caring for him: the mother's face, voice and smell are all preferred to those of another woman within a week of birth (McFarlane, 1975; Field, 1985; De Casper and Fifer, 1980).

A series of studies has been conducted to explore infant sensitivities to the quality of adult communication. In this research the mother's normal inter-actions with her infant, in which a whole range of adaptations to infant sensitivities are unconsciously made, are experimentally disrupted as, for example, when she is instructed to cease responding and adopt a still, blank-faced expression. Under these conditions infants as young as six weeks first protest, and then become distressed and eventually withdraw. If a qualitatively different disruption is arranged, for instance if the timing of the mother's communication is put out of phase with infant behaviour but form is held constant, a different pattern of infant response is seen, with the baby appearing to be confused. In each case the particular form of infant behaviour, such as withdrawal or confusion, seems appropriate to the ongoing disruption (Murray, 1980; Murray and Trevarthen, 1985).

This body of research attests to the infant being drawn, firstly, simply to engage with other people, and secondly, to develop particular attachments. In addition, it appears that early on infants are highly sensitive to the form of their interpersonal contacts; interactions of a particular kind are sought, and if these are not forthcoming, reactions are provoked that entail significant alterations in affective state and attention.

This work, using experimental distortions of maternal communication to explore infant sensitivities, has been developed in recent years specifically to explore the effects of disturbed communication arising in the context of depression. In an initial study, Cohn and Tronick (1983) examined the effects of simulated depression on the infant. As in the experiments in which the mother was required to become blank-faced and unresponsive, three-month-old infants reacted by protesting and becoming wary and avoidant when their mothers behaved as though depressed.

Clinical populations

Field and colleagues (Field, 1984; Field et al, 1985, 1988) have conducted a series of studies comparing brief (three-minute sequences) videotaped interactions between depressed and non-depressed mothers and their three-month-old babies. Although the scoring procedures differed somewhat between the various studies, a consistent pattern of results emerged. Depressed mothers were far less active, making fewer vocalizations, touch-ing the baby less and showing fewer positive facial expressions. Further-more, their behaviour was less contingent on that of the infants and there was little game-play. The infants of the depressed mothers themselves showed 'depressed' behaviour: they were fussy, discontented and avoidant, and, like their mothers, made fewer positive facial expressions and vocaliza-tions and were less active. In the most recent study in this series it was found that the depressed mothers' infants generalized this interactive style to other situations, being less positive and active when presented with a non-depressed adult.

Further work with clinical populations has been carried out by Cohn,

Lyons-Ruth and colleagues (Cohn et al, 1986; Lyons-Ruth et al, 1986). They videorecorded both structured mother–infant interactions (where the mother was asked to play face-to-face with the infant) and those occurring spontaneously in the home. These assessments were carried out from six to twelve months postpartum in a population where women had been identified by health care workers as having significant difficulties in the management of their babies. A large proportion of these women were subsequently identified as being depressed. As in the studies conducted by Field, interactions between the depressed mothers and their infants were, on the whole, less harmonious than those found in the authors' previous research with non-clinical populations. In the six-month structured face-to-face interactions, four styles of depressed maternal interactive behaviour were identified. The first, the 'disengaged' pattern, resembled that already described in the literature: mothers were withdrawn, and 'slouched back in their chairs, turned away from the infant, or spoke to the baby in an expressionless voice with little facial expression' (Cohn et al, 1986, p 36). A second group, described as 'mixed', did attempt to engage with their babies, using many eliciting techniques seen in normal samples. However, like the disengaged group, they showed low levels of positive affect and were not able to play. Unlike previous descriptions of depressed maternal behaviour, almost half the mothers in this sample were categorized as 'intrusive': they showed low proportions of positive expression, and high levels of anger, frequently poking or pulling at their infants. All three of these subgroups of mothers failed to respond contingently to infant behaviours. Finally, there were depressed women who appeared to have positive relations with their infants.

The infants of the depressed women were themselves withdrawn and showed very little positive affective expression during the interactions; it was also found that the particular form of infant response related to maternal style. Thus, infants of 'disengaged' mothers showed a great deal of protest behaviour, whereas maternal intrusiveness tended to provoke infant avoidance. The authors found that both maternal and infant styles seen in the structured interactions carried over to a large extent to their spontaneous behaviour, although the intrusive mothers tended to become somewhat withdrawn when left to determine the extent of their involvement with the infant.

In a follow-up study of these same mother–infant pairs, along with additional cases from the same population, assessments were made of infant development, the quality of interactions and of attachment to the mother. In naturalistic observations of the mothers' behaviour at home at 12 months postpartum it was found that the depressed women were significantly more angry and controlling in relation to their infants than non-depressed controls. Maternal depression was also significantly related to lowered infant scores on both the physical and mental indices of the Bayley Scales of Development, even after controlling for the effects of maternal IQ. The effects of depression on infant attachment were less clear-cut. Severely depressed women had infants who were insecure and ambivalent. However, the infants of mildly depressed women tended to be securely attached. It should be noted that some caution is required when considering these data, since the population was not a random community sample but was specifically selected on the basis of problems identified in the mother–child relationship. Nevertheless, this work is important in providing detailed documentation of the variability in the quality of relations between depressed mothers and their infants, and of the links between maternal interactive style and infant behaviour.

Preliminary data from an ongoing prospective study of depressed and control women and their infants, drawn from a large random community sample in Cambridge (L. Murray and H. Marwick, unpublished data), also reveal significant effects of depression on the quality of the mother's communication with her infant. An analysis of the content of the mother's 'baby-talk' at two months showed that, compared with non-depressed mothers, those who were depressed were far more self-oriented, critical and controlling. These features of baby-talk were independent of the severity of symptoms and timing of onset; however, they were far more likely to occur where the episode of depression was the first in the woman's experience, where the feelings of depression seemed to centre on difficulties in adapting to motherhood rather than on stresses unrelated to child-bearing. Voice quality was also altered in depressed women, who showed far fewer of the specific features that normally occur in maternal speech to infants. As in the work of Cohn, Lyons-Ruth and colleagues outlined above, there were also indications that, within the case group, there was a relation between the style of interaction at three months and later performance on developmental tasks; thus infants were successful on tests of object constancy at nine months where maternal speech during the three-month interactions had been focused on infant experience, but failed where speech had been mother-centred (Murray, 1989).

The role of infant variables

It is clear from this review of studies that have made direct observations of relations between depressed mothers and their infants that in a large proportion of cases the adaptations to infant characteristics that are normally made by mothers when interacting with their babies do not occur. In turn, infant behaviour departs from the usual pattern of responsive and positive engagement. One issue raised by this evidence of early deviations in the profile of infant behaviour is that of the possible role of infant temperament. It might be argued, for example, that infants who are inherently 'difficult' and unresponsive contribute both to deviations in maternal interactive style and even to depression in the mother. Indeed, with regard to the impact on interactive style, it was found in the study carried out by Field et al (1988) that when the non-depressed experimenter interacted with infants of depressed mothers, their own behaviour became less positive and expressive than when interacting with infants of non-depressed mothers. Murray and Trevarthen (1986) found that if infant behaviour was set out of phase with the mother's, maternal speech style came to resemble that found in depressed populations.

Evidence consistent with the impact of difficult infant temperament on depression itself derives from several sources. Cutrona and Troutman (1986) assessed infant temperament at three months, using crying records, maternal reports and direct observations of the infants in the home. They found that maternal depression was far more likely to persist where the infant was difficult to soothe and cried excessively. Similarly, Whiffen and Gotlib (1989) found that depressed mothers perceived their two-month-old infants as being more difficult to care for and more bothersome than did non-depressed mothers, and independent assessments by the experimenter showed the depressed mothers' infants to be more tense and less content, and to deteriorate more quickly during cognitive testing. This evidence alone is not, of course, conclusive, since it could be the case that these infants became 'difficult' over the first two to three months through the process of being with a depressed mother, and direct assessments of infants are required in the neonatal period in order to resolve this issue.

Other researchers have found that stressful postpartum events specifically related to the infant are predictors of maternal depression and depressive symptomatology. O'Hara et al (1984) carried out a prospective study of postnatal depression and found that events such as the baby having health problems during the first few months of life were the only significant life-stress variables to predict depression. However, not all perinatal problems pose risks for later depression; other studies have found that complications occurring in the immediate perinatal period that are short-lived play little or no role in the aetiology of postpartum depression (Stein et al, 1989).

IMPLICATIONS FOR OBSTETRIC STAFF

It is clear from the above review of the effects of postnatal depression on the infant that although frank psychiatric and behavioural disturbance in the child is not a likely outcome, relations between depressed mothers and their babies are, on the whole, markedly different from those occurring in non-clinical populations. Although the particular form of disengagement may vary, interactions are generally characterized by a lack of positive affect and mutual responsiveness. Furthermore, there is evidence to suggest that the infant's cognitive development and security of attachment to the mother may be adversely effected in the longer term as a function of the early impaired relationship. It should be stressed, however, that these difficulties between postnatally depressed mothers and their infants are not inevitable, and that a proportion of these mothers adapt well and form close and secure bonds with their babies.

Antenatal identification of vulnerable women

Epidemiological research suggests that it may be possible to identify those at risk of postnatal depression before delivery, a cluster of risk factors having been found in a number of studies. Thus a poor marital relationship, severe social and economic stress, the lack of a close, confiding relationship and a previous psychiatric history consistently have been found to be as. ociated with episodes of postnatal depression (see Chapter 11; also reviewed in O'Hara and Zekoski, 1988; Cooper et al, 1989), thus affording the obstetric team some opportunity for allocating resources to those who are identified as vulnerable at the time of antenatal clinic contact. One key area for future research is the development of a suitable tool for accurate, routine identification of those at risk on the basis of antenatal factors.

Postnatal identification

No matter how refined the instruments developed for antenatal clinic administration, predictions based on antenatal risk factors will never be wholly accurate. Furthermore, as noted above, events following the child's birth may play a significant role in the onset of maternal emotional disturbance. Close attention is still required therefore on the postnatal ward, where many of the difficulties experienced by the woman who is vulnerable to depression may become evident, before the onset of a full clinical episode. Thus, in addition to the factors that can be identified during the antenatal period and stresses relating to infant health, the areas considered below may be worthy of particular attention.

Maternal response to the infant at delivery

Although it is now acknowledged that a large minority of women do not experience an immediate rush of intense positive feeling for their infant at delivery, but develop such affection gradually over the first few days (Robson and Kumar, 1980), it has been found that those who become postnatally depressed are far more likely to have responded negatively to their infants at birth. For example, in the study carried out by Murray (L. Murray, unpublished data), 47% of those who had a postnatal depressive episode, compared with 22% of those who did not, experienced feelings about their infants at this time which ranged from ambivalent to strongly negative. This association was found to hold independently of the method of delivery. These moments of first contact, therefore, may serve to provide the obstetric team with information that is pertinent to the future progress of the mother's relationship with her baby. Clearly, it would be very misguided to make judgements about a mother's capacity to form a warm and close relationship with her child solely on the basis of the response at the time of birth; however, strong adverse maternal reactions to the infant at delivery may alert staff to maternal vulnerability. Such identification could be of benefit if follow-up is sensitively managed.

Feeding difficulties

While just as many women who later become depressed intend to breast-feed their infants as do other mothers, the majority give up by eight weeks (P. J. Cooper et al, unpublished data; L. Murray, unpublished data). Although it has been suggested by some researchers (Alder and Cox, 1983;

Alder and Bancroft, 1988) that hormonal changes implicated in weaning may provoke the depressive episodes, evidence for this interpretation of the association between ceasing to feed and depression is unconvincing. Both the study of Cooper et al and that of Murray showed that in the majority of cases the onset of full depressive symptoms preceded weaning. However, although weaning itself may not be causal in relation to depression, difficulties associated with feeding that culminate in weaning may well play a role in contributing to its onset, as do other difficulties associated with infant care. The inception of problems of this nature may well be detectable on the postnatal ward, where feeding difficulties in those who later become depressed are frequently experienced.

Severe 'blues'

Several studies have found that severe feelings of low mood and tearfulness, usually experienced in mild form on about the fourth day after delivery by a large proportion of mothers, is associated with the occurrence of a full depressive episode postpartum (Paykel et al, 1980). As with response at delivery and the presence of feeding difficulties, such reactions may be detectable by obstetric staff during routine care on the postnatal ward.

Absence of confiding relationships

As noted above, one of the most important risk factors for postnatal depression is the absence of social support and, in particular, a close, confiding relationship. In addition to any information that the mother might give at the point of antenatal contact, the lack of visitors on the postnatal ward, or a strained quality of contact when visits are made, may provide vigilant staff with indications of difficulties in this area.

Secondary prevention

Clinical trials remain to be conducted to establish the most effective means of intervention in cases of postnatal depression and its concomitant disruptions to the mother–infant relationship. A study has recently been published in which health visitors were trained to give non-directive counselling to depressed mothers rather than routine care (Holden et al, 1989). Maternal depressive symptoms remitted significantly more quickly in women who received counselling, although the effects on the mother–infant relationship and on infant development were not evaluated. This preliminary work may carry useful implications for obstetric staff, who are in a unique position, working with women around the time of delivery and the subsequent postpartum days. It suggests that a supportive, counselling approach may very profitably complement the practical advice and training that constitutes the core of routine postnatal care. Such an approach, which could be directed in particular to those who are identified as vulnerable, could address the very difficulties which have been found to be predictors of depression, such as feelings of failure and helplessness when having difficulties feeding, or abandonment when there are no visitors. All this, of course, requires commitment on the part of the relevant professions to give emotional aspects of childbirth their place in the clinical agenda and therefore the training curriculum.

CONCLUSION

The rapidly developing infant is entirely dependent upon, and experiences the world through, those who care for him. In our culture this care is usually undertaken by the mother. If the mother becomes depressed it is very likely that the way in which she handles her infant and presents the world to him will be altered. Research conducted to date suggests that, while frank psychiatric disorder is unusual amongst these children in their later years, there is a significantly increased risk of difficulties in the relationship with the mother and of problems in the child's attachments in general. The possibility of some effects on cognitive development has also been raised.

It is therefore important for obstetric staff to be aware both of the possibility of postnatal depression and of risk factors for the condition; in particular, the lack of social support, especially a confiding relationship, socioeconomic hardship, early difficulties between mother and infant, a temperamentally difficult infant and possibly persistent feeding difficulties may all act as provoking factors. Recent research suggests that the provision of support and counselling may be beneficial to mothers, and may thus help to protect the infant. However, further research is required to establish how best to assist vulnerable women in the context of routine obstetric care.

REFERENCES

Alder EM & Bancroft J (1988) The relationship between breastfeeding persistence, sexuality and mood in postpartum women. *Psychological Medicine* **18:** 389–396.

Alder EM & Cox JC (1983) Breastfeeding and post-natal depression. *Journal of Psychosomatic Research* **27:** 139–144.

Caplan H, Cogill SR, Alexandra H, Robson KM, Katz R & Kumar R (1989) Maternal depression and the emotional development of the child. *British Journal of Psychiatry* **154:** 818–823.

Cogill SR, Caplan HR, Alexandra H, Robson KM & Kumar R (1986) Impact of maternal postnatal depression on cognitive development of young children. *British Medical Journal* **292:** 1165–1167.

Cohler BJ, Grunebaum HU, Weiss JL, Garner E & Gallant DH (1977) Disturbance of attention among schizophrenic, depressed and well mothers and their young children. *Journal of Child Psychology and Psychiatry and Allied Disciplines* **18:** 115–135.

Cohn JF & Tronick EZ (1983) Three month-old infants' reaction to simulated maternal depression. *Child Development* **54:** 185–193.

Cohn JF, Matias R, Tronick EZ, Connell D & Lyons-Ruth D (1986) Face-to-face interactions of depressed mothers and their infants. In Tronick EZ & Field T (eds) *Maternal Depression and Infant Disturbance*, pp 31–45. San Francisco: Jossey-Bass.

Cooper PJ, Campbell EA, Day A, Kennerley H & Bond A (1988) Non-psychotic psychiatric disorder after childbirth: a prospective study of prevalence, incidence, course and nature. *British Journal of Psychiatry* **152:** 799–806.

Cooper PJ, Murray L & Stein A (1989) Postnatal depression. In Seva A (ed.) *European Handbook of Psychiatry and Mental Health.*

Cox AD, Puckering C, Pound A & Mills M (1987) The impact of maternal depression on young children. *Journal of Child Psychology and Psychiatry and Allied Disciplines* **28:** 917–928.

Cutrona CE & Troutman BR (1986) Social support, infant temperament and parenting self efficacy: a mediational model of postpartum depression. *Child Development* **57:** 1507–1518.

De Casper AJ & Fifer WP (1980) Of human bonding: newborns prefer their mothers' voices. *Science* **208:** 1174–1176.

Eisenberg RB (1975) *Auditory Competence in Early Life. The Roots of Communicative Behavior.* Baltimore: University Park Press.

Field TM (1984) Early interactions between infants and their post partum depressed mothers. *Infant Behaviour and Development* **7:** 517–522.

Field TM (1985) Neonatal perception of people: motivational and individual differences. In Field TM & Fox NA (eds) *Social Perception in Infants*, pp 31–52. Norwood, New Jersey: Ablex.

Field T, Sandberg D, Garcia R, Vega Lahr N, Goldstein S & Guy L (1985) Prenatal problems, postpartum depression and early mother–infant interactions. *Developmental Psychology* **12:** 1152–1156.

Field T, Healy B, Goldstein S, Perry S & Bendell D (1988) Infants of depressed mothers show 'depressed' behaviour even with nondepressed adults. *Child Development* **59:** 1569–1579.

Friedlander B (1970) Receptive language development in infancy. *Merrill Palmer Quarterly* **16:** 7–51.

Gamer E, Gallant D, Grunebaum HU & Cohler BJ (1977) Children of psychotic mothers. *Archives of General Psychiatry* **34:** 592–597.

Ghodsian M, Zajicek E & Wolkind S (1984) A longitudinal study of maternal depression and child behaviour problems. *Journal of Child Psychology and Psychiatry and Allied Disciplines* **25:** 91–109.

Goren CG, Sarty M & Wu PYK (1975) Visual following and pattern discrimination of face-life stimuli by newborn infants. *Pediatrics* **56:** 544–549.

Grunebaum HU, Cohler BJ, Kauffman C & Gallant D (1978) Children of depressed and schizophrenic mothers. *Child Psychiatry and Human Development* **8:** 219–228.

Holden JM, Sagovsky R & Cox JL (1989) Counselling in a general practice setting: controlled study of health visitor intervention in treatment of postnatal depression. *British Medical Journal* **298:** 223–226.

Kumar R & Robson KM (1984) A prospective study of emotional disorders in childbearing women. *British Journal of Psychiatry* **144:** 35–47.

Lyons-Ruth K, Zoll D, Connell D & Grunebaum HU (1986) The depressed mother and her one-year-old infant. In Tronick EZ & Field T (eds) *Maternal Depression and Infant Disturbance*, pp 61–82. San Francisco: Jossey-Bass.

McFarlane J (1975) Olfaction in the development of social preferences in the human neonate. In Hofer M (ed.) *Parent–Infant Interaction.* Amsterdam: Elsevier.

McKnew PH, Cytryn L, Efron AM, Gershon ES & Bunney WE (1979) The offspring of parents with affective disorders. *British Journal of Psychiatry* **134:** 148–152.

Murray L (1980) *The sensitivities and expressive capacities of young infants in communication with their mothers.* PhD thesis, University of Edinburgh.

Murray L & Carothers AD (1989) Postnatal depression in 702 Cambridge mothers: estimation of prevalence and validation of the Edinburgh Postnatal Depression Scale (EPDS). *British Journal of Psychiatry* (in press).

Murray L & Trevarthen CB (1985) Emotional regulation of interactions between two month olds and their mothers. In Field TM & Fox NA (eds) *Social Perception in Infants*, pp 177–197. Norwood, New Jersey: Ablex.

Murray L & Trevarthen CB (1986) The infant's role in mother–infant communications. *Journal of Child Language* **13:** 15–29.

Nott PN (1987) Extent, timing and persistence of emotional disorders following childbirth. *British Journal of Psychiatry* **151:** 523–527.

O'Hara MW & Zekoski EM (1988) Postpartum depression: a comprehensive review. In Kumar R & Brockington IF (eds) *Motherhood and Mental Illness*, pp 17–63. London: John Wright.

O'Hara MW, Neunaber DJ & Zekoski EM (1984) A prospective study of postpartum depression: prevalence, course and predictive factors. *Journal of Abnormal Psychology* **93:** 158–171.

Paykel ES, Emms EM, Fletcher J & Rassaby EJ (1980) Life events and social support in puerperal depression. *British Journal of Psychiatry* **136:** 339–346.

Robson K & Kumar R (1980) Delayed onset of maternal affection after childbirth. *British Journal of Psychiatry* **136:** 347–353.

Stein A, Cooper PJ, Campbell EA, Day A & Altham PEM (1989) Social adversity and perinatal complications: their relation to postnatal depression. *British Medical Journal* **298:** 1073–1074.

Uddenberg N & Englesson I (1978) Prognosis of postpartum mental disturbance. A prospective study of primiparous women and their 4-year-old children. *Acta Psychiatrica Scandinavica* **58:** 201–212.

Weissman MM, Paykel ES & Klerman GL (1972) The depressed woman as a mother. *Social Psychiatry* **7:** 98–108.

Weissman MM, Prusoff BA, Gammon GD, Merinkangas KR, Leckman JF & Kid KK (1984) Psychopathology in the children (6–18) of depressed and normal parents. *Journal of the American Academy of Child Psychiatry* **23:** 78–84.

Welner Z, Welner A, Donald M, McCrany BA & Leonard MA (1977) Psychopathology in children of inpatients with depression. *Journal of Nervous and Mental Disease* **164:** 408–413.

Whiffen VE & Gotlib IH (1989) Infants of postpartum depressed mothers: temperament and cognitive status. *Journal of Abnormal Psychology* **98(3):** 1–6.

Williams H & Carmichael A (1985) Depression in mothers in a multi-ethnic urban industrial municipality in Melbourne. Aetiological factors and effects on infants and pre-schoolchildren. *Journal of Child Psychology and Psychiatry and Allied Disciplines* **26:** 277–288.

Wrate RM, Rooney AC, Thomas PF & Cox JL (1985) Postnatal depression and child development: a 3-year follow-up study. *British Journal of Psychiatry* **146:** 622–627.

Zajicek E & De Salis W (1979) Depression in mothers of young children. Family Research Unit. *Child Abuse and Neglect* **146:** 622–627.

14

Perinatal death

EMANUEL LEWIS
STANFORD BOURNE

THE DANGERS

There may be immediate serious sequelae after a perinatal death, but some of the most important effects occur later—following a subsequent pregnancy or in the next generation of children when they grow up.

Effects on the mother

There is a tendency for bewilderment and distress to continue instead of fading normally, so that mourning appears to turn into persistent depression or a variety of psychiatric syndromes such as hypochondria or phobic states (Giles, 1970; Wolff et al, 1970; Cullberg, 1972). Puerperal psychosis is not common and it is not quite clear, from epidemiological studies, whether or not the incidence is somewhat increased (Kendall et al, 1987).

Some women seem to 'get over it surprisingly well', but it is our clinical impression that the birth of the next baby is a dangerous time, especially where there has been minimal distress and little mourning. Pathological mourning (see later), including abnormal states of complaint and grievance, is also a danger sign. The trauma may be reactivated after a latent period of seeming recovery at anniversaries (Pollock, 1975), birthdays or at any later bereavement or crisis such as divorce, the menopause or retirement. The stress on parents when their children leave the nursery to go to school or leave home to get married may be times of added danger.

Effects on family life

Emotional tension and sexual disturbances strain marriage and fragile marriages can crack. As perinatal death is often associated with the suspicion of blame or guilt, partners reproach themselves and easily quarrel. It is difficult to know what to tell the children, who may themselves develop difficulties which further stresses parents. It seems paradoxical but we believe that child abuse is provoked in some cases (Lewis, 1979a). Although most of the distress falls upon the mother, sometimes the father has the worst reactions. An added danger is that these distressed fathers pass unnoticed and unhelped, which generates isolation and more grievance. Pathological jealousy or other bizzare disturbances may ensue.

Effects on other children—the future adults

Siblings

Because of their immaturity, reality testing in young children is precarious, and normal development depends on the interchange of perception with healthy parents. Devastated parents may be little able to facilitate the child's thinking and the testing of reality. The difficulties are usually compounded because children seldom see the body of the dead baby, which adds to difficulty in correcting disturbing fantasies and misconceptions.

The sense of magic and mystery about the making of a baby is intensified by the sudden disappearance of the baby from inside the mother—possibly imagined as taken away or stolen. These ideas, magnified by mirroring in the mother's own fears and guilt, can lead to phobic reactions. Some children have run away from home, others become intensely clinging.

Death in utero will especially activate fantasies that babies are made from faeces and this can lead to such symptoms as constipation and soiling, tummy-ache and other hypochondriacal or hysterical syndromes.

Rivalry with the mother's baby-making capacity, or the idea that the lost baby was stolen, generate delinquent acts. We also see these as a cry for help, but the help may be improved if the delinquency can be more exactly understood.

The next baby

The next baby is commonly conceived in haste, as a replacement for the child that died. Whilst consciously maintaining that no child can replace the dead one, parents find the idea difficult to avoid. Often the new baby is born around the same birthday a year later and is saddled with bewildered parental expectations. The baby is confused with the previous dead baby and the parents are very unsure of his identity and his vitality. He is half-expected to be somebody else. In psychiatric practice, we commonly see these babies as grown-ups, years later—people with personality problems, inhibitions and lack of confidence. Disturbingly, there is a tendency for trouble to follow into the next generation, when they become parents themselves. A legacy of confusion and anxiety from their early nurturing, from the sad look in their mother's eyes when they were babes-in-arms, may disturb the rearing of their own children.

The survivor of twins

When one twin dies, the survivor has parents who are bereft at their birth. The mother has the very difficult contradictory task of celebrating and nurturing the newborn child whilst preoccupied with the thoughts and feelings about her dead baby. The single survivor of twins is left with 'survivor guilt' and a tendency to inhibition, self-destructive behaviour and impaired or driven ambition throughout life.

Effects on doctors and nurses

Perinatal loss generates blame, guilt and bewilderment which hospital staff find hard to cope with and sometimes react to by avoiding the problem and forgetting it. Previously, these patients were usually isolated and quickly sent home for compassionate reasons but also because it is painful to approach them. There used to be virtually nothing in the medical literature about the psychology of stillbirth, as if the problem were taboo. Doctors find it difficult to know, notice or remember anything of these cases and tend to become blank, even regarding the medical facts, let alone any emotional reactions (Bourne, 1968). Case notes tend to get mislaid.

These patients tend to cling to grievances almost as if the grievance becomes a substitute for the lost baby. Since there is quite often a suspicion of mismanagement after a perinatal death, the patients frequently become embattled if not actually litigious. This places further strain on the doctor–patient relationship and staff tend to avoid sharing the problem amongst themselves. Many of these patients change their family doctor or obstetrician after a stillbirth, which helps keep the grievances buried, unresolved and festering.

SOME CLINICAL SYNDROMES

Death in utero, intrapartum death and neonatal death have different kinds of impact.

Stillbirth

Bewildering contradictions form the predominant effects as birth and death are fused. Something grave, horrid and somehow defiling has happened yet there is nothing to see. The tremendous build-up of pregnancy leads to an almost unbelievable non-event. The belly is flat and there is no baby. Instead, there is a legacy of perplexing and conflicting feelings. These afflict the mother directly but also spread around the family. There is bereavement, yet no known living person has died. Some mothers are angered by such a view for they feel they did 'know' the baby moving inside them, but the more fervently this is believed, the more bewildered and aggrieved are the reactions. A fetus is not known in the way a living baby is known in your arms, and the 'person' who dies has existed, as yet, only in the imagination. The bewildering sense of unreality is compounded by the swift disappearance of the baby's body and, commonly, the lack of a funeral or a marked grave. Until recent changes in UK regulations the baby could not even have a registered name.

Mixed up with the disappointment and bewilderment are feelings of guilt and shame, even though there is usually no sensible reason to feel guilty and nothing of which to feel ashamed. There are often inappropriate reasons for guilt, e.g. acts of carelessness or 'doing the wrong things' during pregnancy, that may be imagined to have harmed the baby. Guilty rumination may become hooked on to such 'reasons'. Shame is exacerbated by the frequent reaction of repugnance and avoidance. Doctors, nurses and friends do not know what to say—and keep away. There is a feeling of being diseased even though there is usually no illness, and the mother's feelings of defilement are easily made worse by the reactions of hospital staff and even by some acts of kindly intent, like offering privacy in a side-ward and avoiding talking about babies.

Neonatal death

This is, generally, not so thought-stopping as stillbirth. The longer the baby survives, the less the bewilderment of a non-event. Survival, however briefly, of a live baby means that there is not quite the same feeling of defilement and nightmare that are associated with death in utero. There may also be less feeling of failure and recrimination for the mother and the obstetrician than after many intrapartum deaths. It makes a difference for the parents to have been able to see and hold a live baby. Registration and certificates of birth and death and a funeral with religious ceremony all help to make the death like other deaths. The neonatal death of a live baby has its own special poignancy which gives the loss a reality, very different from the painful uphill work required to make stillbirth a real experience instead of a bad dream. The death of an older child is generally more distressing for the family but, because grieving is easier (in the sense of being more clear and comprehensible), there is usually less risk of failed mourning.

There are appalling stresses on the families of very premature babies. It is difficult for parents to relate to a tiny scrap of humanity, connected to wires and tubes under glass, and who appears to belong to the nurses rather than to themselves. They have little chance to get to know him and to establish a realistic sense of a baby held in the arms who has lived and died. The baby is not really felt to have lived properly (Kennell et al, 1970).

Congenital abnormalities

If there is severe congenital abnormality or other reason to believe that the baby is unlikely to develop into a normal child, few people could avoid thoughts and wishes that the baby might die. Such thoughts may make it easier to accept the death on a rational basis, that this baby is better off dead. Nevertheless, such thoughts feel wrong and carry an undercurrent of intense unease, with the risk of a guilty depressive reaction. Such reactions may go underground and await reactivation at some later loss or, perhaps, at a subsequent birth. Adult ideas about the reason for a malformed baby link up with unconscious memories of childhood fantasy about how babies are made and unmade. Reactivated childhood anxiety adds to the adult's confusion and worry, undermines the bereaved parent's reality testing, and is associated with severe reactions when the baby is congenitally malformed, such as excessive guilt or shame, repugnance or denial (Klaus and Kennell, 1982).

Early miscarriages

Fundamentally, the reactions might well be similar in fetal loss, whatever the stage of pregnancy. Many individual factors may determine an unexpectedly severe reaction to an early miscarriage, e.g. if the pregnancy is either desperately desired or hated, or if there is a bad family history of failed pregnancy. Severe reactions to an early miscarriage are personal, whereas everybody finds a stillbirth to be a quite appalling experience. In contrast to early miscarriage, clothes have been prepared and names chosen, whilst the arms, the breasts and the mind are given over to a receptive state in late pregnancy in a way which helps ensure devotion to a newborn baby but will make the mother vulnerable to his loss. Late pregnancy becomes public and the expectation is shared, whereas an early miscarriage is a more private affair. Early abortions are common, whereas stillbirths make the mother feel more of an odd case, more shamed by failure. Repeated miscarriage, especially in the childless, is of course extremely hurtful and undermining. With quickening a mother 'knows' she has a baby inside, though scans now increase early awareness. From then, she becomes psychologically pregnant and, if the baby dies, she has what is for her, a stillbirth.

THEORETICAL CONSIDERATIONS

Pregnancy and delivery are liable to be bewildering, magical and painful experiences, even at the best of times. These feelings complicate the difficulties of mourning any death in the family during pregnancy. Perinatal deaths are bewildering as birth and death are fused into one experience that feels as if reality has been turned upside-down.

Normal mourning and its difficulties

Mourning a loss means taking in what has happened and sorting out all the mixed feelings and lost hopes so that eventually memories of the dead recede to a healthy perspective (Freud, 1917). Eventually there will be normal forgetting and normal remembering. If mourning fails, the forgetting is more of a desperate blocking out, a no-go area in the mind, and the remembering is more a troubled preoccupation, a haunted state of mind. At first, the loss is taken in with difficulty. The bereaved person's inner world is occupied with conscious and unconscious images of the body and mind and illness of the dead, all of which contribute to the malaise, heaviness and deadness, and may develop into hypochondria or psychosomatic illness. In failed or interrupted mourning such symptoms may become chronic or, after an apparent facile recovery, there is a hidden vulnerability to subsequent traumas.

Difficulties arise when the loss is hard to take in because of uncertain and bewildering circumstances, especially where the body is missing as in drowning accidents or in battle. Other difficulties arise from entangled good and bad feelings about the dead person and any unusual horror or revulsion concerned with the surrounding events of the death (Parkes and Weiss, 1983). Further difficulty is caused by the reactivation of previous losses from the past just as later losses will be liable to reactivate this one. The re-emergence, in an adult, of long-forgotten infantile reactions to loss is bewildering. Infantile thoughts and feelings, recurring in adults, are difficult to accept and accommodate (Klein, 1963).

The psychopathology of death in pregnancy

Not all pregnancies are planned, but even when pregnancy is passionately desired, the impulses and ideas involved are complicated and ambivalent (Bibring et al, 1961; Benedek, 1970; Kestenberg, 1977; Blum, 1980). It is commonplace for an 'unwanted' baby to turn out to be the favourite of the family. Other babies, long-awaited, can arrive as a hostile stranger to a mother perplexed by her own feelings of distance or rejection. Reactions to a new baby, alive or dead, are governed by a mixture of conscious and unconscious hopes, expectations and fears. It is probably normal or universal for children to envy their mother's baby-making capacity, resent their siblings and harbour thoughts of harming rival babies inside their mothers (Klein, 1932; Segal, 1973). These anxious-making thoughts seem to be 'confirmed' by a stillbirth. This is of immediate relevance to our under-standing of the predicament of the sibling of a stillbirth. However, as adult attitudes to babies are influenced by unconscious residues from childhood, a stillbirth can reinforce psychosexual or hypochondriacal anxiety. There are deeply rooted primitive quasi-magical ideas of a life for a life and this can give an anxious tone to the state of mind in which a baby is expected. Such ideas crowd back in if the baby dies and it is as if the parents' own dead die over again. A stillbirth can be felt as mocking the act of procreation, placing a further strain on a couple's sexuality and marriage.

The wish for pregnancy is not always the same as the wish to have a child. Some men find it irresistible to impregnate women yet seem to have no evident wish to be the father of a child. Some women are compulsively pregnant and become depressed when they have to stop, and these do not tend to make the most devoted mothers. Sometimes, the addiction is to having a baby-in-arms, a baby at the breast, and this baby is dropped when a new one arrives. Giving birth is always an ending (of pregnancy) as well as the start of something new. Many women sense sadness within their delight at having the new baby in their arms—sadness at the loss of the one known differently inside. There is an inner emptiness which may be unexpectedly painful, mixed up with other unexpected difficult painful feelings, ubiquitous in the puerperium. A baby may represent wealth to the impoverished or an insurance for old age, and parenthood may be required for acceptance as an adult. Having a big family may appeal to a certain kind of pride. None of this is to devalue the essential human devotion in mother-love, but simply to recognize the presence of other impulses and feelings that can cause trouble. All may be well if the baby is well, but if the baby dies the worst problem may not always be the direct sense of loss of a loved person, nor even of the person that might have been. Some of the gravest disturbance comes from the collapse of a system of hopes and ideas in which the birth of the baby was paramount. In such a case, we may be dealing with something more like a crumbling edifice, the collapse of a personality and its defences, rather than merely seeing a person mourning a death.

For those who seem to need a baby as reassurance regarding their own health and self-esteem, such vulnerability may often be rooted in a preceding history of other losses, including losses in the preceding generation. Nevertheless, vulnerable people may also be those who are subtle, imaginative and creative. The need to have children is probably akin to those other defences and sublimations which are the source of civilization.

The inhibition of mourning in pregnancy is discussed later in this chapter.

Special mourning difficulties after perinatal death

Unreality

The opposing realities of birth and death are difficult to hold in the mind at the same time. Moreover, bewilderment is increased by abnormal circumstances such as congenital malformation, general anaesthetics and caesarean section. Feelings of unreality are also compounded by mismanagement.

Anger

Anger complicates mourning, whether it appears reasonable or unreasonable. Old wells of hatred are reactivated and old grievances, possibly unrelated to the dead, are simultaneously aroused and confused together. Clinical examples include fruitless recrimination or litigation against hospitals and the escalation of family quarrels.

Jealousy or possessive fury

Bereaved people can feel intensely betrayed, almost as if the dead ('the departed') have gone off with somebody else. A perinatal death is often felt like a broken promise or a robbery. A clinical example is the woman who had no obvious reaction at the time of her stillbirth but who became psychotic after the birth of her next baby, believing that a gang of baby stealers had moved in next door.

Envy

Envy of other people who are happy with their families may occur, but also less comprehensible feelings of envy for the dead, for anything enviable they might ever have had or now enjoy beyond the grave. This envy complicates the factors that make it hard to mix with people who have babies, and may also cause phobias of harming or stealing other people's babies.

Shame

Feelings of inferiority, humiliation and defilement may occur. The tendency of others to avoid bereft people reinforces the sensation of being an outcast. Shame exaggerates the withdrawal that is normally necessary in mourning. Withdrawal may be a healthy need for space and privacy to think things out, but it may also be due to the fear of showing one's face—like the irrational shame some people may have about being poor. A clinical example is the nurse who, following stillbirth, developed a fixed idea that she was 'put in a side-ward because they thought I had been a prostitute'. She became frigid and agoraphobic.

Guilt

Guilt differs from shame in being more closely related to a morality of right and wrong and to ideas of punishment, even if this is only the bad time our own conscience can give us. Shame is related to the fear of being seen as defective or inferior, whether or not it includes having done wrong. Shame leads to hiding whereas guilt sometimes leads to a provocation of punishment. For example, getting caught shoplifting after a perinatal death may be unconsciously intended to invite more punishment, as well as being a cry for help. Other syndromes of guilt are exaggerated self-reproach for real or imaginary failures or offences, or the self-accusation of psychotic depression. Sometimes, guilt is re-directed onto complaints about others, inflaming grievances against doctors and hospitals.

Triumph

The joy of being alive may feel illicit and tricky. It can provide some of the energy to do the work of mourning but it can lead to a vicious circle of more guilt and more manic over-activity to get over it. Clinical examples include the rush too soon into an ill-conceived next pregnancy, or a three-year-old child whose sister was recently stillborn who spent much of a family consultation singing 'I'm the king of the castle . . .'.

MANAGEMENT

The aim is to reduce the unreality and bewilderment and to resist the temptation to avoid the bereft parents. The mother does not know whether to feel diseased, ashamed, guilty, angry, envious or what. She feels humiliated by something that is not her fault, angry but often without anybody appropriate to blame. She feels a failure, empty of good things and defiled. The great problem is how to make contact with any of this and how to join in facing reality with tact and compassion. Support from a family similarly bereaved can be most helpful, so the parents should be told of the Stillbirth And Neonatal Death Society (SANDS), which supports a network of self-help groups.

The obstetric team—a structure required

Whatever we do will probably seem wrong in some way and this may be part of the task of sharing feelings of pain and failure with patients. It is hard to enable patients to ask all their most awkward questions.

Unless precautions are built in, the stress on staff will adversely affect the care of patients (Menzies, 1960). The welfare of staff themselves is threatened, with the risk of minor ill health, absenteeism and discontent. Obstetric and nursing work are generally stressful, but the problems posed by perinatal death require special attention. Perinatal death is too uncommon for trainees to have acquired enough experience of it to know where they are. Staff dysfunction, often manifested in fragmentation of care and responsibility, is particularly likely to exacerbate the professional deafness, blindness and amnesia that tend to mark the stillbirth case. Units require a regular forum where each perinatal death can be discussed. Information and awareness are brought together so that patients do not fall into a web of silence and evasion; shared experiences promote clinical knowledge and the strength and welfare of doctors and nurses struggling with these problems. Guidelines produced by the Royal Colleges, the Health Education Council and the Stillbirth and Neonatal Death Society, and schedules or checklists prepared to ensure that inexperienced staff know what to do are all potentially helpful. The report of the Royal College of Obstetricians and Gynaecologists working party on the management of perinatal deaths (1985) should be available in all obstetric units. However, it requires particular effort by senior staff in obstetric and special care baby units if such documents and routines are not to become a substitute for their own close engagement with these problems.

Disclosing bad news

When, who and what to tell when death in utero has been diagnosed seem like dreadful questions. In reality, women carrying a dead baby either already know or are quick to pick up the fear and guess the truth. It is a sensible principle to think of sharing as much of the truth as soon as the people involved feel able to handle it. Patients will suspect evasiveness but respect good reason for it and often feel sorry for the staff who have to share their misery. A little delay may be acceptable if it conveys the sense of something thoughtful and supportive and a staff organization where matters are not merely settled impulsively or by age or rank.

There is room for different styles of tact and judgement and different people may be of use to different patients at different times. We can reduce exaggerated responses about the exact way bad news is broken if staff continue to remain accessible thereafter. Sometimes one person is designated as the one who is good at talking to upset patients but this is probably not a good arrangement as it overburdens one person whilst the others are vaguely uncomfortable about avoiding the painful, though rewarding task. Of course, when there is a need for on-going counselling or psychotherapy later, a specialist may be necessary. However, the staff involved at the birth and death have a special role which is based on sharing experience in a direct way, which will not occur with a different specialist counsellor later.

There are no reliable guidelines to tell us whether the father, the mother or both together would be best to face. There are no right and wrong answers and whatever is done will be wrong in some way. It will help to have thought about these questions beforehand and to be alive to the grievances that fester but, in a good setting, may be ventilated and shared. To await the arrival of the father may involve delay, and can be misunderstood as devaluing women or to reflect fear of facing the mother on her own. To tell the mother by herself may seem to leave the father out, to deprive the women of her essential partner and to be over-hasty. A difficult concurrent problem is how the other children should be told for, so often, the parents are too upset to be able to explain things to their children. The general practitioner, health visitor or community midwife should be informed and consulted for guidance as well as to ensure that there is no hiatus in support.

The decision about induction of labour is delicate. Some mothers describe the ghastliness of 'feeling like a walking coffin' and feel tortured if induction is delayed. Others will want to stay a little longer with their burden and this may help them to initiate the mourning process. Aside from the obstetric indications, it is a question of sensing the needs of the particular family.

The delivery room

The delivery room will seem a gloomy place when death in utero has been diagnosed. Some effort should be made to facilitate the presence of the father in most instances as fathers so often allow themselves to be nudged out of the way when their wives need them most. Intrapartum death occurring unexpectedly poses fresh dilemmas.

The management now widely recommended is intended to maximize the clarity of the experience so as to avoid exacerbating the dangerous sense of residual bewilderment following a 'non-event' (Lewis, 1976; Forrest et al, 1981). The corpse used to be hustled away, supposedly to spare the mother unnecessary grief and the sight of something she cannot bear to see. However, such behaviour is mistaken. It springs partly from our own wish to avoid pain and confusion. The danger is that we communicate and then attribute our own revulsion to the patient.

Considerable experience suggests that parents of dead babies find precious moments to be captured even in the stillness. Formerly, they have felt further violated by the well-meant clumsiness of professional staff, too anxious and embarrassed to see what they need. On the other hand, patients who have at first been afraid to look at the dead baby have, subsequently, been permanently grateful for the support and encouragement they received from doctors and midwives who persuaded them to seize the chance. To have seen yet never held their dead baby is tantalizing and much regretted. The baby should not be bundled away, although there may now be some danger of staff rushing in with a new dogma which demands that every parent obediently inspects and holds every stillbirth immediately. A different danger is that such procedures become institutionalized, rigid and stripped of meaning. Tact and patience are important in all these matters, but unfortunately there is often an atmosphere of anxious noise and rush in the delivery room so that people do not have the space to think. Even malformed babies may not be as ghastly as we imagine at first; what mothers imagine their unseen malformed baby looks like is nearly always worse than the reality (Shokeir, 1979). With tactful sensitive concern, the normal body and limbs have given a deep sad solace for the mother of an anencephalic fetus; they commonly say; 'What lovely hands and feet!' (Klaus and Kennell, 1982). And, when looking is unbearable, the wrapped body may yet be felt and this can help to give some sense of reality in the emptiness. Often, such mothers will gently go on to unwrap the covers and explore her baby, and we have never heard this to be regretted afterwards.

Professional staff also have an important role in acting as memory-containers. The parents may be overwhelmed at the time of delivery and unable to look or to see, but the professional staff may be able to register the scene and make themselves available to talk later. Most of these parents will ask then to see and hold their dead baby.

Obstetric intervention and intrapartum death

There are special dangers of bewildered unreality when instruments and anaesthetics are involved even when a baby is alive. To wake up from an anaesthetic to be told the baby is dead compounds the perplexity and it is especially weird then not to see or hold the baby. There will be suppressed fury at what feels like having been robbed and vandalized and this may inflame other more justified grievances. Patients should be encouraged to air searching questions in anaesthetic cases so that the family may eventually patch their memories together as well as having the chance to voice concealed suspicions about what happened when they were asleep. Moreover, with intrapartum death, the midwife or obstetrician may feel vulnerable or responsible, blaming themselves, and this can make them defensive and less available to their patients.

Photographs and mementos

The dead baby should be photographed so that there is as much as possible to see and salvage from the nightmare. This aids reality testing in the mourning process as well as often being found to be a comfort for bereft parents. Unfortunately, this is not always the case if the photographs are stupidly of a kind prepared by the pathology department for a record of post mortem specimens. Ideally, photographs of several kinds should be kept as an available record, but there should certainly be at least some photographs of the baby dressed or wrapped, so as to present the most agreeable appearance. Ideally, the labour ward should possess a Polaroid type of camera, so that it is possible to verify that satisfactory photographs have been taken.

A picture of the naked whole body, preferably in black and white as well as in colour (discoloration can look worse than it need in colour prints) should be included. It will be available to help the parents hold the idea of the whole body in their minds when they are struggling to think things through.

With twins, several types of photograph are desirable—taken separately and together, clothed and naked—to provide the most complete record possible.

As well as these post-mortem photographs, it may also be useful to assemble other mementos such as antenatal ultrasound pictures, a lock of hair or a name band. Parents have sometimes been driven to 'steal' such items when they have not been provided by staff.

After the death—the puerperium

Hospital or home? Side-ward or open ward? Burial arrangements? Ideally, flexible arrangements will enable the patient to share some issues with attuned staff and other mothers. Space and privacy are essential for the family to share their grief and the inclusion of other children surviving in the family should be actively encouraged. There should be room for privacy and a side-ward should be available, but it is most important that these patients should not be isolated, which would reinforce the feeling of ostracism and irrational feelings of shame and humiliation may prevail. The encounter between the mothers of live and dead babies will be anxious and difficult, but the problem is not solved nor even really hidden by having a bereft person shut away in a side-room. Fruitful exchanges of experience often occur between mothers and the encounter can be mutually enriching, even if there is a price to pay in terms of risking other pain. Bereft mothers will usually be helped if they can confront and test out some of their complicated feelings about women with live babies rather than being encouraged to repress these feelings. Bereft mothers are usually glad to be allowed near other babies or especially to hold them since their confidence, as mothers, has been badly bruised. This can help prevent the phobia of live babies that some bereaved mothers experience.

The mothers should be warned that they may lactate. Perhaps lactation can be suppressed but some women might appreciate the experience of contributing to a breast-milk bank. Knowledge has been lost that would once have been commonplace when wet-nurses were part of normal experience. It could be reassuring for the mother of a dead baby to know that her milk is still good, and knowing requires more than just being told.

Funerals and registration

In neonatal deaths, the registration of the birth and the death and the funeral are conducted as for any other death, and the statutory Death Grant covers some of the cost. Stillbirths (death after 28 weeks of pregnancy) are legally required to be registered and buried or cremated in properly authorized places. The status of late miscarriages is now ambiguous and the demarcation will probably soon be shifted to some date earlier than 28 weeks. Of course, the ambiguity will remain in psychological terms, but there is an inevitable necessity for a legal cut-off point differentiating miscarriage from stillbirth. At present, viable fetuses are born, live and die at the end of the middle trimester. If the neonate lives and dies, it is of course registered as a live birth and a death like any other. If the baby is born dead before 28 weeks the parents have very little official way of noting the existence of the child as the birth cannot be registered. Previously, many families who found their baby to be consigned to the hospital incinerator took their own steps to bury the child themselves. A late miscarriage, before 28 weeks, may now be buried or cremated if the doctor or midwife writes a note, detailing that the baby was born before 28 weeks' gestation, without any signs of life, and recommending disposal by an undertaker. The situation is even more complex with twins born before 28 weeks' gestation where one is born dead (miscarriage) and the other born alive, maybe to die later (Gabrielczyk, 1987).

Although there is statutory provision to take responsibility for the burial or cremation of a stillbirth, this usually involves burial in a common grave, with no marked place, all of which exacerbates the difficulty of reality testing and overcoming some of the bad feelings that make mourning so difficult. A decent burial with some simple religious or other ceremony is far preferable, and parents should be encouraged to think along those lines. Undertakers and clergy are beginning to be more helpful than has sometimes been the case hitherto. Legalistic obstacles at cemeteries and obscure theological obstacles to decent burial in a marked grave are not really as rigid as people appeared to believe and previously have probably reflected the difficulty of the subject for everybody.

Congenital abnormalities and genetic counselling

Understanding parents' feelings will facilitate the task of asking permission for an autopsy. Photographs and post mortem X-ray pictures help in genetic diagnosis and the recording of scientific data, but are also sometimes useful aids to discussion. Congenital abnormalities involve parents in conflicts of revulsion and attachment towards the dead baby, towards themselves and each other. Spooky feelings about heredity and the power of bad thoughts are intensified and some daylight will help. Genetic counselling provides the opportunity to bring such difficult feelings and irrational fears into the open and should not be confined to a narrow discussion of risk, nor to the contraceptive or obstetric issues that are possibly the primary task.

Including the other children

Bereaved parents may be too incapacitated to talk to siblings without some help. Young children, because of their precarious reality testing, benefit from seeing or touching the stillborn; they should certainly see photographs and, preferably, attend the funeral. Mystery and secretiveness should be avoided, so far as possible. We believe that siblings, even more than their parents, may be in need of psychotherapeutic help in the hope of avoiding or minimizing the emotional difficulties these children can experience, especially when they are grown up and become parents themselves.

Twins

The perinatal death of one twin creates exceptional difficulties in mourning for the parents and carries risk of serious difficulties in later life for the surviving twin. There is a baffling conflict of emotions to encompass with one live baby and one dead one; there is pressure to push the dead baby away beyond memory to make space for the surviving infant, and yet the presence of the living baby is a constant reminder of the fact that there was another baby who died. The risks of failed mourning, survivor guilt and the replacement child are all present, and all these are liable to be compounded by other factors such as abnormal births, prematurity and congenital mal-formations. Further complicated thoughts may arise when the twins are the product of treatment for infertility, when there is guilt and grievance about the treatment which caused life and death to occur. The normal pride in pregnancy that makes the fall of perinatal death so painful, with its attendant guilt and humiliation, is magnified in a twin pregnancy. With multiple pregnancy there will usually be expectant pride of a special kind, with its darker side of grandiosity and unconscious triumph over other people, and extra feelings of humiliation, apart from sadness, occur if one of the babies should die. The parents have to recover from failing to become the parents of live twins as well as having to recover from the loss of the baby. They always see themselves as parents of twins and resent being tactlessly offered consolation with congratulations on being lucky to have the one live baby (Lewis and Bryan, 1988).

There will be a shadow across the cradle of the single live baby. Parents find it difficult to allow themselves to enjoy the child and may need encouragement to do so. They should have a 'good enough' (Winnicott, 1965) experience of the dead twin, sufficient to establish as clearly as possible in their minds the reality of the life and death of the baby. Future grief work will then be facilitated by having a more secure base in the psychic reality of the dead twin. The mother can then try to give the live baby her unhampered attention, to return periodically to her work of mourning. Sometimes fathers and mothers can alternate their tasks of caring and grieving. Sometimes a grandmother, sister or friend can help care for the live twin to provide some necessary time and space for grief. As this is an unusual and difficult problem to manage, help may be available from specialists, to advise those caring for the family or to help the family directly. The bereaved parents will benefit from contact with others who have had a similar experience. The Twins and Multiple Births Association or The Stillbirth and Neonatal Death Society put people in touch with one another and may know local professional advisors.

Vanishing twin syndrome

Ultrasound scans in the first trimester show that as many as half of twin conceptions end up as single deliveries. The disappearance of one twin can be complete, but a fetus papyraceous may give rise to considerable anxiety. Specialists in ultrasound scanning wonder whether or when to disclose these early findings to the parents. Misinformation and secretiveness will usually be counter-productive and most people would prefer to know.

Later, the surviving twin may sense there was something odd or hidden, unexplained and distressing about his birth. Vagueness may prove more troublesome to the surviving twin than a proper knowledge of the lost fetus.

Selective fetocide

The option for uterine killing of a fetus in a multiple pregnancy poses problems which feel bizarre or even horrifying to many doctors and parents. Uncomfortable ethical issues are perhaps too complicated to explore here, but the emotional issues abound. In addition to the soul-searching and guilt that must occur in these cases, there are other weird disturbing ideas. There will be thoughts of the live baby lying for many weeks by the side of a dead twin. With the survival of the live baby, it is not so easy to forget and forgive oneself as it is after a simple termination of pregnancy. The reminder is always there. The fate of the dead fetus is worrying and puzzling, whether relics persist and are delivered as a fetus papyraceous or whether it vanishes altogether. Maternity ward staff will also be inclined to forget the dead twin if they can and this failure to acknowledge and respect the dead baby may cause distress to the parents. A photograph of the ultrasound scan showing both babies may be a precious and unique proof for parents to keep.

THE NEXT BABY

If mourning is achieved, another pregnancy will offer consolation and fulfilment. Unfortunately, a new pregnancy very often cuts short the mourning process, predisposing to mental disturbance (Bourne and Lewis, 1984).

Timing—normal and abnormal mourning

It is not easy to suggest a minimum interval before embarking on another pregnancy, nor is it easy to differentiate normal grieving from an abnormal mourning reaction. Danger signals are intensity or rigidity of symptoms rather than any specific features. If, in either parent, there are persistent immoderate grievances, persistent psychiatric disability or an unrealistic idealization of the dead baby or of the cure a new one will bring, then it is probably too soon for another pregnancy. We may, however, be reassured if there is sadness and thoughtfulness in more ordinary proportions and also if there is a capacity to recognize some irrational ideas, where they do exist, and to speak of them sensibly rather than becoming possessed by them. Special alertness is indicated where the reaction to the perinatal death seems to have been slight and where the next pregnancy supervenes in a few months. The rush is hard to resist, especially for older women with time running out. A gap of at least several months would usually be sensible, and it is particularly important to avoid such timing as will bring the next baby's birthday close to the anniversary of the death.

Pregnancy and the inhibition of mourning

Pregnancy tends to cut mourning short. Of course it is quite possible to be miserable or depressed during pregnancy and to be troubled by various symptoms including hypochondria. It is also true that pregnancy appears to offer some protection from mental breakdown and suicide or, at any rate, postponement of it. Psychiatric disturbances can certainly occur during pregnancy, but they should not be mistaken for a continuation of the normal mourning process.

There are various theoretical reasons why pregnancy will block mourning (Lewis, 1979b). Most obviously, the general mental stance in preparation for the arrival of the new baby is in collision with the stance required for preoccupation with the death, which is required for the mourning process. Actually, the obvious clash between mourning and optimistic expectation is only half the problem. The other half resides in certain important paradoxical similarities between mourning and 'primary maternal pre-occupation', a term introduced to describe the state of mind in expectant mothers (Winnicott, 1958). Both in mourning and in primary maternal preoccupation, the thoughts are turned inwards towards an inner world occupied on the one hand by a new baby developing and on the other hand by a dead one being laid to rest. The process of mourning a dead baby (or indeed any other dead person) involves this internalization of images of the dead who are then subjected to an intense process that is very difficult to conduct at the same time as a mother is trying to make physical and mental space for a new baby due to arrive. Unconsciously, she is liable to feel that the new baby is endangered by the mourning processes going on so closely or simultaneously, if indeed she allows such processes to continue. Mostly, the mourning process is stopped short as too dangerous or simply impossible.

Hence, the problem is not only to consider whether the mother has mourned sufficiently and got over the previous loss so as to be in a reasonable state for a new pregnancy. The problem is also the risk of the new pregnancy cutting mourning short and leaving the woman with a permanent fragility, with the disturbance liable to be reactivated at any future times of stress—in addition to possible reactivation when the new baby is born.

Reassurance and antenatal care

After a perinatal death, obstetric care will usually be attentive during the next pregnancy, which is reassuring, but the anxieties of the mother and her family should not be smothered. Rather, they should be helped to express their specific anxieties. Questions persistently repeated despite comprehensive answers should suggest that other anxieties, or grievances, lie behind the questions and are being missed. The obstetric history should be taken with particular care and should include the wider family obstetric history, which generally gets meagre attention. Inattention to these facts may collude with trends in precisely those inauspicious families where trouble gets ignored and old hidden traumas then await reactivation. Children grow up with a confusing mixture of half-knowledge in families where there has been a perinatal death in their own sibship or in their parents' sibship. Such results may be lessened by improving parents' awareness of this potential legacy. Discussion may help a mother-to-be to differentiate herself from her own mother and to free events in this generation from those of the preceding one.

General anaesthesia and caesarean section

Bewilderment and unreality which are so pathogenic will have been intensified if the stillbirth occurred during general anaesthesia. After caesarean section the dead baby and the obstetrician are both the subjects of irrational resentment over the fruitless wound, and this will aggravate any unresolved problems now reactivated in the next pregnancy. Also, the irrational sense of being diseased after stillbirth are made worse by the way a mother is turned into 'a patient' by surgery. The licence to be ill and cared for may be temporarily comforting, but it can be disabling if it persists into this next pregnancy when another caesarean section may often be anticipated. The previous experience should be clarified and discussed during pregnancy. Such matters are not disposed of by a few questions and answers; anxiety and memories change focus. If obstetric intervention is required now, general anaesthesia is best avoided, especially if there is significant likelihood of a next baby dying too.

The puerperium: the replacement child

Children born after any bereavement are at risk of becoming 'replacement children' (Cain and Cain, 1964; Poznanski, 1972). It may be dangerous for the next baby to be saddled with the name formerly intended for one who died, adding to the risk that the new baby is only precariously differentiated from the dead one. Ideas that the new baby looks 'just like' the dead baby may be usefully dispelled by reference to photographs. Ideas of reincarnation add to expectations that the new baby will make up for the old one. Doctors and midwives are in a good position to pick up these dangers early and to use their influence to stop the name being recycled.

Feeding and rearing the baby who follows a perinatal death can be difficult and the pleasure may be spoiled. Mothering may be unexpectedly difficult and either parent may feel some rejection of the new child. Such difficulties may be less overwhelming if the patients are warned during the pregnancy to expect to be puzzled by some of their reactions to their new live baby. They expect to be over-anxious, but need warning of some sadness which may otherwise take them by surprise; painful memories of the dead baby will be reawakened. People often need 'permission' to be confused and afraid, and preparation may help them to be less frightened by their unexpected muddled thoughts and feelings.

DEATH OF OTHER RELATIVES SHORTLY BEFORE OR DURING PREGNANCY

It is common folk-wisdom (perhaps a little ignored by obstetricians and psychiatrists) that people often embark on pregnancy as part of their response to a death, either recent or impending, especially the demise of their own parents. This is a deeply rooted human response and may be an important part of whatever the normal promptings are that lead to procreation. Unfortunately, the pregnancy may be started as a defence against depression, a phenomenon which is also very well-known. In such case, the omens are complicated for two reasons, both fairly obvious in the context of this chapter. Firstly, a pregnancy which is motivated by a fear of depression has a heavy threat hanging over it if anything goes wrong. Secondly, the juxtaposition of the pregnancy and new baby with the underlying bereavement (actual or anticipated) causes many of the mental problems emphasized in the preceding pages discussing perinatal deaths of infants, i.e. the problems of a birth and a death occurring at the same time. The overriding problem is the fact, not at all well recognized, that pregnancy usually blocks the mourning process. This is also liable to be a serious danger when any important bereavement occurs in the course of a pregnancy.

When mourning is cut short by pregnancy the bereaved person is left with unfinished business and residual fragility. The baby born in that context is exposed to many of the dangers described for the replacement child, the baby born after the perinatal death of a sibling, since his parents are liable to be in the same perplexed state of mind, with divided attention and vague haunting sadness in the atmosphere.

REFERENCES

Benedek T (1970) The psychobiology of pregnancy. In Anthony EJ & Benedek T (eds) *Parenthood: Its Psychology and Psychopathology*, pp 137–152. Boston: Little, Brown & Co.

Bibring GL, Dwyer TF, Huntington DS & Valenstein AF (1961) A study of the psycho-social processes in pregnancy and of the earliest mother–child relationship. *Psychoanalytic Study of the Child* **16:** 9–24.

Blum H (1980) The maternal ego ideal and the regulation of maternal qualities. In Greenspan S & Pollock GH (eds) *The Course of Life: Psychoanalytic Contributions toward Understanding Personality Development, Vol 111: Adulthood and the Ageing Process*, pp 91–141. Washington, DC: US Government Printing Office.

Bourne S (1968) The psychological effects of stillbirth on women and their doctors. *Journal of the Royal College of General Practitioners* **16:** 103–112.

Bourne S & Lewis E (1984) Pregnancy after stillbirth or neonatal death. *Lancet* **ii:** 31–33.

Cain AC & Cain PC (1964) On replacing a child. *Journal of the American Academy of Child Psychiatry* **3:** 443–455.

Cullberg J (1972) Mental reactions of women to perinatal death. In Morris N (ed.) *Psychosomatic Medicine in Obstetrics and Gynaecology*, pp 326–329. Basel: Karger.

Freud S (1917) *Mourning and Melancholia*, Standard edn, vol. 14. London: Hogarth Press and Institute of Psychoanalysis.

Forrest GC, Claridge RS & Baum JD (1981) Practical management of perinatal death. *British Medical Journal* **282:** 31.

Gabrielczyk MR (1987) Personal view. *British Medical Journal* **295:** 205–209.

Giles PFH (1970) Reactions of women to perinatal death. *Australian and New Zealand Journal of Obstetrics and Gynaecology* **10:** 207.

Health Education Council. *The Loss of Your Baby*.

Kendall RE, Chalmers JC & Platz C (1987) Epidemiology of puerperal psychoses. *British Journal of Psychiatry* **150:** 662–673.

Kennell JH, Slyter H & Klaus MH (1970) The mourning response of parents to the death of a newborn infant. *New England Journal of Medicine* **283**: 344.

Kestenberg JS (1977) Regression and reintegration in pregnancy. In Blum HP (ed.) *Female Psychology: Contemporary Psychoanalytic Views*, pp 213–250. New York: International Universities Press.

Klaus MH & Kennell JH (1982) *Parent–Infant Bonding* 2nd edn. St Louis: CV Mosby.

Klein M (1932) *The Psychoanalysis of Children*. London: Hogarth.

Klein M (1963) *Our Adult World and other Essays*. London: Heinemann Medical Books.

Lewis E (1976) The management of stillbirth: coping with an unreality. *Lancet* **ii**: 619–620.

Lewis E (1979a) Two hidden predisposing factors in child abuse. *International Journal of Child Abuse* **3**: 327–330.

Lewis E (1979b) Inhibition of mourning by pregnancy: psychopathology and management. *British Medical Journal* **ii**: 27–28.

Lewis E & Bryan E (1988) Management of perinatal loss of a twin. *British Medical Journal* **297**: 1321–1323.

Menzies IEP (1960) A case study in the functioning of social systems as a defence against anxiety. *Human Relations* **13**: 95–121.

Parkes CM & Weiss RS (1983) *Recovery from Bereavement*. New York: Basic Books.

Pollock GH (1975) On anniversary suicide and mourning. In Benedek T & Anthony EJ (eds) *Depression and Human Existence*, pp 369–394. Boston: Little, Brown & Co.

Poznanski EO (1972) The 'replacement child': a saga of unresolved parental grief. *Journal of Pediatrics* **81**: 1190.

Royal College of Obstetricians and Gynaecologists (1985) *Report of the RCOG Working Party on the Management of Perinatal Deaths*. London: RCOG.

Segal H (1973) *Introduction to the Work of Melanie Klein*. London: Hogarth Press and Institute of Psychoanalysis.

Shokeir M (1979) Managing the family of the abnormal newborn. In Hall BD (ed.) *Proceedings of the 1978 Birth Defects Conference, National Foundation*. March of Dimes, New York.

Winnicott DW (1958) Primary maternal preoccupation. In *Collected Papers: Through Paediatrics to Psycho-analysis*, pp 300–305. London: Tavistock.

Winnicott DW (1965) The theory of the parent–infant relationship. In *The Maturational Processes and the Facilitating Environment*, pp 37–55. London: Hogarth Press.

Wolff JR, Nielson PE & Schiller P (1970) The emotional reactions to a stillbirth. *American Journal of Obstetrics and Gynecology* **108(1)**: 73–77.

Index